NASH and NAFLD

Editor

DAVID E. BERNSTEIN

CLINICS IN
LIVER DISEASE

www.liver.theclinics.com

Consulting Editor
NORMAN GITLIN

February 2018 • Volume 22 • Number 1

ELSEVIER

1600 John F. Kennedy Boulevard • Suite 1800 • Philadelphia, Pennsylvania, 19103-2899

http://www.theclinics.com

CLINICS IN LIVER DISEASE Volume 22, Number 1
February 2018 ISSN 1089-3261, ISBN-13: 978-0-323-56986-6

Editor: Kerry Holland
Developmental Editor: Meredith Madeira

Clinics in Liver Disease (ISSN 1089-3261) is published quarterly by Elsevier Inc., 360 Park Avenue South, New York, NY 10010-1710. Months of issue are February, May, August, and November. Business and Editorial Offices: 1600 John F. Kennedy Blvd., Ste. 1800, Philadelphia, PA 19103-2899. Customer Service Office: 3251 Riverport Lane, Maryland Heights, MO 63043. Periodicals postage paid at New York, NY and additional mailing offices. Subscription prices are $292.00 per year (U.S. individuals), $100.00 per year (U.S. student/resident), $509.00 per year (U.S. institutions), $403.00 per year (international individuals), $200.00 per year (international student/resident), $631.00 per year (international instituitions), $338.00 per year (Canadian individuals), $200.00 per year (Canadian student/resident), and $631.00 per year (Canadian institutions). Foreign air speed delivery is included in all *Clinics* subscription prices. All prices are subject to change without notice. **POSTMASTER:** Send address changes to *Clinics in Liver Disease*, Elsevier Health Sciences Division, Subscription Customer Service, 3251 Riverport Lane, Maryland Heights, MO 63043. **Customer Service: Telephone: 1-800-654-2452 (U.S. and Canada); 314-447-8871 (outside U.S. and Canada). Fax: 314-447-8029. E-mail: journalscustomer service-usa@elsevier.com (for print support); journalsonlinesupport-usa@elsevier.com (for online support).**

Reprints. For copies of 100 or more of articles in this publication, please contact the Commercial Reprints Department, Elsevier Inc., 360 Park Avenue South, New York, NY 10010-1710. Tel.: 212-633-3874; Fax: 212-633-3820; E-mail: reprints@elsevier.com.

Clinics in Liver Disease is covered in *MEDLINE/PubMed (Index Medicus)*, Science Citation Index Expanded, Journal Citation Reports/Science Edition, and Current Contents/Clinical Medicine.

Contributors

CONSULTING EDITOR

NORMAN GITLIN, MD, FRCP (LONDON), FRCPE (EDINBURGH), FAASLD, FACP, FACG
Formerly, Professor, Department of Medicine, Chief of Hepatology, Emory University, Currently, Consultant, Atlanta Gastroenterology Associates, Atlanta, Georgia

EDITOR

DAVID E. BERNSTEIN, MD, FAASLD, FACG, FACP, FAGA
Vice Chair of Medicine for Clinical Trials, Chief, Division of Hepatology and Sandra Atlas Bass Center for Liver Diseases, Northwell Health, Professor of Medicine and Educational Sciences, Donald and Barbara Zucker School of Medicine at Hofstra/Northwell, Manhasset, New York

AUTHORS

DAVID E. BERNSTEIN, MD, FAASLD, FACG, FACP, FAGA
Vice Chair of Medicine for Clinical Trials, Chief, Division of Hepatology and Sandra Atlas Bass Center for Liver Diseases, Northwell Health, Professor of Medicine and Educational Sciences, Donald and Barbara Zucker School of Medicine at Hofstra/Northwell, Manhasset, New York

HENRY C. BODENHEIMER Jr, MD
Professor of Medicine, Department of Medicine, Donald and Barbara Zucker School of Medicine at Hofstra/Northwell, Sandra Atlas Bass Center for Liver Diseases, Northwell Health, Manhasset, New York

HALEY BUSH, MPH
Betty & Guy Beatty Center for Integrated Research, Inova Health System, Falls Church, Virginia

DANIELLE CARTER, MD
Viral Hepatitis Fellow, Division of Liver Diseases, Icahn School of Medicine at Mount Sinai, New York, New York

NAGA CHALASANI, MD
Division of Gastroenterology and Hepatology, Indiana University School of Medicine, Indianapolis, Indiana

CHARISSA CHANG, MD
Assistant Professor of Medicine, Division of Liver Diseases, Icahn School of Medicine at Mount Sinai, New York, New York

MICHAEL CHARLTON, MD, FRCP
Professor of Medicine, Division of Gastroenterology and Hepatology, The University of Chicago, Center for Liver Diseases, The University of Chicago Biological Sciences, Chicago, Illinois

DOUGLAS T. DIETERICH, MD
Professor of Medicine, Division of Liver Diseases, Icahn School of Medicine at Mount Sinai, New York, New York

YONAH B. ESTERSON, MD, MS
Department of Radiology, Northwell Health, Donald and Barbara Zucker School of Medicine at Hofstra/Northwell, Manhasset, New York

SAMER GAWRIEH, MD
Division of Gastroenterology and Hepatology, Indiana University School of Medicine, Indianapolis, Indiana

NIDHI P. GOYAL, MD, MPH
Assistant Physician, Division of Gastroenterology, Hepatology, and Nutrition, Department of Pediatrics, UC San Diego, La Jolla, California; Department of Gastroenterology, Rady Children's Hospital San Diego, San Diego, California

GREGORY M. GRIMALDI, MD
Assistant Professor, Department of Radiology, Northwell Health, Donald and Barbara Zucker School of Medicine at Hofstra/Northwell, Manhasset, New York

NADEGE T. GUNN, MD
Pinnacle Clinical Research, Rollingwood, Texas

PRIYA HANDA, PhD
Liver Care Network and Organ Care Research, Swedish Medical Center, Seattle, Washington

LINDA HENRY, PhD
Center for Outcomes Research in Liver Disease, Washington, DC

CHUN KIT HUNG, MD
Fellow, Division of Gastroenterology, Department of Medicine, Northwell Health, New Hyde Park, New York

DONGHEE KIM, MD, PhD
Division of Gastroenterology and Hepatology, Stanford University School of Medicine, Stanford, California

W. RAY KIM, MD
Division of Gastroenterology and Hepatology, Stanford University School of Medicine, Stanford, California

ALEXANDER J. KOVALIC, MD
Department of Internal Medicine, Wake Forest School of Medicine, Winston-Salem, North Carolina

KRIS V. KOWDLEY, MD
Liver Care Network and Organ Care Research, Swedish Medical Center, Seattle, Washington

TAI-PING LEE, MD
Associate Professor, Department of Internal Medicine, Division of Hepatology, Sandra Atlas Bass Center of Liver Diseases, Northwell Health, Manhasset, New York

HUEI-WEN LIM, MD
Internal Medicine Resident, Department of Internal Medicine, Northwell Health, Manhasset, New York

CHRISTINA C. LINDENMEYER, MD
Department of Gastroenterology and Hepatology, Cleveland Clinic, Clinical Instructor, Cleveland Clinic Lerner College of Medicine of Case Western Reserve University, Cleveland, Ohio

VIGNAN MANNE, MD
Liver Care Network and Organ Care Research, Swedish Medical Center, Seattle, Washington

OMAR MASSOUD, MD
Associate Professor of Medicine, Division of Gastroenterology and Hepatology, The University of Alabama, Birmingham, Alabama

ARTHUR J. McCULLOUGH, MD
Departments of Gastroenterology and Hepatology, and Pathobiology, Transplantation Center, Cleveland Clinic, Professor, Cleveland Clinic Lerner College of Medicine of Case Western Reserve University, Cleveland, Ohio

ALITA MISHRA, MD
Department of Medicine, Center for Liver Diseases, Inova Fairfax Hospital, Falls Church, Virginia

PUNEET PURI, MBBS, MD
Associate Professor of Medicine, Division of Gastroenterology, Department of Internal Medicine, School of Medicine, Virginia Commonwealth University, Richmond, Virginia

ARUN J. SANYAL, MBBS, MD
Professor of Medicine, Physiology and Molecular Pathology, Division of Gastroenterology, Department of Internal Medicine, School of Medicine, Virginia Commonwealth University, Richmond, Virginia

SANJAYA K. SATAPATHY, MBBS, MD, DM, FACG, FASGE
Associate Professor of Surgery, Transplant Hepatologist, Transplantation, Methodist University Hospital Transplant Institute, Division of Surgery, The University of Tennessee Health Sciences Center, Memphis, Tennessee

JEFFREY B. SCHWIMMER, MD
Professor of Pediatrics, Division of Gastroenterology, Hepatology, and Nutrition, Department of Pediatrics, UC San Diego, La Jolla, California; Department of Gastroenterology, Rady Children's Hospital San Diego, San Diego, California

MITCHELL L. SHIFFMAN, MD
Liver Institute of Virginia, Bon Secours Health System, Newport News, Virginia; Liver Institute of Virginia, Bon Secours Health System, Richmond, Virginia

ALEXIS TOUROS, BA
Division of Gastroenterology and Hepatology, Stanford University School of Medicine, Stanford, California

EUGENIA TSAI, MD
Fellow, Department of Internal Medicine, Division of Gastroenterology and Hepatology, Tulane Medical Center, New Orleans, Louisiana

ZOBAIR M. YOUNOSSI, MD, MPH
Department of Medicine, Center for Liver Diseases, Inova Fairfax Hospital, Betty & Guy Beatty Center for Integrated Research, Inova Health System, Falls Church, Virginia

Contents

Preface: Nonalcoholic Fatty Liver Disease: An Expanding Health Care Epidemic　　xiii

David E. Bernstein

**Clinical and Economic Burden of Nonalcoholic Fatty Liver Disease and
Nonalcoholic Steatohepatitis**　　1

Zobair M. Younossi, Linda Henry, Haley Bush, and Alita Mishra

> Nonalcoholic fatty liver disease (NAFLD) is a chronic liver disease with an increasing global prevalence associated with tremendous clinical, economic, and health-related quality-of-life burden. Clinically, NAFLD is considered the liver manifestation of metabolic syndrome. However, diagnosing NAFLD presents significant challenges due to the limited noninvasive and accurate diagnostic tools available to not only accurately diagnose nonalcoholic steatohepatitis but also to stage hepatic fibrosis, the major predictor of long-term outcomes, including mortality.

The Natural History of Nonalcoholic Fatty Liver Disease—An Evolving View　　11

Christina C. Lindenmeyer and Arthur J. McCullough

> Nonalcoholic fatty liver disease (NAFLD) is a major cause of chronic liver disease worldwide, and its clinical and economic burden will continue to grow with parallel increases in rates of obesity, diabetes, and the metabolic syndrome. Evolving understanding of the natural history of NAFLD suggests that these patients are at risk for disease progression to steatohepatitis, fibrosis, and cirrhosis. Recent studies also suggest that these patients are at elevated risk for cardiovascular-, malignancy-, and liver-related morbidity and mortality, although their risk for progression, decompensation, and hepatocellular carcinoma may be less than that of patients with alternative causes of chronic liver disease.

Pathophysiology of Nonalcoholic Fatty Liver Disease/Nonalcoholic Steatohepatitis　　23

Vignan Manne, Priya Handa, and Kris V. Kowdley

> Nonalcoholic fatty liver disease (NAFLD) encompasses a spectrum of liver disorders ranging from hepatic steatosis to nonalcoholic steatohepatitis (NASH) and ultimately may lead to cirrhosis. Hepatic steatosis or fatty liver is defined as increased accumulation of lipids in hepatocytes and results from increased production or reduced clearance of hepatic triglycerides or fatty acids. Fatty liver can progress to NASH in a significant proportion of subjects. NASH is a necroinflammatory liver disease governed by multiple pathways that are not completely elucidated. This article describes the main mechanisms that have been reported to contribute to the pathophysiology of NAFLD and NASH.

Risk Factors for the Development of Nonalcoholic Fatty Liver Disease/Nonalcoholic
Steatohepatitis, Including Genetics   39

Huei-Wen Lim and David E. Bernstein

Nonalcoholic fatty liver disease is emerging as the most common cause of chronic liver disease worldwide. This trend is, in part, secondary, to the growing incidence of obesity, type 2 diabetes, and metabolic syndrome. Other risk factors include age, gender, race/ethnicity, genetic predisposition, and polycystic ovarian disease. With the introduction of genome-wide association studies, genetic mutations contributing to inherited susceptibility to steatosis have been identified, which hold keys to future improvement in diagnosis and management. This article expands on the aforementioned risk factors and summarizes the current available data on genetic and environmental factors associated with this common entity.

The Genetics of Pediatric Nonalcoholic Fatty Liver Disease   59

Nidhi P. Goyal and Jeffrey B. Schwimmer

Nonalcoholic fatty liver disease (NAFLD) is the leading cause of chronic liver disease in children. Severe fibrosis and cirrhosis are potential consequences of pediatric NAFLD and can occur within a few years of diagnosis. Observations suggest that genetics may be a strong modifying factor in the presentation, severity, and natural history of the disease. There is increasing interest in determining at-risk populations based on genetics in the hope of finding genotypes that correlate to NAFLD phenotype. Ultimately, the hope is to be able to tailor therapeutics to genetic predispositions and decrease disease morbidity in children with NAFLD.

Diagnosis and Evaluation of Nonalcoholic Fatty Liver Disease/Nonalcoholic
Steatohepatitis, Including Noninvasive Biomarkers and Transient Elastography   73

Eugenia Tsai and Tai-Ping Lee

The incidence and prevalence of nonalcoholic fatty liver disease (NAFLD) are increasing and identification of people at risk of disease progression is extremely important. The current gold standard for diagnosing NAFLD/ nonalcoholic steatohepatitis (NASH) is by liver biopsy, but it has several limitations. Noninvasive tests via biomarkers and transient elastography to assess NAFLD/NASH are being used in clinical practice. The most validated diagnostic panels include the NAFLD fibrosis score, Fibrosis-4, and FibroMeter. Transient elastography is very useful in evaluating advanced fibrosis and cirrhosis.

Radiologic Imaging in Nonalcoholic Fatty Liver Disease and Nonalcoholic
Steatohepatitis   93

Yonah B. Esterson and Gregory M. Grimaldi

The article reviews the multimodality (ultrasound, computed tomography, and magnetic resonance [MR]) imaging appearance of nonalcoholic fatty liver disease (NAFLD) and discusses the radiologic diagnostic criteria as well as the sensitivity and specificity of these imaging methods. The authors review the role of both ultrasound and MR elastography for the diagnosis of fibrosis and for the longitudinal evaluation of patients following therapeutic intervention. Last, the authors briefly discuss the screening and diagnosis of hepatocellular carcinoma in patients with NAFLD, as there are special considerations in this population.

The Use of Liver Biopsy in Nonalcoholic Fatty Liver Disease: When to Biopsy and in Whom   109

Nadege T. Gunn and Mitchell L. Shiffman

Nonalcoholic fatty liver disease (NAFLD) is a common liver disorder that can be divided into benign steatosis or nonalcoholic fatty liver (NAFL) and nonalcoholic steatohepatitis (NASH). Elastography and scoring systems based on clinical features and routine biochemical testing can be used to assess fibrosis in patients with NAFLD. Patients with fibrosis are thought to have NASH. However, only a liver biopsy can reliably diagnose NAFLD and differentiate NAFL from NASH. Because medical therapy for NASH is not available, it is not necessary to perform a liver biopsy in all patients. Patients suspected of having NASH should undergo liver biopsy.

The Intestinal Microbiome in Nonalcoholic Fatty Liver Disease   121

Puneet Puri and Arun J. Sanyal

Nonalcoholic fatty liver disease is the most common cause of chronic liver disease in North America and is growing as a cause of chronic liver disease in many other parts of the world as well. It has 2 principal clinical-pathologic phenotypes: (1) nonalcoholic fatty liver and (2) nonalcoholic steatohepatitis. The development of both phenotypes is tightly linked to excess body weight and insulin resistance. This review discusses the emerging tools for the analysis of the microbiome, their limitations, and the existing literature with respect to the intestinal microbiome and their role in nonalcoholic fatty liver.

Nonalcoholic Fatty Liver Disease and Metabolic Syndrome   133

Donghee Kim, Alexis Touros, and W. Ray Kim

Nonalcoholic fatty liver disease (NAFLD) and metabolic syndrome (MS) are highly prevalent, affecting approximately one-third of the US population. The relationship between NAFLD and MS is complex and may be bidirectionally associated. NAFLD is strongly associated with MS, the components of which include abdominal obesity, hyperglycemia, hypertension, and dyslipidemia. NAFLD associated with certain genetic factors, such as the PNPLA3 G allele variant, is not accompanied by insulin resistance and MS. Lifestyle modification, including diet and physical activity targeting visceral adiposity, remains the standard of care for patients with NAFLD and MS.

The Role of Nonalcoholic Fatty Liver Disease on Cardiovascular Manifestations and Outcomes   141

Alexander J. Kovalic and Sanjaya K. Satapathy

Cardiovascular disease has been postulated as the leading cause of mortality among patients with nonalcoholic fatty liver disease (NAFLD), rather than from sequalae of liver disease specifically. Although there is ample evidence validating the association between NAFLD and increased cardio-vascular comorbidities, events, and mortality, current data present a chal-lenge in attributing this effect solely due to NAFLD given the rampant presence of insulin resistance and type 2 diabetes mellitus (T2DM). End-points of increased cardiovascular risk remain tightly linked to the concomitant presence of insulin resistance and T2DM. Prospective studies accentuating early detection of NAFLD are imperative to institute early intervention and prevent future cardiovascular events.

Current Treatment of Nonalcoholic Fatty Liver Disease/Nonalcoholic Steatohepatitis   175

Chun Kit Hung and Henry C. Bodenheimer Jr

Treatment of nonalcoholic fatty liver disease (NAFLD)/nonalcoholic steato-hepatitis (NASH) is focused on patients with NASH because they are at high-est risk for progressive liver disease. Current first-line treatment consists of lifestyle modifications. Patients should lose at least 7% to 10% of body weight via a combination of physical exercise and calorie restriction dieting. Surgical or endoscopic surgery for weight loss can be considered in obese patients, depending on degree of excess body weight and comorbidities. There is no currently approved pharmacotherapy for NASH. Vitamin E and pioglitazone have the most evidence of therapeutic efficacy but have limita-tions. The treatment modality chosen should be individualized.

Emerging Treatments for Nonalcoholic Fatty Liver Disease and Nonalcoholic Steatohepatitis   189

Samer Gawrieh and Naga Chalasani

This article discusses completed phase II randomized clinical trials with high-quality published results for compounds that demonstrate effects on nonalcoholic steatohepatitis histology (obeticholic acid, elafibranor, and liraglutide). The authors also review the available preliminary data on cenicriviroc and selonsertib, with or without simtuzumab's phase II studies. Finally, the authors briefly discuss compounds that have been tested but did not achieve the primary end point of histologic improvement and appeared in high-quality published articles (cysteamine bitartrate and long-chain polyunsaturated fatty acids).

Nonalcoholic Fatty Liver Disease/Nonalcoholic Steatohepatitis and Hepatocellular Carcinoma   201

Omar Massoud and Michael Charlton

Although hepatocellular carcinoma (HCC) is more common in the setting of cirrhosis, there is increasing evidence that it can develop in the setting of noncirrhotic nonalcoholic fatty liver disease (NAFLD)/nonalcoholic steato-hepatitis (NASH) and that steatosis alone can promote carcinogenesis. In addition, obesity, diabetes, and metabolic syndrome are recognized risks for the development of HCC. A better understanding of the mechanisms involved in the development of NAFLD/NASH-related HCC will allow the discovery of new targets for therapeutic and preventive intervention. The surveillance for HCC in the setting of noncirrhotic NAFLD/NASH, obesity, diabetes, and metabolic syndrome remains an area of uncertainty.

Nonalcoholic Fatty Liver Disease/Nonalcoholic Steatohepatitis in Liver Transplantation   213

Danielle Carter, Douglas T. Dieterich, and Charissa Chang

The number of transplants caused by nonalcoholic fatty liver disease/ nonalcoholic steatohepatitis (NASH) has been progressively increasing and this is expected to become the most common indication for liver transplantation in the United States. Patients with NASH show many features of the metabolic syndrome and, as a result, are at higher risk for postoperative cardiovascular morbidity and mortality. Despite this, patients with NASH have long-term graft and patient survival rates comparable with other causes of chronic liver disease. Posttransplant metabolic syndrome is a common occurrence that increases the risk of steatosis in the graft liver.

NASH and NAFLD

CLINICS IN LIVER DISEASE

FORTHCOMING ISSUES

May 2018
Acute Liver Failure
Nikolaos T. Pyrsopoulos, *Editor*

August 2018
Primary Biliary Cholangitis
Cynthia Levy and Elizabeth J. Carey,
Editors

November 2018
Pediatric Liver Disease
Philip Rosenthal, *Editor*

RECENT ISSUES

November 2017
Consultations in Liver Disease
Steven L. Flamm, *Editor*

August 2017
Hepatitis C Infection as a Systemic Disease:
Extra-Hepatic Manifestation of Hepatitis C
Zobair M. Younossi, *Editor*

May 2017
Liver Transplantation
Roberto J. Firpi, *Editor*

THE CLINICS ARE AVAILABLE ONLINE!
Access your subscription at:
www.theclinics.com

Preface

Nonalcoholic Fatty Liver Disease: An Expanding Health Care Epidemic

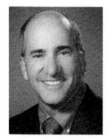

David E. Bernstein, MD
Editor

Nonalcoholic fatty liver disease (NAFLD) has become a common worldwide condition, the prevalence of which continues to increase with the worldwide surge in the incidence of obesity and diabetes. In the United States alone, NAFLD affects between 60 and 100 million people, including 10% of American children. The spectrum of disease ranges from simple, nonclinically significant hepatic steatosis to steatohepatitis (NASH) to cirrhosis, hepatocellular carcinoma, and decompensated liver disease. In 2016, NAFLD was reported to surpass hepatitis C as the leading indication for liver transplantation among adults under the age of 50, and it is predicted to be the leading indication for liver transplantation in the next decade (Banini and Sanyal, Am J Gastroenterol 2016, Vol 111; Abstract 46).

NAFLD/NASH is the hepatic manifestation of the metabolic syndrome and therefore associated with hypertension, hyperlipidemia, diabetes, and obesity. Despite this association, NAFLD may occur in nondiabetic, nonobese individuals, suggesting that multiple mechanisms may exist for its development. Over the past decade, there have been significant advances in our understanding of the prevalence, natural history, genetics, evaluation, and treatment of NAFLD.

This issue of *Clinics in Liver Disease* provides an update to our current understanding of NAFLD as presented by a cadre of distinguished experts in the field. The first section reviews its clinical and economic burden, discusses the implication of NAFLD in children, and reviews the natural history of the disease. The second section discusses the diagnosis and evaluation of NAFLD/NASH, focusing on noninvasive serological markers, the role of liver biopsy, and an in-depth discussion of the use of radiological imaging. The third section concentrates on the pathophysiology, risk factors, genetics, and the role of intestinal microbes in the disease. The final section discusses

Clin Liver Dis 22 (2018) xiii–xiv
https://doi.org/10.1016/j.cld.2017.10.001
1089-3261/18/© 2017 Published by Elsevier Inc.

associated conditions, reviews current and emerging treatments, and discusses the development of hepatocellular carcinoma and the role of liver transplantation in NAFLD/NASH.

Our understanding of NAFLD/NASH continues to grow at a rapid pace, and keeping up with the latest information can be challenging. The contributors to this issue have worked hard to provide excellent, concise, up-to-date reviews of the topics listed above. I hope you enjoy their work, and I thank them all for their contributions.

David E. Bernstein, MD
Zucker School of Medicine at Hofstra/Northwell
400 Community Drive
Manhasset, NY 11030, USA

E-mail address:
dbernste@northwell.edu

Clinical and Economic Burden of Nonalcoholic Fatty Liver Disease and Nonalcoholic Steatohepatitis

 CrossMark

Zobair M. Younossi, MD, MPH[a,b,*], Linda Henry, PhD[c],
Haley Bush, MPH[b], Alita Mishra, MD[a]

KEYWORDS

- Prevalence - Risk factors - Mortality - Health-related quality of life

KEY POINTS

- The prevalence of nonalcoholic fatty liver disease (NAFLD) and nonalcoholic steatohepatitis (NASH) continues to increase around the world as a result of the increase in obesity and other metabolic disorders.
- The true incidences of NAFLD and NASH are unknown because of the lack of accurate noninvasive diagnostic methods and lack of awareness of this disease outside of gastroenterology and hepatology practices.
- The economic burden of NAFLD/NASH, which is projected to be immense, must be more precisely defined for an effective national and global strategy to deal with the epidemic of NAFLD-related liver disease.

THE EPIDEMIOLOGIC BURDEN OF NONALCOHOLIC FATTY LIVER DISEASE

Nonalcoholic fatty liver disease (NAFLD) is a complex liver disease, which affects up to one-quarter of the adult population in the world.[1,2] In a recent meta-analysis, the worldwide prevalence of NAFLD was estimated to be 25.24% (95% confidence interval [CI]: 22.10–28.65).[2] This prevalence varied across the globe, with the highest prevalence reported in the Middle East and the lowest in Africa.[2] Interestingly, the prevalence of NAFLD in Asian countries seems to follow a rural-to-urban gradient,

Disclosure: Dr Z.M. Younossi is a consultant or advisory board member of Intercept, Gilead, Allergan, BMS, and GSK. Drs L. Henry, H. Bush, and A. Mishra have nothing to disclose.
[a] Department of Medicine, Center for Liver Diseases, Inova Fairfax Hospital, 3300 Gallows Road, Falls Church, VA 22042, USA; [b] Betty and Guy Beatty Center for Integrated Research, Inova Health System, 3300 Gallows Road, Falls Church, VA 22042, USA; [c] Center for Outcomes Research in Liver Disease, 2411 I Street NW, Washington, DC 20037, USA
* Corresponding author. Betty and Guy Beatty Center for Integrated Research, Claude Moore Health Education and Research Building, 3300 Gallows Road, Falls Church, VA 22042.
E-mail address: zobair.younossi@inova.org

Clin Liver Dis 22 (2018) 1–10
http://dx.doi.org/10.1016/j.cld.2017.08.001
1089-3261/18/

with lower prevalence rates reported from the rural areas of India and China and higher prevalence rates from the urban areas.[3–5]

In the United States, the prevalence of NAFLD varies according to ethnicity.[6–15] NAFLD is more common among Mexican Americans when compared with non-Hispanic whites and non-Hispanic blacks.[10] Even within an ethnic group, there are differences according to the country of origin.[8,11–17] In one study, Hispanics of Mexican origin had a significantly higher prevalence of NAFLD compared with the Hispanics of Dominican and Puerto Rican origin.[9] In contrast to Hispanic Americans, African Americans have a lower prevalence of NAFLD despite having a higher rate of metabolic conditions associated with NAFLD (obesity, type 2 diabetes mellitus, and hypertension).[14,15,17] These variations in prevalence rates suggest a dual impact of genetic predisposition coupled with environmental factors playing a role in determining the risk for NAFLD.[18–26]

As previously noted, NAFLD is considered the liver manifestation of metabolic syndrome and is highly associated with obesity, type 2 diabetes mellitus, hypertension, and hyperlipidemia.[18] The data from the meta-analysis revealed that the prevalence of these comorbidities within people with NAFLD were high, which included obesity at 51.34% (95% CI: 41.38–61.20), type 2 diabetes at 22.51% (95% CI: 17.92–27.89), hyperlipidemia at 69.16% (95% CI: 49.91%–83.46%), hypertension at 39.34% (95% CI: 33.15–45.88), and metabolic syndrome at 42.54% (95% CI: 30.06–56.05).[2] As the prevalence of obesity and diabetes increases, the incidence and disease burden from NAFLD will continue to increase.[27–33]

Although most patients with NAFLD are obese, it is important to recognize that some patients with NAFLD are considered lean. A study using the National Health and Nutrition Examination Survey's data suggested that the prevalence of lean NAFLD in the United States general population was about 7.8%, comprising 17% of all NAFLD cases.[34] In contrast, lean NAFLD may be the predominant type of NAFLD in certain geographic areas.[3–5] In one study, from rural India, lean NAFLD subjects comprised more than 50% of all NAFLD cases.[3–5] These data suggest that factors other than obesity, such as environmental factors or gut microbiome, may contribute to the development of lean NAFLD in the Asian countries.

It is important to note that the minority of patients with NAFLD will progress to cirrhosis, hepatocellular carcinoma, and liver-related death. In this context, NAFLD has been divided into different histologic subtypes.[35–38] Most long-term studies of NAFLD suggest that only patients with documented histologic evidence of nonalcoholic steatohepatitis (NASH), which comprises about 20% of NAFLD cases, are at the greatest risk for progression and adverse outcomes.[28–34,39–44] In other words, most patients with NAFLD have non-NASH NAFLD and are primarily at risk for cardiovascular mortality.[16,17,31,45–51] In contrast, about 15% to 20% of patients with NASH can have a progressive liver disease and may succumb to liver-related mortality.[39–44,51] Although mostly nonprogressive, it is important to note that a few patients with non-NASH NAFLD may progress and develop NASH and advanced fibrosis.[40] In contrast, a few patients with NASH and even NASH-related fibrosis can regress.[50] The exact circumstances under which patients with NASH can progress or regress has not been well defined. Nevertheless, in general, the progressive course of NASH has been closely linked to the increasing number of metabolic comorbidities, especially type 2 diabetes mellitus[34,45,47,52] (Figs. 1 and 2).

Finally, it is important to note that the risk of progressive liver disease for an individual patient with NAFLD is relatively small.[2] However, given the considerable prevalence of NAFLD in the United States, the total number of patients with

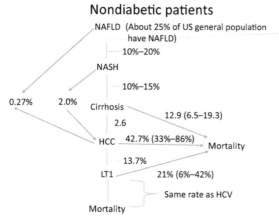

Fig. 1. Transition rates for NAFLD and NAFLD in nondiabetic patients.

NAFLD-related advanced liver disease could be substantial.[1–9] In this context, NAFLD is now considered among the top 3 causes of hepatocellular carcinoma[27] and the second leading indication for liver transplantation in the United States.[28] Given the current epidemic of obesity and diabetes, the expected increase in the incidence of NAFLD, and its potential for progression to cirrhosis, the clinical burden of NAFLD is expected to become enormous.

THE VALUE OF CLINICAL, LABORATORY, AND RADIOLOGIC DATA IN ESTABLISHING THE DIAGNOSIS OF NONALCOHOLIC STEATOHEPATITIS

Because of the complexities of the NASH phenotype, it is difficult to accurately establish the diagnosis solely based on the clinical data. In this context, liver enzymes lack specificity.[53] Ultrasound is a reasonably good method to establish the presence of fatty liver but is unable to distinguish NASH or the stage of fibrosis.[54] The introduction

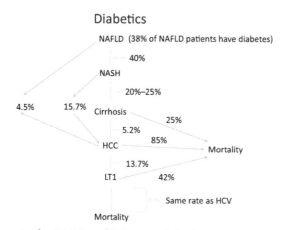

Fig. 2. Transition rates for NAFLD and NAFLD in diabetic patients.

of newer technologies to assess liver stiffness with transient elastography and magnetic resonance elastography have been encouraging but still lack the required performance characteristics to establish the diagnosis of NASH or to document the progression of liver fibrosis over time.[55]

There are several other noninvasive models that rely on clinical data in patients with NAFLD. These models include the Fibrosis-4 index, fatty liver index, NAFLD fibrosis score scoring system, and index of Nash.[56–58] Despite reasonable reliability in predicting the presence of advanced fibrosis in NAFLD, they lack the required predictive capacity to establish the diagnosis of NASH or accurately document earlier stages of fibrosis.[56–58] Nevertheless, these noninvasive modalities are useful in enriching our understanding of the population at risk for NASH and advanced fibrosis, as these are the patients who should be the primary group of patients to consider for further treatment interventions.

In summary, because of the lack of validated noninvasive diagnostic tests, liver biopsy continues to be considered the gold standard for diagnosing and staging NASH.[1] Nevertheless, it is expected that a combination of the next-generation radiologic modalities and noninvasive tests could improve their diagnostic performance, reducing the need for liver biopsy in most patients with NAFLD.

MORTALITY RISKS IN PATIENTS WITH NONALCOHOLIC FATTY LIVER DISEASE

Most patients with NAFLD die of cardiovascular diseases rather than liver disease.[16,17,33,38,48–51,59–63] Nevertheless, liver-related mortality is the second or third leading cause of death in these patients.[28,33,37,39,47] In this context, the initial study of subjects with biopsy-proven NAFLD and 146 months of follow-up reported that 9% of subjects died of liver-related causes.[37,47] A different study from Scandinavia also reported similar data with increased mortality in the NAFLD cohort as compared with the reference population (hazard ratio [HR] 1.29, 95% CI 1.04–1.59).[63] They also reported an increased risk for cardiovascular mortality (HR 1.55, CI 1.11–2.15, $P = .01$) as well as development of hepatocellular carcinoma (HR 6.55, CI 2.14–20.03, $P = .001$) and cirrhosis (HR 3.2, CI 1.05–9.81, $P = .041$).[63]

Given the increased risk of mortality in patients with NAFLD, several studies have carefully assessed liver biopsies of subjects with NAFLD to determine the predictive ability of individual pathologic features. Of the individual pathologic features from liver biopsies, only advanced fibrosis was initially reported as an independent predictor of mortality (adjusted HR = 5.68 [1.50–21.45]).[38] These data were confirmed in another study of subjects with biopsy-proven NAFLD and 12.6 years of follow-up, which showed that the presence of stage 2 fibrosis or higher was independently associated with liver-related mortality.[59] Finally, in a recent study, the risk for all-cause and liver-related mortality increased exponentially with the increasing stage of fibrosis.[49] In fact, liver-related mortality for subjects with NAFLD with fibrosis stage 1 revealed a mortality risk ratio (MMR) of 1.41 (95% CI 0.17–11.95), whereas those with fibrosis stage 4 had MRR of 42.30 (95% CI 3.51–510.34).[49]

In summary, several long-term studies have suggested that cardiovascular mortality is the most common cause of death in patients with NAFLD. Nevertheless, these patients are definitely at risk for excess mortality from liver-related causes. In this context, the presence of advanced fibrosis on the liver biopsy is the most important and independent predictor of mortality. Therefore, the concepts of steatofibrosis (presence of NAFLD of any type with advanced fibrosis) may be the best classification describing patients with NAFLD at the greatest risk for adverse long-term outcomes.[64,65]

QUALITY-OF-LIFE BURDEN OF PATIENTS WITH NONALCOHOLIC FATTY LIVER DISEASE

There is a significant paucity of quality-of-life data for patients with NAFLD. Nevertheless, studies using generic health-related quality of life (HRQL) instruments have suggested that patients with NAFLD have significant impairment of their HRQL when compared with the patients without liver disease. Furthermore, these studies have revealed that the more advanced the liver disease, the more profound the impairment in patients' HRQL.[66–68]

HRQL is an important patient-reported outcome (PRO) in understanding both the natural history of NAFLD and the potential effectiveness of treatments in clinical trials for subjects with NAFLD. Therefore, there was a need for a validated disease-specific HRQL instrument for NAFLD. Such a disease-specific instrument (Chronic Liver Disease Questionnaire-NAFLD/NASH version [CLDQ NAFLD-NASH]) was recently developed and validated.[66] The CLDQ NAFLD-NASH is now being extensively used for the clinical trials of therapeutic regimens for NASH and will be useful in understanding not only the burden of NAFLD but also the impact of its treatment on patients' well-being.

THE ECONOMIC BURDEN OF NONALCOHOLIC FATTY LIVER DISEASE

There are even more limited data related to the economic impact of NAFLD on the society.[68] Nevertheless, a recent analysis of the Medicare database demonstrated growing inpatient and outpatient costs for patients with NAFLD.[69,70] These reports were followed by a formal economic analysis to estimate the clinical and economic burden of NAFLD in the United States and Europe (Germany, France, Italy, and United Kingdom).[71] In this study, 5 models were created (one for the United States and 4 for the European countries) using a series of interlinked Markov chains, each representing age increments of NAFLD and the general populations. In this context, patients with NAFLD were allowed to transition between 9 stages of disease (NAFL, NASH, NASH-fibrosis, NASH-compensated cirrhosis, NASH-decompensated cirrhosis, hepatocellular carcinoma, liver transplantation, post–liver transplant, and death). The study estimated that in the United States, there are more than 64 million people with NAFLD with a potential annual direct medical cost of about $103 billion ($1613 per patient). In Europe, it was estimated that approximately 52 million people may have NAFLD with an annual cost of about €35 billion (from €354 to €1163 per patient). If the analysis had focused only on patients with NASH and fibrosis who are at the greatest for progression, an estimated 3 to 4 million patients in the United States with an annual expenditure of $10 to 15 billion will fall into this category.[71] This segregation of patients with NAFLD at the highest risk for adverse outcomes may provide a better and stepwise approach to addressing this serious form of liver disease in the United States. In this context, the diagnostic modalities must focus on determining steatofibrosis and treatment regimens must be developed for these patients at the greatest risk for mortality and adverse clinical, economic, and PROs.[64]

SUMMARY

In summary, as the prevalence of NAFLD continues to parallel those related to obesity and diabetes, there is a mounting need for new and better diagnostic modalities and treatment regimens. In this context, the currently available noninvasive diagnostic tests lack specificity and precision. Moreover, the current gold standard of liver biopsy is invasive and carries some risks. Despite these shortcomings, there is clear evidence that the clinical, economic, and PRO burden of NAFLD is tremendous and will continue to grow. Therefore, better understanding of the comprehensive (clinical, economic, and PRO) burden of this disease will help inform all important stakeholders, including policymakers, in their decisions to develop a robust strategy to deal with this significant health problem in the United States and the rest of the world.

The prevalence of NAFLD and NASH continues to increase around the world as a result of the increase in obesity and other metabolic disorders. However, the true incidence of NAFLD and NASH are unknown because the lack of accurate noninvasive diagnostic methods and lack of awareness of this disease outside of gastroenterology and hepatology practices. In order to deal with the clinical impact of NAFLD, these barriers must be overcome. Additionally, the economic burden of NAFLD/NASH, which is projected to be immense, must be more precisely defined for an effective national and global strategy to deal with the epidemic of NAFLD-related liver disease.

REFERENCES

1. Chalasani N, Younossi Z, Lavine JE, et al. The diagnosis and management of nonalcoholic fatty liver disease: practice guidance from the American Association for the study of liver diseases. Hepatology 2017. [Epub ahead of print].
2. Younossi ZM, Koenig AB, Abdelatif D, et al. Global epidemiology of nonalcoholic fatty liver disease-meta-analytic assessment of prevalence, incidence, and outcomes. Hepatology 2016;64(1):73–84.
3. Ashtari S, Pourhoseingholi MA, Zali MR. Non-alcohol fatty liver disease in Asia: prevention and planning. World J Hepatol 2015;7(13):1788–96.
4. Zhu JZ, Dai YN, Wang YM, et al. Prevalence of nonalcoholic fatty liver disease and economy. Dig Dis Sci 2015;60(11):3194–202.
5. Chatterjee A, Basu A, Chowdhury A, et al. Comparative analyses of genetic risk prediction methods reveal extreme diversity of genetic predisposition to nonalcoholic fatty liver disease (NAFLD) among ethnic populations of India. J Genet 2015;94(1):105–13.
6. Lazo M, Hernaez R, Eberhardt MS, et al. Prevalence of nonalcoholic fatty liver disease in the United States the third national health and nutrition examination survey, 1988-1994. Am J Epidemiol 2013;178(1):38–45.
7. Browning JD, Szczepaniak LS, Dobbins R, et al. Prevalence of hepatic steatosis in an urban population in the United States: impact of ethnicity. Hepatology 2004; 40:1387–95.
8. Schneider AL, Lazo M, Selvin E, et al. Racial differences in nonalcoholic fatty liver disease in the U.S. population. Obesity (Silver Spring) 2014;22(1):292–9.
9. Saab S, Manne V, Nieto J, et al. Nonalcoholic fatty liver disease in Latinos. Clin Gastroenterol Hepatol 2016;14(1):5–12 [quiz: e9–10].
10. Balakrishnan M, Kanwal F, El-Serag HB, et al. Acculturation and NAFLD risk among Hispanics of Mexican-origin: findings from the National Health and Nutrition Examination Survey. Clin Gastroenterol Hepatol 2016. http://dx.doi.org/10.1016/j.cgh.2016.09.149.
11. Wagenknecht LE, Scherzinger AL, Stamm ER, et al. Correlates and heritability of nonalcoholic fatty liver disease in a minority cohort. Obesity (Silver Spring) 2009; 17:1240–6.
12. Kalia HS, Gaglio PJ. The prevalence and pathobiology of nonalcoholic fatty liver disease in patients of different races or ethnicities. Clin Liver Dis 2016;20(2): 215–24.
13. Pan JJ, Fallon MB. Gender and racial differences in nonalcoholic fatty liver disease [review]. World J Hepatol 2014;6(5):274–83.

14. Kallwitz ER, Guzman G, TenCate V, et al. The histologic spectrum of liver disease in African-American, non-Hispanic white, and Hispanic obesity surgery patients. Am J Gastroenterol 2009;104(1):64–9.

15. Kanwal F, Kramer JR, Duan Z, et al. Trends in the burden of nonalcoholic fatty liver disease in a United States cohort of veterans. Clin Gastroenterol Hepatol 2016; 14(2):301–8.e1-2.

16. Carroll JF, Fulda KG, Chiapa AL, et al. Impact of race/ethnicity on the relationship between visceral fat and inflammatory biomarkers. Obesity (Silver Spring) 2009; 17:1420–7.

17. Morimoto Y, Conroy SM, Ollberding NJ, et al. Ethnic differences in serum adipokine and C-reactive protein levels: the multiethnic cohort. Int J Obes (Lond) 2014; 38(11):1416–22.

18. Smits MM, Ioannou GN, Boyko EJ, et al. Non-alcoholic fatty liver disease as an independent manifestation of the metabolic syndrome: results of a US national survey in three ethnic groups. J Gastroenterol Hepatol 2013;28(4):664–70.

19. Bambha K, Belt P, Abraham M, et al. Nonalcoholic steatohepatitis clinical research network research group ethnicity and nonalcoholic fatty liver disease. Hepatology 2012;55(3):769–80.

20. Stepanova M, Hossain N, Afendy A, et al. Hepatic gene expression of Caucasian and African-American patients with obesity-related non-alcoholic fatty liver disease. Obes Surg 2010;20(5):640–50.

21. Karrar A, Stepanova M, Alaparthi L, et al. Anti-adipocyte antibody response in patients with non-alcoholic fatty liver disease. J Gastroenterol Hepatol 2015; 30(5):900–8.

22. Estep JM, Goodman Z, Sharma H, et al. Adipocytokine expression associated with miRNA regulation and diagnosis of NASH in obese patients with NAFLD. Liver Int 2015;35(4):1367–72.

23. Khan UI, Wang D, Sowers MR, et al. Race-ethnic differences in adipokine levels: the study of Women's Health across the Nation (SWAN). Metabolism 2012;61(9): 1261–9.

24. Fleischman MW, Budoff M, Zeb I, et al. NAFLD prevalence differs among hispanic subgroups: the Multi-Ethnic Study of Atherosclerosis. World J Gastroenterol 2014;20(17):4987–93.

25. Foster T, Anania FA, Li D, et al. The prevalence and clinical correlates of nonalcoholic fatty liver disease (NAFLD) in African Americans: the multiethnic study of atherosclerosis (MESA). Dig Dis Sci 2013;58(8):2392–8.

26. Dongiovanni P, Romeo S, Valenti L. Genetic factors in the pathogenesis of nonalcoholic fatty liver and steatohepatitis. Biomed Res Int 2015;2015:460190.

27. Younossi ZM, Otgonsuren M, Henry L, et al. Association of nonalcoholic fatty liver disease (NAFLD) with hepatocellular carcinoma (HCC) in the United States from 2004 to 2009. Hepatology 2015;62(6):1723–30.

28. Wong RJ, Cheung R, Ahmed A. Nonalcoholic steatohepatitis is the most rapidly growing indication for liver transplantation in patients with hepatocellular carcinoma in the U.S. Hepatology 2014;59(6):2188–95.

29. Mavrogiannaki AN, Migdalis IN. Nonalcoholic fatty liver disease, diabetes mellitus and cardiovascular disease: newer data. Int J Endocrinol 2013;2013:450639.

30. Finucane MM, Stevens GA, Cowan MJ, et al. National, regional, and global trends in body-mass index since 1980: systematic analysis of health examination surveys and epidemiological studies with 960 country-years and 9·1 million participants. Lancet 2011;377:557–67.

31. Anstee QM, Targher G, Day CP. Progression of NAFLD to diabetes mellitus, cardiovascular disease or cirrhosis [review]. Nat Rev Gastroenterol Hepatol 2013; 10(6):330–44.

32. Lonardo A, Sookoian S, Chonchol M, et al. Disease - atherosclerosis as a major player in the natural course of NAFLD. Curr Pharm Des 2013;19:5177–92.

33. Adams LA, Anstee QM, Tilg H, et al. Non-alcoholic fatty liver disease and its relationship with cardiovascular disease and other extrahepatic diseases. Gut 2017; 66(6):1138–53.

34. Younossi ZM, Stepanova M, Negro F, et al. Nonalcoholic fatty liver disease in lean individuals in the United States. Medicine (Baltimore) 2012;91(6):319–27.

35. Ekstedt M, Franzen LE, Mathiesen UL, et al. Long-term follow-up of patients with NAFLD and elevated liver enzymes. Hepatology 2006;44(4):865–73.

36. Matteoni CA, Younossi ZM, Gramlich T, et al. Nonalcoholic fatty liver disease: a spectrum of clinical and pathological severity. Gastroenterology 1999;116(6): 1413–9.

37. Rafiq N, Bai C, Fang Y, et al. Long-term follow-up of patients with nonalcoholic fatty liver. Clin Gastroenterol Hepatol 2009;7(2):234–8.

38. Younossi ZM, Stepanova M, Rafiq N, et al. Pathologic criteria for nonalcoholic steatohepatitis: interprotocol agreement and ability to predict liver-related mortality. Hepatology 2011;53(6):1874–82.

39. Wong RJ, Aguilar M, Cheung R, et al. Nonalcoholic steatohepatitis is the second leading etiology of liver disease among adults awaiting liver transplantation in the United States. Gastroenterology 2015;148(3):547–55.

40. Ertle J, Dechêne A, Sowa JP, et al. Non-alcoholic fatty liver disease progresses to hepatocellular carcinoma in the absence of apparent cirrhosis. Int J Cancer 2011; 128(10):2436–43.

41. Perumpail RB, Wong RJ, Ahmed A, et al. Hepatocellular carcinoma in the setting of non-cirrhotic nonalcoholic fatty liver disease and the metabolic syndrome: US experience. Dig Dis Sci 2015;60(10):3142–8.

42. Yopp AC, Choti MA. Non-alcoholic steatohepatitis-related hepatocellular carcinoma: a growing epidemic? Dig Dis 2015;33(5):642–7.

43. Ferlay JS, Ervik M, Dikshit R, et al. GLOBOCAN 2012 v1.0, cancer incidence and mortality worldwide: IARC CancerBase No. 11. Lyon (France): International Agency for Research on Cancer; 2013.

44. Mittal S, Sada YH, El-Serag HB, et al. Temporal trends of nonalcoholic fatty liver disease-related hepatocellular carcinoma in the veteran affairs population. Clin Gastroenterol Hepatol 2015;13(3):594–601.e1.

45. Younossi ZM, Gramlich T, Matteoni CA, et al. Nonalcoholic fatty liver disease in patients with type 2 diabetes. Clin Gastroenterol Hepatol 2004;2(3):262–5 [Erratum appears in Clin Gastroenterol Hepatol 2004;2(6):522].

46. Otgonsuren M, Stepanova M, Gerber L, et al. Anthropometric and clinical factors associated with mortality in subjects with nonalcoholic fatty liver disease. Dig Dis Sci 2013;58(4):1132–40.

47. Stepanova M, Younossi ZM. Independent association between nonalcoholic fatty liver disease and cardiovascular disease in the US population. Clin Gastroenterol Hepatol 2012;10(6):646–50.

48. McPherson S, Hardy T, Henderson E, et al. Evidence of NAFLD progression from steatosis to fibrosing-steatohepatitis using paired biopsies: implications for prognosis and clinical management. J Hepatol 2015;62(5):1148–55.

49. Dulai PS, Singh S, Patel J, et al. Increased risk of mortality by fibrosis stage in non-alcoholic fatty liver disease: systematic review and meta-analysis. Hepatology 2017;65(5):1557–65.

50. Motamed N, Rabiee B, Poustchi H, et al. Non-alcoholic fatty liver disease (NAFLD) and 10-year risk of cardiovascular diseases. Clin Res Hepatol Gastroenterol 2017;41(1):31–8.

51. Sinn DH, Kang D, Chang Y, et al. Non-alcoholic fatty liver disease and progression of coronary artery calcium score: a retrospective cohort study. Gut 2017; 66(2):323–9.

52. Adams LA, Lymp JF, St Sauver J, et al. The natural history of nonalcoholic fatty liver disease: a population-based cohort study. Gastroenterology 2005;129: 113–21.

53. Golabi P, Sayiner M, Fazel Y, et al. Current complications and challenges in nonalcoholic steatohepatitis screening and diagnosis. Expert Rev Gastroenterol Hepatol 2016;10(1):63–71.

54. Saadeh S, Younossi ZM, Remer EM, et al. The utility of radiological imaging in nonalcoholic fatty liver disease. Gastroenterology 2002;123(3):745–50.

55. Hashemi SA, Alavian SM, Gholami-Fesharaki M. Assessment of transient elastography (FibroScan) for diagnosis of fibrosis in non-alcoholic fatty liver disease: a systematic review and meta-analysis. Caspian J Intern Med 2016;7(4):242–52.

56. Otgonsuren M, Estep MJ, Hossain N, et al. Single non-invasive model to diagnose non-alcoholic fatty liver disease (NAFLD) and non-alcoholic steatohepatitis (NASH). J Gastroenterol Hepatol 2014;29(12):2006–13.

57. Cui J, Ang B, Haufe W, et al. Comparative diagnostic accuracy of magnetic resonance elastography vs. eight clinical prediction rules for non-invasive diagnosis of advanced fibrosis in biopsy-proven non-alcoholic fatty liver disease: a prospective study. Aliment Pharmacol Ther 2015;41(12):1271–80.

58. Goulart AC, Oliveira IR, Alencar AP, et al. Diagnostic accuracy of a noninvasive hepatic ultrasound score for non-alcoholic fatty liver disease (NAFLD) in the Brazilian Longitudinal Study of Adult Health (ELSA-Brasil). Sao Paulo Med J 2015;133(2):115–24.

59. Angulo P, Kleiner DE, Dam-Larsen S, et al. Liver fibrosis, but no other histologic features, is associated with long-term outcomes of patients with nonalcoholic fatty liver disease. Gastroenterology 2015;149(2):389–97.e10.

60. Younossi Z, Henry L. Contribution of alcoholic and nonalcoholic fatty liver disease to the burden of liver-related morbidity and mortality. Gastroenterology 2016; 150(8):1778–85.

61. Haflidadottir S, Jonasson JG, Norland H, et al. Long-term follow-up and liver-related death rate in patients with non-alcoholic and alcoholic related fatty liver disease. BMC Gastroenterol 2014;14:166.

62. Golabi P, Fazel S, Otgonsuren M, et al. Mortality assessment of patients with hepatocellular carcinoma according to underlying disease and treatment modalities. Medicine (Baltimore) 2017;96(9):e5904.

63. Ekstedt M, Hagström H, Nasr P, et al. Fibrosis stage is the strongest predictor for disease-specific mortality in NAFLD after up to 33 years of follow-up. Hepatology 2015;61(5):1547–54.

64. Younossi ZM, Stepanova M, Rafiq N, et al. Non-alcoholic steatofibrosis is independently associated with both overall mortality and liver-related mortality in patients with non-alcoholic fatty liver disease (NAFLD). J of Hepat 2017; 66(1):S598.

65. Younossi Z, Stepanova M, Goodman Z, et al. Improvement of hepatic fibrosis in patients with non-alcoholic steatohepatitis (NASH) treated with selonsertib is associated with improvement of patient-reported outcomes (PROS). [Abstract]. EASL. Amsterdam, Netherlands, April 19-23, 2017.
66. Younossi ZM, Stepanova M, Henry L, et al. A disease-specific quality of life instrument for non-alcoholic fatty liver disease and non-alcoholic steatohepatitis: CLDQ-NAFLD. Liver Int 2017;37(8):1209–18.
67. Golabi P, Otgonsuren M, Cable R, et al. Non-alcoholic fatty liver disease (NAFLD) is associated with impairment of health related quality of life (HRQOL). Health Qual Life Outcomes 2016;14:18.
68. Younossi ZM, Henry L. Economic and quality-of-life implications of non-alcoholic fatty liver disease [review]. Pharmacoeconomics 2015;33(12):1245–53.
69. Sayiner M, Otgonsuren M, Cable R, et al. Variables associated with inpatient and outpatient resource utilization among Medicare beneficiaries with nonalcoholic fatty liver disease with or without cirrhosis. J Clin Gastroenterol 2017;51(3): 254–60.
70. Younossi ZM, Zheng L, Stepanova M, et al. Clinical outcomes and resource utilisation in Medicare patients with chronic liver disease: a historical cohort study. BMJ Open 2014;4(5):e004318.
71. Younossi ZM, Blissett D, Blissett R, et al. The economic and clinical burden of nonalcoholic fatty liver disease in the United States and Europe. Hepatology 2016;64(5):1577–86.

The Natural History of Nonalcoholic Fatty Liver Disease—An Evolving View

Christina C. Lindenmeyer, MD[a], Arthur J. McCullough, MD[b,c],*

KEYWORDS

- Insulin resistance • Metabolic syndrome • Obesity • Nonalcoholic fatty liver disease
- Nonalcoholic steatohepatitis • Fibrosis • Steatosis • Cirrhosis

KEY POINTS

- Nonalcoholic fatty liver disease (NAFLD) is a worldwide epidemic, with global prevalence increasing in parallel with rates of obesity, diabetes, and the metabolic syndrome.
- Understanding of the natural history of NAFLD is evolving; recent studies suggest that both patients with steatosis and with steatohepatitis are at risk for progression.
- Patients with NAFLD experience elevated rates of cardiovascular events and higher-than-expected all-cause mortality; fibrosis is the strongest predictor of liver-related complications and mortality.

INTRODUCTION

Since first described in 1980,[1] nonalcoholic fatty liver disease (NAFLD) is defined as the accumulation of hepatic fat, as evidenced by radiologic or histologic examination, in the absence of a coexisting cause of chronic liver disease or secondary cause of steatosis (including drugs, significant alcohol consumption, or inherited or acquired metabolic states). The spectrum of NAFLD encompasses 2 subtypes: nonalcoholic fatty liver (NAFL) and nonalcoholic steatohepatitis (NASH). Isolated NAFL is characterized by steatosis (which may be associated with mild chronic inflammation) in at least 5% of hepatocytes.

Disclosure Statement: The authors have nothing to disclose. This work is supported in part by NIH grants UDK 505, P50AA024333 and U01 AA021893.
^a Department of Gastroenterology and Hepatology, Cleveland Clinic, Cleveland Clinic Lerner College of Medicine of Case Western Reserve University, 9500 Euclid Avenue, Mail Code A30, Cleveland, OH 44195, USA; ^b Department of Gastroenterology and Hepatology, Transplantation Center, Cleveland Clinic, Cleveland Clinic Lerner College of Medicine of Case Western Reserve University, 9500 Euclid Avenue, Mail Code A30, Cleveland, OH 44195, USA; ^c Department of Pathobiology, Transplantation Center, Cleveland Clinic, Cleveland Clinic Lerner College of Medicine of Case Western Reserve University, 9500 Euclid Avenue, Mail Code A30, Cleveland, OH 44195, USA
* Corresponding author. 9500 Euclid Avenue, Mail Code A30, Cleveland, OH 44195.
E-mail address: MCCULLA@ccf.org

Clin Liver Dis 22 (2018) 11–21
http://dx.doi.org/10.1016/j.cld.2017.08.003
1089-3261/18/Published by Elsevier Inc.

On the other end of the spectrum, NASH is defined by a pattern of characteristics that include steatosis, lobular and portal inflammation, and liver cell injury in the form of hepatocyte ballooning. Lobular inflammation is classically mild, characterized by a mixed inflammatory cell infiltrate. Other potential histologic findings include Mallory–Denk bodies, iron deposition, periportal hepatocytes with vacuolated nuclei, ductular reaction, megamitochondria, lobular lipogranulomas, periodic acid–Schiff–diastase–resistant Kupffer cells, and acinar zone 3 perisinusoidal/pericellular fibrosis, which may be indistinguishable from alcoholic steatohepatitis.[2,3] In recent years, the NAFLD activity score, developed by the Pathology Committee of the NASH Clinical Research Network, has gained wide acceptance for histologically diagnosing NASH.[4] The NAFLD activity score assesses the degree of steatosis, lobular inflammation, hepatocellular ballooning, and fibrosis. The NAS, however, does not supplant a pathologist's overall histologic evaluation.[5]

Histologically, it is important clinically to establish the distinction between NAFL and NASH, because most NAFLD patients have steatosis without necroinflammation or fibrosis and do not require medical therapy. In its more advanced stages, NAFLD can progress to fibrosis, cirrhosis, and end-stage liver disease with related complications, including hepatocellular carcinoma (HCC).[6]

To understand the clinical relevance of NAFLD, define long-term outcomes, and risk-stratify patients for disease-related complications and mortality, it is important to understand the natural history of the disease. Long-term observational studies, paired liver biopsy studies, and high-quality global meta-analysis have better defined the course of NAFLD. Conflicting data among studies persists, however, with resultant persistent ambiguity in the field. This review attempts to add to the current literature by summarizing recent high-quality evidence supporting the elucidation of the natural history of NAFLD.

EPIDEMIOLOGY

A recent systematic review and meta-analysis has estimated the global prevalence of NAFLD, as diagnosed by imaging in the absence of significant alcohol use, to be approximately 25%, with the highest prevalence in the Middle East and South America and the lowest prevalence in Africa. Metabolic comorbidities associated with a diagnosis of NAFLD included obesity (51.34%), type 2 diabetes mellitus (22.51%), hyperlipidemia (69.16%), hypertension (39.34%), and the metabolic syndrome (42.54%).[7] In the United States, data from the National Health and Nutrition Examination Surveys (NHANES) conducted between 1988 and 2008 estimate that the prevalence of NAFLD increased from 5.5% to 11%, with concurrent increased prevalence of obesity, type 2 diabetes mellitus, insulin resistance, and hypertension. By contrast, the prevalence of hepatitis B–related, hepatitis C–related, and alcohol-related chronic liver disease remained stable over the same period of time. NAFLD is increasingly diagnosed in the pediatric population, with studies estimating prevalence rates of 3% to 18%.[8–11]

Based on data collected from the United Network for Organ Sharing and the Organ Procurement and Transplantation Network registry from 2004 through 2013, NAFLD is now the most common form of chronic liver disease in the United States and is the second-most common indication for liver transplantation.[12] The same study identified that new liver transplant waitlist registrants with NASH increased by 170%; however, these same patients experienced higher 90-day waitlist mortality and were less likely to undergo liver transplantation. NAFLD is on track to be the most common indication for liver transplantation by the year 2020.[13]

CLINICAL SIGNIFICANCE OF NONALCOHOLIC FATTY LIVER DISEASE

NAFLD is thought to be the hepatic manifestation of the metabolic syndrome, defined as the presence of 3 or more of the following[1]: abdominal obesity (waist circumference >102 cm in men and >88 cm in women),[2] hypertriglyceridemia (>150 mg/dL),[3] low high-density lipoprotein levels (<40 mg/dL in men and <50 mg/dL in women),[4] hypertension (>130/80 mm/Hg), and[5] high fasting glucose levels (>110 mg/dL).[14,15] The prevalence of NAFLD in patients with the metabolic syndrome,[16] in particular diabetes, is high.[17,18] The global prevalence of obesity among NAFLD patients and among NASH patients is estimated to be 51% and 82%, respectively.[7] In studies of patients with cryptogenic cirrhosis, greater than 60% of patients have been shown to have metabolic risk factors for NAFLD.[19,20] NAFLD has also been associated with hypothyroidism,[21] polycystic ovarian syndrome,[22] and colonic adenomas and neoplasms.[23]

Cardiovascular Disease

Metabolic syndrome is a powerful risk factor for cardiovascular disease, and multiple studies have demonstrated that cardiovascular disease is the leading cause of death in NAFLD patients, with NASH, fibrosis stage, and diabetes being the strongest risk factors for overall and liver-specific mortality.[24–30] An early population study from Olmstead County,[27] Minnesota, of 420 patients with NAFLD with a mean follow-up of 7.6 years, observed that patients with NAFLD have a higher all-cause mortality rate than age-matched and gender-matched patients without NAFLD (standardized mortality ratio, 1.34; 95% CI, 1.003–1.76; $P = .03$).[27] The 3 leading causes of death in patients with NAFLD were malignancy, ischemic heart disease, and liver disease, with higher mortality rates observed in older patients and in patients with impaired fasting glucose and cirrhosis.

In a population-based study from NHANES III[30] of 12,822 patients between 1988 and 1994, 80 patients with NAFLD (defined by elevated serum aminotransferases in the absence of other chronic liver disease) died, consistent with higher overall mortality (hazard ratio [HR] 1.038; 95% CI, 1.036–1.041; $P<.0001$) and liver-related mortality (HR 9.32; 95% CI, 9.21–9.43; $P<.0001$) than patients without NAFLD. Cardiovascular events were the leading cause of death in patients with suspected NAFLD, followed by nonhepatic malignancy and liver-related death.

In a follow-up study of NHANES III, suspected NAFLD (based on similar inclusion criteria), especially in the 45-year-old to 54-year-old age group, was demonstrated to be an independent risk factor for cardiovascular event-related death, although the HR of 1.37 (95% CI, 0.98–1.91) for all-cause mortality was found to be of borderline statistical significance.[31]

A recent meta-analysis and systematic review of 16 observational or retrospective studies of patients with suspected NAFLD (based on either radiological imaging or histology) found that patients with NAFLD were at higher risk of fatal and nonfatal cardiovascular events than those without NAFLD (random effect odds ratio 1.64; 95% CI, 1.26–2.13).[32] In addition, patients with severe NAFLD, that is, NASH with or without fibrosis, were also at elevated risk for fatal and nonfatal cardiovascular events (odds ratio 2.58; 1.78–3.75). Patients with NAFLD also have higher rates of cardiovascular disease than patients with hepatitis C virus (HCV). In a long-term follow-up study comparing the natural history of cirrhosis in patients with NASH to patients with HCV, patients with NASH had a significantly higher risk of cardiovascular-related mortality than their matched controls with HCV (8/152 vs 1/150; $P<.03$).[33] The observational nature of these studies included in this systematic review falls short of establishing causality with respect to cardiovascular disease but prompts the need for intensified guidelines regarding cardiovascular screening strategies in patients with NAFLD.

Liver-Related Morbidity

In terms of histologic progression, dogma endures that NAFL carries a more favorable prognosis than NASH, which can histologically progress to fibrosis and, in up to 25% of patients, to cirrhosis.[34,35] The evolution of fibrosis carries secondary risks, including complications associated with portal hypertension (ascites, variceal hemorrhage, and hepatic encephalopathy), end-stage liver disease, and HCC. Liver-related death is the third leading cause of death in patients with NAFLD.[27,28] In developed Western nations, between 4% and 22% of cases of HCC are now attributed to NAFLD.[36] Lack of awareness about risk factors for NAFLD and its progression, combined with insufficient or unreliable screening and surveillance modalities, may contribute to a delay in diagnosis and may explain why many patients present in the later stages of the disease.[37] The burden of NAFLD is associated with worldwide increased health care costs and resource utilization as well as with decreased health-related quality of life.[38]

RISK FACTORS FOR PROGRESSION
Steatosis

Hepatic steatosis occurs in the setting of insulin resistance and the metabolic syndrome modulated by visceral adipose tissue. This alteration of lipid and glucose metabolism can result in dysregulation of hepatic transcription factors and nuclear receptors, resulting in hepatic fat accumulation. Hepatic steatosis can create a proinflammatory environment, leading to cellular injury and necroinflammation.[39,40]

In keeping with the hypothesis that NAFLD is the hepatic manifestation of the metabolic syndrome, weight gain has been associated with the development of NAFLD, and, conversely, weight loss has been associated with regression of hepatic steatosis. In a subsample prospective ultrasound study of the first Israeli national health and nutrition examination survey (MABAT), 19% of patients who did not have imaging evidence of NAFLD at baseline were found to have NAFLD at a 7-year follow-up. Weight gain (5.8 ± 6.1 vs 1.4 ± 5.5 kg) was significantly higher in patients who developed NAFLD compared with those who did not. Of the patients who were found to have NAFLD at baseline, 36.4% had no imaging evidence of NAFLD after 7 years, associated with weight loss of 2.7 kg $\pm$ 5.0 kg, or a 5% decrease from baseline weight.[41]

Pooled data from a recent global meta-analysis estimated the incidence rate for NAFLD in Asia and Israel were 52.34 per 1000 (95% CI, 28.31–96.77) and 28.01 per 1000 person-years (95% CI, 19.34–40.57), respectively.[7] Whereas early studies suggested that simple steatosis was a benign condition that followed an indolent course,[42] recent histologic paired liver biopsy studies of patients with baseline NAFL suggest that NAFL is more progressive than originally thought.[43] In a prospective longitudinal study of 52 patients who underwent liver biopsy, 13 patients had simple steatosis at baseline. On follow-up biopsy at 26 months, 39% developed borderline NASH and 23% developed NASH. Weight loss (specifically, reduced BMI and waist circumference) was independently associated with disease stability and nonprogression to fibrosis.[44] In a study of 108 patients with NAFLD over a median interval of 6.6 years, 27 patients had NAFL (steatosis alone or associated with mild inflammation). Of the patients with NAFL at baseline, 44% of patients developed NASH, 27% of patients developed fibrosis, and 22% of patients had bridging fibrosis on follow-up liver biopsy. A similar proportion of patients with NAFL at baseline had progressive fibrosis as patients with NASH on index biopsy.[45] In a similar study of patients who underwent paired liver biopsies with a mean follow-up of 3.7 years, among 25 patients with NAFL, 64% progressed to NASH and 24% developed bridging fibrosis.[46] In a 2015 meta-analysis of paired liver biopsy studies, Singh and colleagues[47] found that patients with NAFL and stage 0 fibrosis at baseline progressed 1 stage of fibrosis over 14.3 years. By comparison, patients with NASH and stage 0 fibrosis at baseline demonstrated an accelerated rate of progression, advancing 1 stage of fibrosis over 7.1 years.

Steatohepatitis and Evolution of Fibrosis

In comparison to isolated hepatic steatosis, the evolution of NASH and the associated risk factors for progression have been widely investigated. In a recent meta-analysis of patients with NAFLD who underwent liver biopsy, the global prevalence of NASH in NAFLD patients has been estimated to be 59%.[7] Male gender, age, weight, total cholesterol, insulin resistance, hypertension, metabolic syndrome, thyroid-stimulating hormone levels, vitamin D levels, hyperuricemia, and certain genetic polymorphisms are predictors of histologic findings diagnostic of NASH.[48–55] Furthermore, factors associated with progression of fibrosis in patients with NASH include age, inflammation at index biopsy, hypertension, and low aspartate aminotransferase-to-alanine aminotransferase ratio.[47,56]

Argo and colleagues[56] conducted a systematic review of 10 studies inclusive of 221 patients in 2009, finding that 37.6% of patients with NASH had progressive fibrosis over a mean follow-up interval of 5.3 years. A recent meta-analysis of 4 studies of patients with biopsy-proven NASH estimated a pooled mean fibrosis progression rate 0.09 (95% CI, 0.06–0.12); meta-analysis of 6 studies of patients with histologic NASH estimated a percent fibrosis progression of 40.76% (95% CI, 34.69–47.13). Alarmingly, however, 1 of every 5 patients who experienced progression were identified as "rapid progressors"—patients who progressed from stage 0 fibrosis on initial biopsy to bridging fibrosis or cirrhosis at follow-up.[7] Unfortunately, due to the nature of the analysis, factors associated with rapid progression could not be distinguished, which identifies an important gap in understanding of the natural history of NAFLD and related fibrosis, and calls for further investigation.

The presence and stage of fibrosis seem the most important predictors of cardiovascular and liver-related complications. In a long-term study of 229 patients with NAFLD, Ekstedt and colleagues[24] discerned that patients with fibrosis stages 3 to 4, irrespective of the histologic NAS, had increased mortality (HR 3.3; CI, 2.27–4.76; P<.001) compared with a reference population from the Swedish National Registry of Population. These data are supported by a retrospective analysis of 619 patients with NAFLD from 1975 through 2005 at medical centers in the United States, Europe, and Thailand.[57] Angulo and colleagues[57] observed that the presence of fibrosis, independent of steatohepatitis, was associated with the need for liver transplantation, liver-related complications, and overall mortality.

Advanced Fibrosis and Cirrhosis

Overall, there is more limited information on long-term outcomes and the natural history of advanced fibrosis and cirrhosis due to NAFLD. The global incidence of advanced fibrosis in NASH patients has been estimated in meta-analysis to be 67.95 in 1000 person-years, with 41% of NASH patients experiencing fibrosis progression (average annual progression rate of 0.09%).[7] Up to 25% of patients with NAFLD progress to cirrhosis[35,58] and 7% to end-stage liver disease.[34] Advanced fibrosis and cirrhosis secondary to NAFLD have also been observed in the pediatric population, in up to 8% of patients with histologic NASH.[59] Obesity, diabetes, and carotid artery disease are predictive of advanced fibrosis and cirrhosis in patients with NASH.[60–62] In addition, a systematic review of 10 studies encompassing 221 patients with NASH identified age and inflammation on initial liver biopsy as independent factors associated with progression to advanced fibrosis.[56] In an early longitudinal study of 42 patients with NAFLD, Powell and colleagues[63] observed that fibrosis progression to cirrhosis was associated with loss of steatosis and inflammation histologically.

Patients with NAFLD-related cirrhosis seem to have lower rates of liver-related morbidity and mortality than patients with HCV-related cirrhosis. In a prospective, international study of 247 patients with histologically proved NAFLD-related advanced fibrosis (grade 3) or cirrhosis, patients with NAFLD had lower rates of liver-related complications than age-matched and gender-matched patients with HCV-related advanced fibrosis or cirrhosis, including HCC. Rates of cardiovascular events and overall mortality were similar between the 2 groups.[64] In a prospective study of 152 patients with NASH-related cirrhosis compared with 150 matched patients with HCV-related cirrhosis, at a 10-year follow-up, patients with Child-Pugh class A cirrhosis secondary to NASH had a significantly lower mortality than patients with similar patients with HCV (3/74 vs 15/75; P<.004) as well as a lower risk of decompensation (P<.007). Similar mortality rates were observed in patients with Child-Pugh class B or C cirrhosis across groups. Patients with NASH had lower rates of ascites development, hyperbilirubinemia, and HCC than comparable HCV patients.[33] An earlier, similar study from Hui and colleagues[65] observed similar liver-related complication and overall mortality rates between patients with NASH-related cirrhosis and HCV-related cirrhosis but also observed a lower rate of HCC in patients with NASH-related cirrhosis.

Powell and colleagues'[63] early findings can support reclassifying a large proportion of patients originally labeled as having cryptogenic cirrhosis as "burned-out NASH." A large proportion of these patients have risk known factors for the metabolic syndrome,[19,20] and histologically, although they may lack recognized features of NASH, these findings may have regressed concurrently with fibrosis progression.[19,66] This is supported by the high prevalence of NASH in liver transplant recipients who were transplanted for cryptogenic cirrhosis.[67]

Hepatocellular Carcinoma

Compared with alternative causes of chronic liver disease (for example, viral hepatitis and autoimmune or metabolic liver disease) that contribute to the global burden of HCC, patients with HCC attributed to NAFLD tend to be older and female. The development of HCC in NAFLD patients has been associated with age, obesity, diabetes, the PNPLA3 I148 M polymorphism, dietary habits, and drugs.[66,68] The annual incidence of HCC in NAFLD patients has been estimated to be 0.44 per 1000 person-years in a global meta-analysis. By comparison, the annual HCC incident rate in patients with NASH was 5.29 per 1000 person-years.[7] A recent Surveillance, Epidemiology, and End Results database study demonstrated a 9% annual increase (over a 6-year period, 2004–2009) in the number of HCC cases attributed to NAFLD. The investigators also observed that patients with NAFLD and HCC had a shorter survival time after diagnosis, more cardiovascular events, and were more likely to experience liver cancer–related mortality than patients without NAFLD.[69] Finally, and distressingly, HCC in patients with metabolic syndrome and NAFLD has been observed in the absence of significant fibrosis or cirrhosis.[70,71] As a result, HCC is frequently diagnosed at a more advanced stage than in patients with viral hepatitis, possibly the consequence of insufficient surveillance, which may contribute to the poorer prognosis observed in several studies.[72]

RECURRENCE AFTER LIVER TRANSPLANTATION

Recurrence of NAFLD and NASH has been reported in patients who have received liver transplantation, associated with persistence of the metabolic syndrome post–liver transplantation and negatively associated with weight loss after liver transplantation.[73–75] In an early series of 622 liver transplant recipients,[73] 8 female patients had histologic features of NAFLD pre–liver transplantation. At a median follow-up of 15 months, 6 patients developed steatosis, 3 of whom had features consistent with NASH, and 2 patients progressed from mild steatosis to NASH within 2 years of liver transplantation. In a case-control single-center study of patients undergoing liver transplantation from 1997 to 2008,[74] 98 patients were transplanted for NASH. Recurrent NAFLD, NASH, and advanced fibrosis were seen in 70%, 25%, and 18%, respectively, of patients at a mean follow-up of 18 months. Patients with recurrent NASH did not develop graft failure or require retransplantation at a mean follow-up of 3 years. In a study comparing post–liver transplantation outcomes between patients transplanted for NASH and patients transplanted for alcoholic liver disease,[75] steatohepatitis post–liver transplantation was more common in patients transplanted for NASH (33 vs 0%), but there was no statistically significant difference in rates of graft failure or retransplantation or in post–liver transplantation survival.

SUMMARY

NAFLD is a burgeoning epidemic in the United States and worldwide, and its clinical and economic impact will continue to grow with parallel increases in rates of obesity, diabetes, and the metabolic syndrome. Evolving understanding of the natural history of NAFLD suggests that patients with steatosis may be at a higher risk for disease progression to steatohepatitis and subsequently to fibrosis and cirrhosis than previously thought. Recent studies also suggest that these patients are at elevated risk for cardiovascular-related, malignancy-related, and liver-related morbidity and mortality, although their risk for progression, decompensation, and development of HCC may be less than that of patients with HCV. Continued study of the natural history of NAFLD and its complications through the conduction of high-quality, prospectively designed studies is needed. An improved understanding of the natural history of NAFLD, with definition of factors associated with progression and long-term outcomes, will lend itself to the development of enhanced prevention, screening, surveillance, and treatment modalities.

REFERENCES

1. Ludwig J, Viggiano TR, McGill DB, et al. Nonalcoholic steatohepatitis: Mayo Clinic experiences with a hitherto unnamed disease. Mayo Clin Proc 1980; 55(7):434–8.
2. Brunt EM, Janney CG, Di Bisceglie AM, et al. Nonalcoholic steatohepatitis: a proposal for grading and staging the histological lesions. Am J Gastroenterol 1999; 94(9):2467–74.
3. Sheth SG, Gordon FD, Chopra S. Nonalcoholic steatohepatitis. Ann Intern Med 1997;126(2):137–45.
4. Kleiner DE, Brunt EM, Van Natta M, et al. Design and validation of a histological scoring system for nonalcoholic fatty liver disease. Hepatology 2005;41(6): 1313–21.

5. Brunt EM, Kleiner DE, Wilson LA, et al, NASH Clinical Research Network (CRN). Nonalcoholic fatty liver disease (NAFLD) activity score and the histopathologic diagnosis in NAFLD: distinct clinicopathologic meanings. Hepatology 2011; 53(3):810–20.

6. Chalasani N, Younossi Z, Lavine JE, et al. The diagnosis and management of non-alcoholic fatty liver disease: practice guideline by the American Gastroenterological Association, American Association for the Study of Liver Diseases, and American College of Gastroenterology. Gastroenterology 2012;142(7):1592–609.

7. Younossi ZM, Koenig AB, Abdelatif D, et al. Global epidemiology of nonalcoholic fatty liver disease-Meta-analytic assessment of prevalence, incidence, and outcomes. Hepatology 2016;64(1):73–84.

8. Huang R-C, Beilin LJ, Ayonrinde O, et al. Importance of cardiometabolic risk factors in the association between nonalcoholic fatty liver disease and arterial stiffness in adolescents. Hepatology 2013;58(4):1306–14.

9. Ayonrinde OT, Olynyk JK, Beilin LJ, et al. Gender-specific differences in adipose distribution and adipocytokines influence adolescent nonalcoholic fatty liver disease. Hepatology 2011;53(3):800–9.

10. Browning JD, Szczepaniak LS, Dobbins R, et al. Prevalence of hepatic steatosis in an urban population in the United States: impact of ethnicity. Hepatology 2004; 40(6):1387–95.

11. Welsh JA, Karpen S, Vos MB. Increasing prevalence of nonalcoholic fatty liver disease among United States adolescents, 1988-1994 to 2007-2010. J Pediatr 2013;162(3):496–500.e1.

12. Wong RJ, Aguilar M, Cheung R, et al. Nonalcoholic steatohepatitis is the second leading etiology of liver disease among adults awaiting liver transplantation in the United States. Gastroenterology 2015;148(3):547–55.

13. Charlton MR, Burns JM, Pedersen RA, et al. Frequency and outcomes of liver transplantation for nonalcoholic steatohepatitis in the United States. Gastroenterology 2011;141(4):1249–53.

14. Expert Panel on Detection, Evaluation, and Treatment of High Blood Cholesterol in Adults. Executive summary of the third report of the National Cholesterol Education Program (NCEP) Expert Panel on Detection, Evaluation, and Treatment of high blood cholesterol in adults (Adult Treatment Panel III). JAMA 2001;285(19): 2486–97.

15. Ford ES, Giles WH, Dietz WH. Prevalence of the metabolic syndrome among US adults: findings from the third National Health and Nutrition Examination Survey. JAMA 2002;287(3):356–9.

16. Liangpunsakul S, Chalasani N. Unexplained elevations in alanine aminotransferase in individuals with the metabolic syndrome: results from the third National Health and Nutrition Survey (NHANES III). Am J Med Sci 2005;329(3):111–6.

17. Chan W-K, Tan AT-B, Vethakkan SR, et al. Non-alcoholic fatty liver disease in diabetics–prevalence and predictive factors in a multiracial hospital clinic population in Malaysia. J Gastroenterol Hepatol 2013;28(8):1375–83.

18. Portillo-Sanchez P, Bril F, Maximos M, et al. High prevalence of nonalcoholic fatty liver disease in patients with Type 2 diabetes mellitus and normal plasma aminotransferase levels. J Clin Endocrinol Metab 2015;100(6):2231–8.

19. Caldwell SH, Oelsner DH, Iezzoni JC, et al. Cryptogenic cirrhosis: clinical characterization and risk factors for underlying disease. Hepatology 1999;29(3):664–9.

20. Poonawala A, Nair SP, Thuluvath PJ. Prevalence of obesity and diabetes in patients with cryptogenic cirrhosis: a case-control study. Hepatology 2000 Oct; 32(4 Pt 1):689–92.

21. Liangpunsakul S, Chalasani N. Is hypothyroidism a risk factor for non-alcoholic steatohepatitis? J Clin Gastroenterol 2003;37(4):340–3.
22. Baranova A, Tran TP, Birerdinc A, et al. Systematic review: association of polycystic ovary syndrome with metabolic syndrome and non-alcoholic fatty liver disease. Aliment Pharmacol Ther 2011;33(7):801–14.
23. Lee YI, Lim Y-S, Park HS. Colorectal neoplasms in relation to non-alcoholic fatty liver disease in Korean women: a retrospective cohort study. J Gastroenterol Hepatol 2012;27(1):91–5.
24. Ekstedt M, Hagström H, Nasr P, et al. Fibrosis stage is the strongest predictor for disease-specific mortality in NAFLD after up to 33 years of follow-up. Hepatology 2015;61(5):1547–54.
25. Rafiq N, Bai C, Fang Y, et al. Long-term follow-up of patients with nonalcoholic fatty liver. Clin Gastroenterol Hepatol 2009;7(2):234–8.
26. Stepanova M, Rafiq N, Makhlouf H, et al. Predictors of all-cause mortality and liver-related mortality in patients with non-alcoholic fatty liver disease (NAFLD). Dig Dis Sci 2013;58(10):3017–23.
27. Adams LA, Lymp JF, St Sauver J, et al. The natural history of nonalcoholic fatty liver disease: a population-based cohort study. Gastroenterology 2005;129(1): 113–21.
28. Söderberg C, Stål P, Askling J, et al. Decreased survival of subjects with elevated liver function tests during a 28-year follow-up. Hepatology 2010;51(2):595–602.
29. Haflidadottir S, Jonasson JG, Norland H, et al. Long-term follow-up and liver-related death rate in patients with non-alcoholic and alcoholic related fatty liver disease. BMC Gastroenterol 2014;14:166.
30. Ong JP, Pitts A, Younossi ZM. Increased overall mortality and liver-related mortality in non-alcoholic fatty liver disease. J Hepatol 2008;49(4):608–12.
31. Dunn W, Xu R, Wingard DL, et al. Suspected nonalcoholic fatty liver disease and mortality risk in a population-based cohort study. Am J Gastroenterol 2008; 103(9):2263–71.
32. Targher G, Byrne CD, Lonardo A, et al. Non-alcoholic fatty liver disease and risk of incident cardiovascular disease: a meta-analysis. J Hepatol 2016;65(3): 589–600.
33. Sanyal AJ, Banas C, Sargeant C, et al. Similarities and differences in outcomes of cirrhosis due to nonalcoholic steatohepatitis and hepatitis C. Hepatology 2006; 43(4):682–9.
34. Ekstedt M, Franzén LE, Mathiesen UL, et al. Long-term follow-up of patients with NAFLD and elevated liver enzymes. Hepatology 2006;44(4):865–73.
35. McCullough AJ. The clinical features, diagnosis and natural history of nonalcoholic fatty liver disease. Clin Liver Dis 2004;8(3):521–33, viii.
36. Michelotti GA, Machado MV, Diehl AM. NAFLD, NASH and liver cancer. Nat Rev Gastroenterol Hepatol 2013;10(11):656–65.
37. Ratziu V, Cadranel J-F, Serfaty L, et al. A survey of patterns of practice and perception of NAFLD in a large sample of practicing gastroenterologists in France. J Hepatol 2012;57(2):376–83.
38. Younossi ZM, Henry L. Economic and quality-of-life implications of non-alcoholic fatty liver disease. Pharmacoeconomics 2015;33(12):1245–53.
39. Rinella ME. Nonalcoholic fatty liver disease: a systematic review. JAMA 2015; 313(22):2263–73.
40. Ballestri S, Nascimbeni F, Romagnoli D, et al. The role of nuclear receptors in the pathophysiology, natural course, and drug treatment of NAFLD in humans. Adv Ther 2016;33(3):291–319.

41. Zelber-Sagi S, Lotan R, Shlomai A, et al. Predictors for incidence and remission of NAFLD in the general population during a seven-year prospective follow-up. J Hepatol 2012;56(5):1145–51.
42. Teli MR, James OF, Burt AD, et al. The natural history of nonalcoholic fatty liver: a follow-up study. Hepatology 1995;22(6):1714–9.
43. Adams LA, Ratziu V. Non-alcoholic fatty liver - perhaps not so benign. J Hepatol 2015;62(5):1002–4.
44. Wong VW-S, Wong GL-H, Choi PC-L, et al. Disease progression of non-alcoholic fatty liver disease: a prospective study with paired liver biopsies at 3 years. Gut 2010;59(7):969–74.
45. McPherson S, Hardy T, Henderson E, et al. Evidence of NAFLD progression from steatosis to fibrosing-steatohepatitis using paired biopsies: implications for prognosis and clinical management. J Hepatol 2015;62(5):1148–55.
46. Pais R, Charlotte F, Fedchuk L, et al. A systematic review of follow-up biopsies reveals disease progression in patients with non-alcoholic fatty liver. J Hepatol 2013;59(3):550–6.
47. Singh S, Allen AM, Wang Z, et al. Fibrosis progression in nonalcoholic fatty liver vs nonalcoholic steatohepatitis: a systematic review and meta-analysis of paired-biopsy studies. Clin Gastroenterol Hepatol 2015;13(4):643–54.e1-9 [quiz: e39–40].
48. Ballestri S, Nascimbeni F, Romagnoli D, et al. The independent predictors of nonalcoholic steatohepatitis and its individual histological features: insulin resistance, serum uric acid, metabolic syndrome, alanine aminotransferase and serum total cholesterol are a clue to pathogenesis and candidate targets for treatment. Hepatol Res 2016;46(11):1074–87.
49. Dixon JB, Bhathal PS, O'Brien PE. Nonalcoholic fatty liver disease: predictors of nonalcoholic steatohepatitis and liver fibrosis in the severely obese. Gastroenterology 2001;121(1):91–100.
50. Carulli L, Canedi I, Rondinella S, et al. Genetic polymorphisms in non-alcoholic fatty liver disease: interleukin-6-174G/C polymorphism is associated with non-alcoholic steatohepatitis. Dig Liver Dis 2009;41(11):823–8.
51. Petta S, Cammà C, Cabibi D, et al. Hyperuricemia is associated with histological liver damage in patients with non-alcoholic fatty liver disease. Aliment Pharmacol Ther 2011;34(7):757–66.
52. Petta S, Grimaudo S, Cammà C, et al. IL28B and PNPLA3 polymorphisms affect histological liver damage in patients with non-alcoholic fatty liver disease. J Hepatol 2012;56(6):1356–62.
53. Carulli L, Ballestri S, Lonardo A, et al. Is nonalcoholic steatohepatitis associated with a high-though-normal thyroid stimulating hormone level and lower cholesterol levels? Intern Emerg Med 2013;8(4):297–305.
54. Dasarathy J, Periyalwar P, Allampati S, et al. Hypovitaminosis D is associated with increased whole body fat mass and greater severity of non-alcoholic fatty liver disease. Liver Int 2014;34(6):e118–27.
55. Italian Association for the Study of the Liver (AISF), Lonardo A, Nascimbeni F, Targher G, et al. AISF position paper on nonalcoholic fatty liver disease (NAFLD): updates and future directions. Dig Liver Dis 2017;49(5):471–83.
56. Argo CK, Northup PG, Al-Osaimi AMS, et al. Systematic review of risk factors for fibrosis progression in non-alcoholic steatohepatitis. J Hepatol 2009;51(2):371–9.
57. Angulo P, Kleiner DE, Dam-Larsen S, et al. Liver fibrosis, but no other histologic features, is associated with long-term outcomes of patients with nonalcoholic fatty liver disease. Gastroenterology 2015;149(2):389–97.e10.

58. Önnerhag K, Nilsson PM, Lindgren S. Increased risk of cirrhosis and hepatocellular cancer during long-term follow-up of patients with biopsy-proven NAFLD. Scand J Gastroenterol 2014;49(9):1111–8.
59. Schwimmer JB, Behling C, Newbury R, et al. Histopathology of pediatric nonalcoholic fatty liver disease. Hepatology 2005;42(3):641–9.
60. Koehler EM, Plompen EPC, Schouten JNL, et al. Presence of diabetes mellitus and steatosis is associated with liver stiffness in a general population: the Rotterdam study. Hepatology 2016;63(1):138–47.
61. You SC, Kim KJ, Kim SU, et al. Factors associated with significant liver fibrosis assessed using transient elastography in general population. World J Gastroenterol 2015;21(4):1158–66.
62. Roulot D, Czernichow S, Le Clésiau H, et al. Liver stiffness values in apparently healthy subjects: influence of gender and metabolic syndrome. J Hepatol 2008;48(4):606–13.
63. Powell EE, Cooksley WG, Hanson R, et al. The natural history of nonalcoholic steatohepatitis: a follow-up study of forty-two patients for up to 21 years. Hepatology 1990;11(1):74–80.
64. Bhala N, Angulo P, van der Poorten D, et al. The natural history of nonalcoholic fatty liver disease with advanced fibrosis or cirrhosis: an international collaborative study. Hepatology 2011;54(4):1208–16.
65. Hui JM, Kench JG, Chitturi S, et al. Long-term outcomes of cirrhosis in nonalcoholic steatohepatitis compared with hepatitis C. Hepatology 2003;38(2):420–7.
66. Bugianesi E, Leone N, Vanni E, et al. Expanding the natural history of nonalcoholic steatohepatitis: from cryptogenic cirrhosis to hepatocellular carcinoma. Gastroenterology 2002;123(1):134–40.
67. Ong J, Younossi ZM, Reddy V, et al. Cryptogenic cirrhosis and posttransplantation nonalcoholic fatty liver disease. Liver Transpl 2001;7(9):797–801.
68. Singal AG, Manjunath H, Yopp AC, et al. The effect of PNPLA3 on fibrosis progression and development of hepatocellular carcinoma: a meta-analysis. Am J Gastroenterol 2014;109(3):325–34.
69. Younossi ZM, Otgonsuren M, Henry L, et al. Association of nonalcoholic fatty liver disease (NAFLD) with hepatocellular carcinoma (HCC) in the United States from 2004 to 2009. Hepatology 2015;62(6):1723–30.
70. Paradis V, Zalinski S, Chelbi E, et al. Hepatocellular carcinomas in patients with metabolic syndrome often develop without significant liver fibrosis: a pathological analysis. Hepatology 2009;49(3):851–9.
71. Piscaglia F, Svegliati-Baroni G, Barchetti A, et al. Clinical patterns of hepatocellular carcinoma in nonalcoholic fatty liver disease: a multicenter prospective study. Hepatology 2016;63(3):827–38.
72. Giannini EG, Marabotto E, Savarino V, et al. Hepatocellular carcinoma in patients with cryptogenic cirrhosis. Clin Gastroenterol Hepatol 2009;7(5):580–5.
73. Kim WR, Poterucha JJ, Porayko MK, et al. Recurrence of nonalcoholic steatohepatitis following liver transplantation. Transplantation 1996;62(12):1802–5.
74. Malik SM, Devera ME, Fontes P, et al. Recurrent disease following liver transplantation for nonalcoholic steatohepatitis cirrhosis. Liver Transpl 2009;15(12): 1843–51.
75. Bhagat V, Mindikoglu AL, Nudo CG, et al. Outcomes of liver transplantation in patients with cirrhosis due to nonalcoholic steatohepatitis versus patients with cirrhosis due to alcoholic liver disease. Liver Transpl 2009;15(12):1814–20.

Pathophysiology of Nonalcoholic Fatty Liver Disease/Nonalcoholic Steatohepatitis

Vignan Manne, MD[1], Priya Handa, PhD[1], Kris V. Kowdley, MD*

KEYWORDS

- Nonalcoholic fatty liver disease (NAFLD) • Nonalcoholic steatohepatitis (NASH)
- Inflammation • Fibrosis • Genetic factors

KEY POINTS

- Hepatic steatosis is a consequence of impaired lipid metabolism in the liver. Major contributing factors are hepatic insulin resistance and increased influx of free fatty acids in the liver.
- Impaired adipose tissue function, dysbiosis of the gut microbiome, and recently identified genetic factors influence the development of nonalcoholic fatty liver disease.
- Although fatty liver progresses to nonalcoholic steatohepatitis (NASH) in a significant proportion of patients, the underlying mechanisms are not completely elucidated.
- Inflammation in the liver is triggered by the production of proinflammatory cytokines and chemokines by adipocytes, hepatic macrophages, and lipid-laden hepatocytes, which promote activation of stellate cells, the key cell type responsible for fibrogenesis in the liver.
- NASH is a common liver disease that is associated with progression to hepatocellular carcinoma and cirrhosis; therefore, there is an urgent need to discover drug targets and develop effective therapies.

INTRODUCTION

Nonalcoholic fatty liver disease (NAFLD) is a major public health concern because of its increased prevalence worldwide and potentially severe sequelae.[1] NAFLD is a hepatic manifestation of metabolic syndrome and a risk factor for type 2 diabetes mellitus, dyslipidemia, and hypertension.[1] NAFLD encompasses a broad spectrum

Disclosure: Dr K.V. Kowdley receives grants/research from Allergan, Galectin, Gilead, Immuron, Intercept, NGM Biopharma; serves on the advisory board of Allergan, Conatus, Enanta, Gilead, Intercept, Verlyx; is a consultant at Conatus, Gilead, Intercept, NGM Biopharma, Verlyx; and serves on the speaker's bureau of Gilead, Intercept.
Swedish Liver Care Network and Organ Care Research, Swedish Medical Center, 1124 Columbia Street, Suite 600, Seattle, WA 98104, USA
[1] Equal first coauthors.
* Corresponding author.
E-mail address: kris.kowdley@swedish.org

of liver disorders, ranging from simple steatosis to the more severe form, nonalcoholic steatohepatitis (NASH), that may progress to cirrhosis or hepatocellular carcinoma.[1] The hallmark of NAFLD is triglyceride (TG) accumulation in the cytoplasm of hepatocytes. This arises from an imbalance between lipid acquisition (ie, fatty acid uptake and de novo lipogenesis [DNL]) and removal (ie, mitochondrial fatty acid oxidation [FAO] and export as a component of very low-density lipoprotein [VLDL] particles).[2]

NASH, the more severe form of the disease, is characterized by steatosis, hepatic inflammation, and hepatocellular ballooning and may include varying degrees of fibrosis.[3] The understanding of the pathophysiology of NASH has evolved substantially from the original 2-hit hypothesis wherein a first hit, such as insulin resistance (IR), resulted in hepatic steatosis, and a subsequent second hit, such as oxidative stress, was required to develop NASH.[4] It is now apparent that the 2-hit hypothesis is not sufficient to describe the multiple pathways that may be interrelated and contribute to NASH. Thus, a multihit model has been proposed more recently for the pathophysiology of NASH, with multiple parallel hits occurring to cause NASH.[5]

The purpose of this article is to present an overall review of the most recent pathophysiologic concepts related to NAFLD and NASH.

PATHOPHYSIOLOGY OF NONALCOHOLIC FATTY LIVER DISEASE
Adipose Tissue Dysfunction and Increased Free Fatty Acid Flux to the Liver

Adipose tissue is the systemic site for storage of energy in the form of TGs.[6] Furthermore, it is an important endocrine organ involved in the secretion of hormones, cytokines, and chemokines, called adipokines.[7] Obesity as a result of overnutrition and/or underexertion commonly results in adipose tissue dysfunction.[6] Adipose tissue dysfunction has been thought to play a pivotal role in the development of metabolic disorders, such as IR and NAFLD (**Fig. 1**).[8] In an obese state, excess free fatty acids (FFAs) can enter the liver through the portal circulation. Increased levels of hepatic FFAs induce increased lipid synthesis and gluconeogenesis.[9] Studies from both animal models and human subjects have shown that increased levels of circulating FFAs can also lead to peripheral IR.[9,10] In addition, FFAs can contribute to

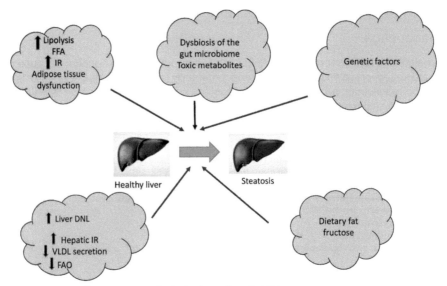

Fig. 1. Factors influencing nonalcoholic fatty liver (NAFL).

inflammation by serving as ligands for Toll-like receptor (TLR) 4 and inducing cytokine production, thereby contributing to NAFLD.[11,12]

Dysregulation of Adipokines

During obesity, the enlarged adipose tissue experiences a dysregulation of adipokine production.[13] Inflammatory chemokines and cytokines, such as monocyte chemotactic protein (MCP)-1, tumor necrosis factor (TNF)-α, interleukin (IL)-6, and IL-8, are increased and have been demonstrated to cause IR.[14] Furthermore, the macrophage content of adipose tissue is significantly associated with both adipocyte size and body mass and contributes significantly to the secretion of inflammatory cytokines.[15] Obesity also induces a phenotypic switch in macrophages from an anti-inflammatory M2 polarization to a proinflammatory M1 polarization.[16] In contrast, the expression of the beneficial anti-inflammatory insulin-sensitizing hormone, adiponectin, is decreased. Adiponectin is a adipocyte-specific adipokine that regulates FAO and attenuates lipid accumulation in the adipose tissue and the liver.[17] Furthermore, it regulates whole-body glucose homeostasis and hepatic insulin sensitivity.[18] Several studies have reported that adiponectin levels are lower in the serum of NAFLD patients relative to healthy controls.[19]

Leptin is yet another important adipokine that contributes to NAFLD.[6,7] Although leptin is important for regulating appetite and augmenting energy expenditure, its levels are increased in obesity, presumably due to leptin resistance.[6,7] A positive association has been documented between circulating leptin levels and serum alanine aminotransferase or hepatic steatosis.[20] In addition, leptin has been documented to promote fibrogenesis in stellate cells by stimulating the production of fibrogenic genes and inflammation in T cells.[21,22]

EXCESS FREE FATTY ACID UPTAKE BY THE LIVER

Plasma FFAs are usually derived from white adipocytes via lipolysis.[23] A study reported the importance of fatty acid uptake in the pathogenesis of NAFLD, that approximately 60% of hepatic TGs in human subjects result from nonesterified fatty acids in the plasma.[24] These data are in keeping with the finding that nonesterified fatty acid concentrations are increased in NAFLD subjects due to increased rates of fatty acid release from adipose tissue.[25] NAFLD is significantly correlated with obesity, and increased fat mass contributes significantly to higher fatty acid release from adipose tissue.[26] Peripheral IR in NAFLD patients also leads to higher rates of fatty acid release from adipose tissue.[27] Hepatic expression levels of a fat transporter protein, CD36, have been reported to be increased in NAFLD and are thought to stimulate increased uptake of nonesterified fatty acids.[28]

DEFECTS IN HEPATIC LIPID PRODUCTION AND PROCESSING

The end-product of hepatic DNL is triacylglycerols (TAGs) that are stored in lipid droplets.[24] TAG production during NAFLD is affected by a variety of factors, including hepatic IR, diet, resident hepatic macrophages, and even genetic factors that promote increased DNL,[29–33] discussed in this section. Relative to healthy subjects, where DNL contributes 5% to the accumulation of TGs, DNL in NAFLD patients contributes 26% to the increase TGs.[34]

De Novo Lipogenesis

Insulin plays a dual role in the liver by stimulating glucose and lipid metabolism. Insulin promotes lipogenesis and glycogenesis while simultaneously decreasing hepatic gluconeogenesis.[35] Hepatic IR manifests as a change in carbohydrate metabolism without any change in lipid metabolic pathways.[35] The resulting hyperinsulinemia to overcome hepatic IR in the carbohydrate pathway leads to increased DNL. In the setting of hyperinsulinemia, the transcriptional factor, sterol-regulatory element binding protein 1c (SREBP1c), is considered a primary driving force.[36] This is because SREBP1c controls many downstream lipogenic genes involved in DNL and is highly sensitive to insulin.[36]

Diet

Specific dietary patterns have been associated with increased hepatic steatosis. In addition to increased caloric intake, multiple nutrients are independently linked to the development of NAFLD.[37] High-calorie diets are associated with hepatic steatosis in part due to hypertrophy of adipose tissue, in particular the accumulation of visceral adipose tissue.[38] High-calorie diets are also associated with the development of IR, further increasing circulating FFAs.[39]

Fructose, a commonly consumed sugar in the standard American diet, promotes hepatic IR.[34,40] Fructose is not easily absorbed through the gastrointestinal tract[34] because the cells of the gut do not express adequate levels of glucose transporter-5, the transporter responsible for the uptake of fructose.[34] Fructose is absorbed from the intestine through the portal vein and delivered to the liver first-pass metabolism.[41,42] In the liver, fructose augments its own metabolism through upregulation of ketohexokinase, the first step of fructose metabolism. In addition, fructose stimulates the expression of lipogencic enzymes involved in DNL and is utilized as a substrate for DNL.[34,42] The stimulation of DNL and accumulation of lipids in the liver itself may further increase hepatic insulin IR. In addition, fructose is also known to inhibit the production and release of adiponectin, further promoting hepatic IR as well as whole-body IR and therefore potentiating hepatic steatosis.[43]

The effect of high-fat diets on hepatic steatosis has been demonstrated in animal studies and humans.[44] The effects of high-fat diets on NAFLD histology are different depending on the composition of the diet.[45,46] Specifically, it has been reported that saturated fatty acids (SFAs) stimulate obesity and hepatic steatosis,[47] whereas polyunsaturated fatty acids are reported to increase insulin sensitivity and improve hepatic steatosis.[48] The action of SFAs on hepatic steatosis is believed to be due to impaired insulin signaling as well as a multitude of other effects that fall under the term, *lipotoxicity*,[49] discussed in detail later.

Kupffer Cells

Resident hepatic macrophages, known as Kupffer cells (KCs), were previously thought to play a role in the progression of NASH, but recent studies have reported that they can contribute to hepatic steatosis.[50,51] When activated, KCs are polarized to have 2 phenotypes: the proinflammatory M1 subtype or the anti-inflammatory M2 subtype.[29] A polarization of macrophages to the M1 phenotype can lead to increased hepatic steatosis via increased activity of diacylglycerol transferase, which converts diacylglycerol to TAG.[50]

DEFECTS IN HEPATIC CLEARANCE OF LIPIDS
Fatty Acid Oxidation

The liver can clear TGs through either FAO in the mitochondria of hepatocytes or through secretion of TGs in the form of VLDL.[31] There is evidence suggesting that both reduced FAO and increased TG production play important roles in NAFLD pathogenesis.[31] It has been reported that KCs also play an important role in modulating FAO.[51] The macrophage M1 phenotype is not only known to promote TG synthesis but also to inhibit FAO.[51] This occurs via inhibition of peroxisome proliferator-activated receptor-α, a nuclear factor (NF) highly expressed in tissues where FAO occurs.[51] The clinical implications of impaired mitochondrial FAO on NAFLD progression are not conclusive and more studies are needed.

Triglyceride Secretion

In the liver, TG assembly and secretion occur through the synthesis of VLDL in the hepatic rough endoplasmic reticulum (ER). Once a particle is formed, it is transported to the Golgi bodies to undergo maturation and is subsequently released via exocytosis.[31] The formation and secretion of VLDL are in part mediated by insulin, which has been shown to increase VLDL production.[52] In NAFLD, secretion of VLDL is believed to get overwhelmed by the increased FFA uptake and increased hepatic DNL and, therefore, becomes a rate-limiting step, leading to hepatic steatosis.[31]

Genetic Factors Involved in Nonalcoholic Fatty Liver Disease Pathogenesis

Patatin-like phospholipase domain-containing protein 3 (*PNPLA3*) was one of the first genes associated with increased hepatic steatosis.[53] *PNPLA3* is reported to consist of both catabolic and anabolic enzymatic functions, in that it can function as a TG hydrolase or transacylase.[54] The L148 M mutant of *PNPLA3* is associated with hepatic steatosis, but whether this is due to a loss-of-function mutation decreasing the hydrolytic function of the enzyme or a gain-of-function mutation causing overexpression of the enzyme is not clear. The other well-known gene associated with NAFLD is the enzyme diacylglycerol acyltransferase (DGAT) that catalyzes the final step in TAG synthesis.[55] This enzyme has 2 isoforms, *DGAT1* and *DGAT2*, with the second isoform primarily found in the liver.[55] Genetic variations that cause overexpression of this enzyme cause hepatic steatosis.[55] Intriguingly, both *PNPLA3* and *DGAT2* mutations that cause hepatic steatosis are not associated with IR.[33,55] This suggests that although IR may be sufficient to cause hepatic steatosis, it is not necessary for the development of steatosis. The adipose TG lipase, also known as patatin-like phospholipase domain-containing protein 2 (*PNPLA2*), is a protein that is located in the cytosol of multiple tissues.[56] Decreased expression of adipose TG lipase is associated with steatosis, but the mechanism of steatosis is unclear.[57,58] Additionally, mutations in another gene, known as the transmembrane 6 superfamily 2 (*TM6SF2*), have been linked to reduced hepatic TG secretion causing steatosis.[59,60]

Apolipoprotein B-100 is a liver-specific protein that is critical for the assembly of VLDL.[31] It has been reported that patients who have deficiencies in this protein (hypobetalipoproteinemia) have increased risk of hepatic steatosis.[32] Another genetic defect that has been found to influence VLDL synthesis is a defect in microsomal transfer protein (MTP)-1.[61] The presence of a single nucleotide polymorphism *MTP-493 G/T* in the *MTP* gene has been associated with the risk of NAFLD.[61]

PATHOPHYSIOLOGY OF NONALCOHOLIC STEATOHEPATITIS: LIPOTOXICITY, OXIDATIVE STRESS, AND ENDOPLASMIC RETICULUM STRESS

Lipotoxicity, coined in 1994, is a broad term that describes cellular injury and death caused by fatty acids and their intermediates.[62] Palmitic, oleic, and linoleic acids represent 70% of circulating FFAs.[63] Palmitic acid, an SFA, is known to cause inflammatory activation in endothelial cells and the vasculature.[64] Free cholesterol accumulation in the liver is also lipotoxic and occurs due to unrestricted hepatic salvage receptor uptake of circulating low-density lipoprotein.[65,66]

The metabolism of FFAs occurs through FAO, when they are not packaged into TGs or VLDL. This oxidation can directly lead to the production of reactive oxygen species (ROS) that are usually cleared by antioxidant pathways.[67] In NASH, these pathways can be saturated quickly due to the large influx of FFAs. Oxidative stress can lead to hepatocellular damage through several mechanisms, including lipid peroxidation that can directly activate cell necrosis and activation of the apoptotic Fas-ligand pathway and has even been implicated in causing fibrosis.[68] Studies have also shown that palmitic acid can activate the JNK and the NF-κB proinflammatory pathways and cause mitochondrial dysfunction.[64,69] Free cholesterol can also induce the JNK pathway, causing more generation of ROS further stressing the mitochondrial antioxidative mechanisms as well as increasing mitochondrial dysfunction.[70]

Lipotoxic compounds mediate not only oxidative stress and mitochondrial dysfunction but also ER stress that is also seen in NASH.[71] Palmitic acid has toxic effects on the ER and can stimulate ROS production as well as cause apoptosis.[72] ER stress is also manifested through a specific kind of response called the unfolded protein response (UPR).[73,74] The UPR is triggered by the accumulation of unfolded proteins within the ER and is an adaptive response by the cell.[72] The UPR is characterized by increased proteolytic degradation of the unfolded proteins and translational arrest of protein synthesis.[73] When a cell is unable to cope with ER stress, it triggers the JNK-mediated apoptosis pathway.[74] The accumulation of lipotoxic compounds seems to be one possible link connecting ER stress and NASH.[70]

Intriguingly, the accumulation of TGs by itself is not thought to be hepatotoxic and studies involving genetic defects in DGAT and MTP have shown that TG accumulation and steatosis can occur without liver injury.[5,75,76] The storage of FFAs in TGs in lipid droplets may even be protective by sequestering toxic FFAs into inert TGs.[77] Nonetheless, the excessive accumulation of TGs can still be associated with toxicity because these TGs can still be hydrolyzed to FFA and overwhelm the liver's ability to metabolize them.[78]

CELLULAR MEDIATORS OF INFLAMMATION
Kupffer Cells and Recruited Myeloid Cells in the Liver

KCs and recruited hepatic macrophages have been shown to play a crucial role in the development of NASH through activation of the macrophage M1 phenotype and altered M2 macrophage activation as shown in several rodent studies.[50,51] On M1 activation, these cells produce a variety of cytokines, such as IL-1β, IL-12, and TNF-α.[79,80] These cytokines recruit proinflammatory cells, including other innate immune cells as well as T lymphocytes, and propagate local inflammation.[2] Toxic lipids that are generally stored in hepatocytes can also be phagocytosed by KC and further lead to the generation of a proinflammatory phenotype.[81] The activation of KCs occurs through interactions between pattern-recognition receptors like TLRs and nucleotide oligomerization domain-like receptors (NLRs) and their specific ligands, the pathogen-associated molecular patterns (PAMPs) and damage-associated molecular patterns (DAMPs).[82] PAMPs are exogenous molecules that are generally pathogenic bacterial products, such as lipopolysaccharide (LPS).[83,84] DAMPs are endogenous pieces of damaged cells or ligands that are also immunogenic.[84] TLR4 is believed to be essential for the recognition of LPS by KCs that then mediates inflammation through the NF-κB–mediated inflammatory and apoptotic pathway[85] and causes further release of proinflammatory cytokines.[82] Additional research has also shown a role for TLR2 as well as TLR9 as mediators of NASH.[82]

Activation of NLRs promotes assembly of inflammasome multiprotein complexes, consisting of NLR family caspase activation and recruitment domain (CARD) domain-containing proteins (NLRPs), adaptor proteins such as the apoptosis-associated speck-like protein containing a caspase-recruitment domain (ASC), and the serine protease caspase 1 (Casp1).[82,83] NLRP3 inflammasome activation has been reported to play a prominent role in NASH pathogenesis.[82,83] On sensing of DAMPS and PAMPS by the inflammasome complex, Casp1 is cleaved and activated, inducing the maturation of proinflammatory cytokines, such as IL-1β and IL-18, which contribute to inflammation, fibrosis, and cell death in NASH.[82,83]

Hepatic Stellate Cells

The resident fibroblastic cells of the liver are the hepatic stellate cells (HSCs). These cells generally lay dormant within the liver but are activated by inflammation and promote fibrosis.[80] The activation of KCs, specifically the M1 phenotype, leads to the recruitment of HSCs through the secretion of cytokines, CCL2 and CCL5 (**Fig. 2**).[80] TLRs have also been found on HSCs, specifically TLR4, and are activated by the presence of LPS.[86] The activation of HSCs by TLR4 also seems to potentiate the activation of KCs by HSCs.[86] Another activator of HSCs is the hedgehog (Hh) pathway.[87] In mice, this pathway seems activated by up-regulation of Hh ligands in injured hepatocytes, which occurs in the setting of accumulation of toxic lipids, such as SFA.[88] The HSCs respond to these ligands by differentiating into myofibroblasts.[89] These cells cause fibrogenesis and lead to secretion of proinflammatory cytokines as well as promoting further up-regulation of Hh-ligands.[87] The effect of Hh in causing NASH in mice has strong human correlates, with studies showing that Hh activation parallels severity of NASH.[87]

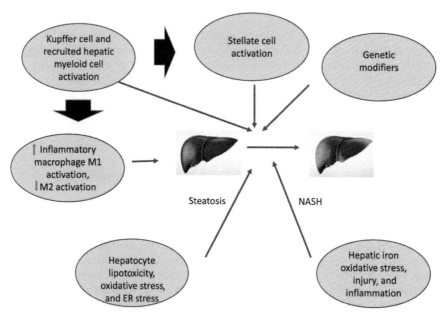

Fig. 2. Factors contributing to the transition from NAFL to NASH.

Gut Microbiome and Nonalcoholic Steatohepatitis Progression

The liver is uniquely positioned to receive a major proportion of blood flow from the gut through the portal system. The liver is generally the first line of defense for gut-derived toxins and, therefore, is exposed to many PAMPs.[2] Studies have shown that in patients with NASH, there are increased levels of circulating endotoxin that, in turn, can activate an innate immune response that can exacerbate NASH.[90] The gut microbiome has also been shown to produce ethanol that is hepatotoxic and alters gut permeability, inducing endotoxemia.[91] Also, small intestinal bacterial overgrowth has been reported to be associated with NAFLD.[92] The exact mechanism for this is unknown but small intestinal bacterial overgrowth is a qualitative change in the host microbiome and seems to alter gut permeability.[92] A prospective study recently demonstrated that specific bacterial metagenomic signatures in the gut microbiome of NAFLD patients are a robust predictor of advanced fibrosis associated with human NASH.[93] Further evidence for bacteria being predictors of NASH and fibrosis was shown by Boursier and colleagues,[94] where patients with biopsy-proved NASH had their microbiomes analyzed. The study showed that *Bacteroides* was independently associated with NASH whereas the genus *Ruminococcus* was associated with fibrosis.[94] The human microbiome is diverse, and the study of the associations of the different organisms that compose the microbiome is still in its infancy and further research is required.

IRON AS A COFACTOR FOR NONALCOHOLIC STEATOHEPATITIS

In a study of 849 patients, more than 34% of patients in the NASH Clinical Research Network had stainable hepatic iron in liver biopsies.[95] In particular, iron in the reticuloendothelial system cells was associated with advanced disease, including increased steatosis, portal and lobular inflammation, and advanced fibrosis in patients with NAFLD (**Fig. 3**).[95] Additionally, it was reported that elevated levels of serum ferritin, a cytokine associated with iron overload, is an independent predictor of histologic severity and advanced fibrosis among patients with NAFLD.[96] Furthermore, iron deposition in the reticuloendothelial system cell compartment was significantly associated with increased levels of oxidative stress and apoptosis in patients with NAFLD.[97] In independent studies, with a large cohort of Italian patients with NAFLD, Valenti and colleagues[98] reported that hepatocellular iron was associated with significantly increased risk of fibrosis compared with those without iron. In vitro studies with iron-loaded KCs have shown that iron causes the activation of NF-κB, a potent inflammatory mediator implicated in the pathogenesis of NASH.[99]

GENETIC FACTORS INVOLVED IN NONALCOHOLIC STEATOHEPATITIS PROGRESSION

Recently, it was reported that polymorphisms in the IL-1β and IL-6 genes are associated with increased severity of NASH.[100] Mutations in the hemochromatosis gene (*HFE*) have been correlated with worsening NASH and advanced fibrosis.[101] Furthermore, Valenti and colleagues[102] reported that *PNPLA3* I148 M allele was significantly associated with NASH progression and fibrosis. More recently, a genome-wide association study reported that genotype rs641738 at the membrane bound O-acyltransferase domain-containing 7 gene and transmembrane channel-like 4 gene (*MBOAT7-TMC4*) locus was associated with increased hepatic steatosis and severe liver damage and increased risk of fibrosis compared with subjects without the variant.[103]

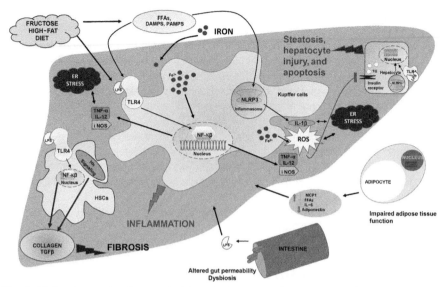

Fig. 3. Molecular mechanisms underlying NASH progression current understanding of the pathophysiology of NAFLD/NASH is that obesity and metabolic syndrome lead to adipose tissue (AT) dysfunction causing the release of excess FFAs from the adipocytes into the portal circulation, which leads to accumulation of excess TGs in the hepatocytes. In addition to FFAs, the adipocytes release increased levels of inflammatory mediators, MCP-1 and IL-6, and decreased levels of adiponectin. Furthermore, the gut releases bacterial products, such as LPS and other PAMPs and DAMPs, which enter the liver and activate pattern recognition receptors, such as the TLR4 and NLRP3 inflammasome, among others, on KCs (and other immune cells), hepatocytes, and HSCs, to produce inflammatory mediators like ROS, IL-1β, TNF-α, Inos, and IL-6, which, in turn, promote hepatocyte injury and IR and inflammation in the hepatic immune cells and activate fibrogenesis in the stellate cells, thereby accelerating NASH progression. In addition, hepatic iron overload leads to oxidative stress and NF-κB–mediated inflammation, promoting NAFLD progression. iNOS, inducible nitric oxide synthase; TGF, transforming growth factor.

SUMMARY

The pathophysiology of NAFL and NASH is complex and numerous intermediaries are involved. Each year brings new and exciting developments as pieces of the pathophysiologic puzzle are put together or new pieces are elucidated. Nonetheless, the task of completing the puzzle seems far in the future. But as the prevalence of this disease continues to increase at an alarming rate, the need for continued research is critical for the discovery of appropriate and novel drug targets and development of effective therapies.

REFERENCES

1. Loomba R, Sanyal AJ. The global NAFLD epidemic. Nat Rev Gastroenterol Hepatol 2013;10:686–90.

2. Caliguri A, Gentilini A, Marra F. Molecular pathogenesis of NASH. Int J Mol Sci 2016;17(9):1575.

3. Cohen JC, Horton JD, Hobbs HH. Human fatty liver disease: old questions and new insights. Science 2011;332:1519–23.

4. Day CP, James O. Steatohepatitis: a tale of two 'hits'? Gastroenterology 1998; 114(4):842–5.

5. Buzzetti E, Pinzani M, Tsochatzis EA. The multiple-hit pathogenesis of non-alcoholic fatty liver disease (NAFLD). Metabolism 2016;65(8):1038–48.

6. Jung UJ, Choi MS. Obesity and its metabolic complications: the role of adipo-kines and the relationship between obesity, inflammation, insulin resistance, dyslipidemia and nonalcoholic fatty liver disease. Int J Mol Sci 2014;15: 6184–223.

7. Kershaw EE, Flier JS. Adipose tissue as an endocrine organ. J Clin Endocrinol Metab 2004;89:2548–56.

8. Wang Y, Rimm EB, Stampfer MJ, et al. Comparison of abdominal adiposity and overall obesity in predicting risk of type 2 diabetes among men. Am J Clin Nutr 2005;81:555–63.

9. Boden G. Role of fatty acids in the pathogenesis of insulin resistance and NIDDM. Diabetes 1997;46:3–10.

10. Kelley DE, Mokan M, Simoneau JA, et al. Interaction between glucose and free fatty acid metabolism in human skeletal muscle. J Clin Invest 1993;92:91–8.

11. Shi H, Kokoeva MV, Inouye K, et al. TLR4 links innate immunity and fatty acid-induced insulin resistance. J Clin Invest 2006;116:3015–25.

12. Suganami T, Nishida J, Ogawa Y. A paracrine loop between adipocytes and macrophages aggravates inflammatory changes: role of free fatty acids and tu-mor necrosis factor alpha. Arterioscler Thromb Vasc Biol 2005;25:2062–8.

13. Skurk T, Alberti-Huber C, Herder C, et al. Relationship between adipocyte size and adipokine expression and secretion. J Clin Endocrinol Metab 2007;92: 1023–33.

14. Rotter V, Nagaev I, Smith U. Interleukin-6 (IL-6) induces insulin resistance in 3T3-L1 adipocytes and is, like IL-8 and tumor necrosis factor-alpha, overex-pressed in human fat cells from insulin-resistant subjects. J Biol Chem 2003; 278:45777–84.

15. Weisberg SP, McCann D, Desai M. Obesity is associated with macrophage accumulation in adipose tissue. J Clin Invest 2003;112:1796–808.

16. Lumeng CN, Bodzin JL, Saltiel AR. Obesity induces a phenotypic switch in ad-ipose tissue macrophage polarization. J Clin Invest 2007;117:175–84.

17. Angulo P. NAFLD, obesity, and bariatric surgery. Gastroenterology 2006;130: 1848–52.

18. Berg AH, Combs TP, Du X, et al. The adipocyte-secreted protein ACRP30 en-hances hepatic insulin action. Nat Med 2001;7:947–53.

19. Masarone M, Federico A, Abenavoli L, et al. Non-alcoholic fatty liver: epidemi-ology and natural history. Rev Recent Clin Trials 2014;9:126–33.

20. Poordad FF. The role of leptin in NAFLD contender or pretender? J Clin Gastro-enterol 2004;38:841–3.

21. Cao Q, Mak KM, Ren C, et al. Leptin stimulates tissue inhibitor of metalloproteinase-1 in human hepatic stellate cells: respective roles of the JAK/STAT and JAK-mediated H2O2-dependent MAPK pathways. J Biol Chem 2004;279:4292–304.

22. Lord GM, Matarese G, Howard JK, et al. Leptin modulates the T-cell immune response and reverses starvation-induced immunosuppression. Nature 1998; 394:897–901.

23. Arner P. Human fat cell lipolysis: biochemistry, regulation and clinical role. Best Pract Res Clin Endocrinol Metab 2005;19:471–82.

24. Donnelly K, Smith CI, Schwarzenburg SJ, et al. Sources of fatty acids stored in liver and secreted via lipoproteins in patients with nonalcoholic fatty liver disease. J Clin Invest 2005;115(5):1343–51.
25. Holt HB, Wild SH, Wood PJ, et al. Non-esterified fatty acid concentrations are independently associated with hepatic steatosis in obese subjects. Diabetologia 2006;49:141–8.
26. Fabbrini E, Sullivan S, Klein S. Obesity and nonalcoholic fatty liver disease: biochemical, metabolic, and clinical implications. Hepatology 2010;51:679–89.
27. Hwang JH, Stein DT, Barzilai N, et al. Increased intrahepatic triglyceride is associated with peripheral insulin resistance: in vivo MR imaging and spectroscopy studies. Am J Physiol Endocrinol Metab 2007;293:E1663–9.
28. Miquilena-Colina ME, Lima-Cabello E, Sanchez-Campos S, et al. Hepatic fatty acid translocase CD36 upregulation is associated with insulin resistance, hyperinsulinaemia and increased steatosis in non-alcoholic steatohepatitis and chronic hepatitis C. Gut 2011;60:1394–402.
29. Marra F, Lotersztajn S. Pathophysiology of NASH: perspectives for a targeted treatment. Curr Pharm Des 2013;19(29):5250–69.
30. Rui L. Energy metabolism in the liver. Compr Physiol 2014;4(1):177–97.
31. Koo SH. Nonalcoholic fatty liver disease: molecular mechanisms for hepatic steatosis. Clin Mol Hepatol 2013;19(3):210–5.
32. Amaro A, Fabbrini E, Kars M, et al. Dissociation between intrahepatic triglyceride content and insulin resistance in familial hypobetalipoproteinemia. Gastroenterology 2010;139:149–53.
33. Kantartzis K, Peter A, Machicao F, et al. Dissociation between fatty liver and insulin resistance in humans carrying a variant of the patatin-like phospholipase 3 gene. Diabetes 2009;58:2616–23.
34. Basanroglu M, Basanroglu G, Bugianesi E. Carbohydrate intake and nonalcoholic fatty liver disease: fructose as a weapon of mass destruction. Hepatobiliary Surg Nutr 2015;4(2):109–16.
35. Sanders F, Griffin JL. De novo lipogenesis in the liver in health and disease: more than just a shunting yard for glucose. Biol Rev Camb Philos Soc 2016; 91(2):452–68.
36. Lin J, Yang R, Tarr PT, et al. Hyperlipidemic effects of dietary saturated fats mediated through PGC-1beta coactivation of SREBP. Cell 2005;120(2):261–73.
37. Yu J, Marsh S, Hu J, et al. The pathogenesis of nonalcoholic fatty liver disease: interplay between diet, gut microbiota, and genetic background. Gastroenterol Res Pract 2016;2016:2862173.
38. Bays HE, Gonzalez-Campoy JM, Bray GA, et al. Pathogenic potential of adipose tissue and metabolic consequences of adipocyte hypertrophy and increased visceral adiposity. Expert Rev Cardiovasc Ther 2008;6(3):343–68.
39. Fan JG, Cao HX. Role of diet and nutritional management in non-alcoholic fatty liver disease. J Gastroenterol Hepatol 2013;28(Suppl 4):81–7.
40. Aerbeli I, Hochuli M, Gerber PA, et al. Moderate amounts of fructose consumption impair insulin sensitivity in healthy young men: a randomized controlled trial. Diabetes Care 2013;36(1):150–6.
41. Basanroglu M, Basanroglu G, Sabuncu T, et al. Fructose as a key player in the development of fatty liver disease. World J Gastroenterol 2013;19:1166–72.
42. Softic S, Cohen DE, Kahn CR. Role of dietary fructose and hepatic de novo lipogenesis in fatty liver disease. Dig Dis Sci 2016;61:1282–93.
43. Basciano H, Federico L, Adeli K. Fructose, insulin resistance, and metabolic dyslipidemia. Nutr Metab (Lond) 2005;2:5.

44. Kucera O, Cervinkova Z. Experimental models of non-alcoholic fatty liver disease in rats. World J Gastroenterol 2014;20(26):8364–76.

45. Rosenstengel S, Stoeppeler S, Bahde R, et al. Type of steatosis influences microcirculation and fibrogenesis in different rat strains. J Invest Surg 2011; 24:273–82.

46. Romestaing C, Piquet MA, Bedu E, et al. Long term highly saturated fat diet does not induce NASH in Wistar rats. Nutr Metab (Lond) 2007;4:4.

47. de Wit N, Derrien M, Bosch-Vermeulen H, et al. Saturated fat stimulates obesity and hepatic steatosis and affects gut microbiota composition by an enhanced overflow of dietary fat to the distal intestine. Am J Physiol Gastrointest Liver Physiol 2012;303(5):G589–99.

48. Summers LK, Fielding BA, Bradshaw HA, et al. Substituting dietary saturated fat with polyunsaturated fat changes abdominal fat distribution and improves insulin sensitivity. Diabetologia 2002;45(3):369–77.

49. Ricchi M, Odoardi MR, Carulli L, et al. Differential effect of oleic and palmitic acid on lipid accumulation and apoptosis in cultured hepatocytes. J Gastroenterol Hepatol 2009;24:830–40.

50. Miura K, Kodama Y, Inokuchi S, et al. Toll-like receptor 9 promotes steatohepatitis by induction of interleukin-1beta in mice. Gastroenterology 2010;139: 323–34.e7.

51. Stienstra R, Saudale F, Duval C, et al. Kupffer cells promote hepatic steatosis via interleukin-1beta-dependent suppression of peroxisome proliferator-activated receptor alpha activity. Hepatology 2010;51:511–22.

52. Ginsberg HN, Fisher EA. The ever-expanding role of degradation in regulation of apolipoprotein B metabolism. J Lipid Res 2009;50(Suppl):S162–6.

53. Browning JD, Cohen JC, Hobbs HH. PNPLA3 and the pathogenesis and progression of pediatric NAFLD. Hepatology 2010;52(4):1189–92.

54. Jenkins CM, Mancuso DJ, Yan W, et al. Identification, cloning, expression, and purification of three novel human calcium-independent phospholipase A2 family members possessing triacylglycerol lipase and acylglycerol transacylase activities. J Biol Chem 2004;279:48968–75.

55. Gaggini M, Morelli M, Buzzigoli E. Non-alcoholic fatty liver disease (NAFLD) and its connection with insulin resistance, dyslipidemia, atherosclerosis and coronary artery disease. Nutrients 2013;5(5):1544–60.

56. Saponaro C, Gaggini M, Carli F, et al. The subtle balance between lipolysis and lipogenesis: a critical point in metabolic homeostasis. Nutrients 2015;7: 9453–74.

57. Ong KT, Mashek MT, Bu SY, et al. Adipose triglyceride lipase is a major hepatic lipase that regulates triacylglycerol turnover and fatty acid partitioning. Hepatology 2011;53(1):116–26.

58. Fuchs CD, Claudel T, Kumari P, et al. Absence of adipose triglyceride lipase protects from hepatic endoplasmic reticulum stress in mice. Hepatology 2012; 56(1):270–80.

59. Kozlitina J, Smagris E, Stender S, et al. Exome-wide association study identifies a TM6SF2 variant that confers susceptibility to nonalcoholic fatty liver disease. Nat Genet 2014;46(4):352–6.

60. Liu YL, Reeves L, Burt AD. TM6SF2 rs58542926 influences hepatic fibrosis progression in patients with non-alcoholic fatty liver disease. Nat Commun 2014;5: 4309.

61. Li L, Wang SJ, Shi K, et al. Correlation between MTP -493G>T polymorphism and non-alcoholic fatty liver disease risk: a meta-analysis. Genet Mol Res 2014;13(4):10150–61.
62. Lee Y, Hirose H, Ohneda M, et al. β-Cell lipotoxicity in the pathogenesis of non-insulin-dependent diabetes mellitus of obese rats: impairment in adipocyte-β-cell relationships. Proc Natl Acad Sci U S A 1994;91:10878–82.
63. Yli-Jama P, Meyer HE, Ringstad J, et al. Serum free fatty acid pattern and risk of myocardial infarction: a case-control study. J Intern Med 2002;251:19–28.
64. Maloney E, Sweet IR, Hockenbery DM, et al. Activation of NF-κB by palmitate in endothelial cells: a key role for NADPH oxidase-derived superoxide in response to TLR4 activation. Arterioscler Thromb Vasc Biol 2009;29(9):1370–5.
65. Puri P, Baillie RA, Wiest M, et al. A lipidomic analysis of nonalcoholic fatty liver disease. Hepatology 2007;46:1081–90.
66. Tomita K, Teratani T, Suzuki T, et al. Free cholesterol accumulation in hepatic stellate cells: mechanism of liver fibrosis aggravation in nonalcoholic steatohepatitis in mice. Hepatology 2014;59:154–69.
67. Neuschwander-Tetri BA. Hepatic lipotoxicity and the pathogenesis of nonalcoholic steatohepatitis: the central role of nontriglyceride fatty acid metabolites. Hepatology 2010;52(2):774–88.
68. Koek GH, Liedrop PR, Bast A. The role of oxidative stress in nonalcoholic steatohepatitis. Clin Chim Acta 2011;412(15–16):1297–305.
69. Win S, Than TA, Le BH, et al. Sab (Sh3bp5) dependence of JNK mediated inhibition of mitochondrial respiration in palmitic acid induced hepatocyte lipotoxicity. J Hepatol 2015;62:1367–74.
70. Caballero F, Fernandez A, De Lacy AM, et al. Enhanced free cholesterol, SREBP-2 and star expression in human NASH. J Hepatol 2009;50:789–96.
71. Puri P, Mirshahi F, Cheung O, et al. Activation and dysregulation of the unfolded protein response in nonalcoholic fatty liver disease. Gastroenterology 2008;134:568–76.
72. Wei Y, Wang D, Topczewski F, et al. Saturated fatty acids induce endoplasmic reticulum stress and apoptosis independently of ceramide in liver cells. Am J Physiol Endocrinol Metab 2006;291:E275–81.
73. Kaufmann RJ. Orchestrating the unfolded protein response in health and disease. J Clin Invest 2002;110(10):1389–98.
74. Schwabe RF, Uchinami H, Qian T, et al. Differential requirement for c-JUN NH2 terminal kinase in TNF-alpha and FAS-mediated apoptosis in hepatocytes. FASEB J 2004;18(6):720–2.
75. Liao W, Hui TY, Young SG, et al. Blocking microsomal triglyceride transfer protein interferes with apoB secretion without causing retention or stress in the ER. J Lipid Res 2003;44:978–85.
76. Monetti M, Levin MC, Watt MJ, et al. Dissociation of hepatic steatosis and insulin resistance in mice overexpressing DGAT in the liver. Cell Metab 2007;6:69–78.
77. Garbarino J, Sturley SL. Saturated with fat: new perspectives on lipotoxicity. Curr Opin Clin Nutr Metab Care 2009;12:110–6.
78. Schaffer JE. Lipotoxicity: when tissues overeat. Curr Opin Lipidol 2003;14:281–7.
79. Tosello-Trampont AC, Landes SG, Nguyen V, et al. Kuppfer cells trigger nonalcoholic steatohepatitis development in diet-induced mouse model through tumor necrosis factor-α production. J Biol Chem 2012;287:40161–72.
80. Marra F, Tacke F. Roles for chemokines in liver disease. Gastroenterology 2014;147:577–94.

81. Leroux A, Ferrere G, Godie V, et al. Toxic lipids stored by Kupffer cells correlates with their pro-inflammatory phenotype at an early stage of steatohepatitis. J Hepatol 2012;57:141–9.

82. Arrese M, Cabrera D, Kalergis AM, et al. Innate immunity and inflammation in NAFLD/NASH. Dig Dis Sci 2016;61:1294–303.

83. Ganz M, Szabo G. Immune and inflammatory pathways in NASH. Hepatol Int 2013;7(Suppl 2):771–81.

84. Barton GM, Medzhitov R. Toll-like receptors and their ligands. Curr Top Microbiol Immunol 2002;270:81–92.

85. Jia L, Vianna CR, Fukuda M, et al. Hepatocyte toll-like receptor 4 regulates obesity-induced inflammation and insulin resistance. Nat Commun 2014;5:3878.

86. Seki E, De Minicis S, Osterreicher CH, et al. TLR4 enhances TGF-beta signaling and hepatic fibrosis. Nat Med 2007;13:1324–32.

87. Verdelho Machado M, Diehl AM. Role of hedgehog signaling pathway in NASH. Int J Mol Sci 2016;17(6) [pii:E857].

88. Kakisaka K, Cazanave SC, Werneburg NW, et al. A hedgehog survival pathway in 'undead' lipotoxic hepatocytes. J Hepatol 2012;57:844–51.

89. Fleig SV, Choi SS, Yang L, et al. Hepatic accumulation of hedgehog-reactive progenitors increases with severity of fatty liver damage in mice. Lab Invest 2007;87:1227–39.

90. Rivera CA, Adegboyega P, van Rooijen N, et al. Toll-like receptor-4 signaling and Kupffer cells play pivotal roles in the pathogenesis of non-alcoholic steatohepatitis. J Hepatol 2007;47:571–9.

91. Cope K, Risby T, Diehl AM. Increased gastrointestinal ethanol production in obese mice: implications for fatty liver disease pathogenesis. Gastroenterology 2000;119:1340–7.

92. Minemura M, Shimizu Y. Gut microbiota and liver diseases. World J Gastroenterol 2015;21:1691–702.

93. Loomba R, Seguritan V, Li W, et al. Gut Microbiome based metagenomic signature for non-invasive detection of advanced fibrosis in human nonalcoholic fatty liver disease. Cell Metab 2017;25(5):1054–62.e5.

94. Boursier J, Mueller O, Barret M, et al. The severity of nonalcoholic fatty liver disease is associated with gut dysbiosis and shift in the metabolic function of the gut microbiota. Hepatology 2016;63(3):764–75.

95. Nelson JE, Wilson L, Brunt EM, et al. Relationship between the pattern of hepatic iron deposition and histological severity in nonalcoholic fatty liver disease. Hepatology 2011;53:448–57.

96. Kowdley KV, Belt P, Wilson LA, et al. Serum ferritin is an independent predictor of histologic severity and advanced fibrosis in patients with nonalcoholic fatty liver disease. Hepatology 2012;55:77–85.

97. Maliken BD, Nelson JE, Klintworth HM, et al. Hepatic reticuloendothelial system cell iron deposition is associated with increased apoptosis in nonalcoholic fatty liver disease. Hepatology 2013;57:1806–13.

98. Valenti L, Fracazani AL, Bugianesi E, et al. HFE genotype, parenchymal iron accumulation, and liver fibrosis in patients with nonalcoholic fatty liver disease. Gastroenterology 2010;138:905–12.

99. Chen L, Xiong S, She H, et al. Iron causes interactions of TAK1, p21ras, and phosphatidylinositol 3-kinase in caveolae to actiave IkappaB kinase in hepatic macrophages. J Biol Chem 2007;282:5582–8.

100. Nelson JE, Handa P, Aouizerat B, et al. Increased parenchymal damage and steatohepatitis in Caucasian non-alcoholic fatty liver patients with common IL1B and IL6 polymorphisms. Aliment Pharmacol Ther 2016;44:1253–64.
101. Nelson JE, Bhattacharya R, Lindor KD, et al. HFE C282Y mutations are associated with advanced hepatic fibrosis in Caucasians with nonalcoholic steatohepatitis. Hepatology 2007;46:723–9.
102. Valenti L, Al-Serri A, Daly AK, et al. Homozygosity for the patatin-like phospholipase-3/adiponutrin I148M polymorphism influences liver fibrosis in patients with nonalcoholic fatty liver disease. Hepatology 2010;51:1209–17.
103. Mancina RM, Dongiovanni P, Petta S, et al. The MBOAT7-TMC4 variant rs641738 increases risk of nonalcoholic fatty liver disease in individuals of European descent. Gastroenterology 2016;150:1219–30.

Risk Factors for the Development of Nonalcoholic Fatty Liver Disease/Nonalcoholic Steatohepatitis, Including Genetics

 CrossMark

Huei-Wen Lim, MD[a], David E. Bernstein, MD[b],*

KEYWORDS

- NAFLD • NASH • Risk factors • Genetics

KEY POINTS

- Nonalcoholic fatty liver disease (NAFLD) and its subtype, nonalcoholic steatohepatitis, are common causes of chronic liver disease with an increasing worldwide prevalence.
- Individuals with NAFLD often have 1 or more components of the metabolic syndrome: obesity, systemic hypertension, dyslipidemia, or insulin resistance.
- Polymorphisms in genes controlling lipid metabolism, proinflammatory cytokines, and fibrotic mediators may be associated with steatohepatitis and/or fibrosis.
- The prevalence of NAFLD is high in people of Asian and Hispanic decent, its prevalence can be explained by the tendency for visceral adiposity and presence of predisposing genetic variants in these cohorts.
- Other risk factors associated with NAFLD are the difference in gender and presence of polycystic ovarian syndrome.

INTRODUCTION

Nonalcoholic fatty liver disease (NAFLD) is prevalent worldwide and is the most common chronic liver disease in Western countries. Its increasing prevalence is associated with major risk factors such as obesity, dyslipidemia, type 2 diabetes mellitus (T2DM), and the metabolic syndrome (MetS).[1] It is estimated that 10% to 46% of Americans

Disclosure: The authors have nothing to disclose.
[a] Department of Internal Medicine, Northwell Health, 400 Community Drive, Manhasset, NY 11030, USA; [b] Department of Gastroenterology and Hepatology, Northwell Health, Center for Liver Diseases, 400 Community Drive, Manhasset, NY 11030, USA
* Corresponding author.
E-mail address: dbernste@northwell.edu

are affected by this epidemic, with data on worldwide prevalence varying from 6% to 35%, depending on the type of diagnostic modalities used.[2–4] NAFLD can present as a spectrum of histologic findings that range from benign steatosis to steatohepatitis, fibrosis, and cirrhosis.[5] Nonalcoholic steatohepatitis (NASH) may be histologically indistinguishable from alcoholic steatohepatitis[6]; patients with NASH are at an increased risk of developing cirrhosis and hepatocellular carcinoma (HCC).[7] Although NAFLD has been associated with obesity and insulin resistance in Western countries, it is common to observe NAFLD at lower body mass indices (BMIs) and without insulin resistance in Asian countries.[8] With the introduction of genome-wide association studies, scientists are able to discern the genetic and geographic differences that shape the prevalence and incidence of NAFLD across the world.[9]

This article expands on the aforementioned risk factors (**Fig. 1**) and summarizes the current data available on genetic and environmental factors associated with this common entity.

METABOLIC SYNDROME

MetS is a clinical entity that is defined as the presence of any 3 of the following 5 traits: (1) serum triglyceride (TG) level of 150 mg/dL or higher, (2) serum high-density lipoprotein (HDL) level of less than 40 mg/dL in men or less than 50 mg/dL in women, (3) systemic blood pressure of 130/85 mm Hg or higher, (4) fasting plasma glucose level of 100 mg/dL or higher, and (5) an increase in waist circumference (this differs based on national or regional cut points).[10]

NAFLD has been associated with MetS owing to its close connection to its cardio-metabolic risk factors. In a study of 3846 subjects using National Health and Nutrition Examination Survey (NHANES) data, the prevalence of NAFLD, measured by ultrasonography, increased as subjects had more MetS criteria, with 90.8% having NAFLD when all 5 criteria were present. More significant abnormal hepatic laboratory values were seen in patients having both NAFLD and MetS, compared with patients with either NAFLD or MetS alone.[11] In a study by Marchesini and colleagues,[12] 304 patients with NAFLD without T2DM who met 3 or more MetS criteria defined by the US National Institutes of Health were studied. patients with NASH had a more severe metabolic disorder and a greater prevalence of MetS compared with subjects with pure fatty liver. MetS was associated with NASH in 88% of patients and simple steatosis in 67% of patients. In Japan, Hamaguchi and colleagues[13] recruited healthy Japanese men and women and conducted biochemical tests for liver function and abdominal ultrasonography. Participants who met criteria for MetS using the modified criteria of the

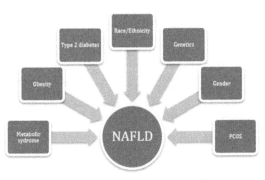

Fig. 1. Risk factors for NAFLD. PCOS, polycystic ovarian syndrome.

National Cholesterol Education Program Adult Treatment Panel III were 4 times more likely to develop NAFLD than their counterparts, and NAFLD was less likely to regress in participants with MetS.

Insulin resistance is the major driving force in the development of NAFLD. There are several proposed mechanisms of MetS-mediated hepatic steatosis and NASH. Increase in visceral adipose tissues increases gluconeogenesis, free fatty acid (FFA) levels, and insulin resistance on peripheral glucose, leading to the deposition of FFA and subsequent accumulation of TGs in the liver, causing hepatic steatosis.[14–16] FFAs promote hepatic lipotoxicity by stimulating tumor necrosis factor alpha (TNF-alpha) expression, causing hepatocyte damage.[17] Subsequently, FFA metabolites such as diacylglycerol and ceramides accumulate in the liver, activating protein kinase C ,which causes phosphorylation of insulin receptor substrate-1 (IRS-1).[16] This phosphorylation inhibits insulin-dependent activation of phosphatidylinositol 3-kinase, which regulates lipid metabolism, leading to hepatic insulin resistance, resulting in increased hepatic gluconeogenesis and shunting of glucose toward the lipogenesis pathway to cause steatosis.[18,19] Another potential mechanism of injury involves toll-like receptors (TLRs), a class of proteins expressed on membranes of leukocytes that play a key role in the innate immune system.[20] Binding of FFA to TLRs activates c-Jun NH_2-terminal kinase (JNK) and IκB kinase (IKK) gene expression, leading to the phosphorylation of IRS-1 and the initiation of the cascade as discussed earlier.[21]

OBESITY

Several studies involving severely obese adults have shown a high correlation between hypertriglyceridemia and NAFLD. Lazo and Clark[22] conducted a literature search and showed that the reported prevalence of NAFLD and NASH in obese patients undergoing bariatric surgery in the studies was 76% (range, 33%–99%) and 37%, respectively. A partner study by Lee and colleagues[23] evaluated 710 obese adults who underwent bariatric surgery at John Hopkins Hospital and showed that, in individuals without diabetes and hypertension, 88% had hepatic steatosis and 7.3% had NASH, suggesting that obesity is modifiable risk factor for NAFLD development in metabolically healthy individuals. In children, studies have shown a similar association between obesity and NAFLD. The largest study, the Teen-Longitudinal Assessment of Bariatric Surgery (TLABS) study, was a prospective multicenter analysis of 148 patients who underwent intraoperative biopsy between 2007 and 2012. The prevalence of NAFLD in these severely obese teenagers was 59%, with 34.5% having borderline or definite NASH.[24] Doycheva and colleagues[25] described the prevalence of NAFLD in adolescents undergoing bariatric surgery to be 59% to 83%. This study reported that NAFLD among young adults has risen by almost 2.5 times since 1994 (9.6% in 1988–1994 to 24% in 2005–2010 based on NHANES data) and that 57.4% of morbidly obese young adults had NAFLD. A meta-analysis of cohort studies performed by Li and colleagues[26] showed that obesity independently led to a 3.5-fold increased risk of developing NAFLD, with a dose-dependent relationship between BMI and NAFLD risk.

Obesity results in the increased accumulation of TGs, derived from glycerol and long-chain fatty acid (FA), throughout the body. Steatosis develops when the rate of FA input (uptake and synthesis with subsequent TG production) is greater than the rate of FA output (oxidation and secretion).[27] The rate of FA released from subcutaneous adipose tissue into the systemic circulation, which is then transported to the liver, is greater in obese than lean patients.[28] Higher expression levels of hepatic lipase and hepatic lipoprotein lipase leading to hepatocellular FA accumulation in obese individuals also contributes to the increase in intrahepatic TG content.[29,30] De novo lipogenesis is regulated independently by insulin and glucose, and hyperinsulinemia promotes hepatic overexpression of SREBP-1 (sterol regulatory element binding protein 1), a protein that regulates genes related to the stimulation lipogenesis.[31] In addition, patients with NAFLD have evidence of hepatic mitochondrial structural and functional abnormalities that affect FA oxidation, leading to intrahepatic TG accumulation.[32]

TYPE 2 DIABETES MELLITUS

T2DM and insulin resistance have contributed to the development of NAFLD. Several studies have described a higher prevalence of NAFLD among patients with T2DM compared with nondiabetics, with prevalence estimated to be 40% to 69.5%.[33,34] Lazo and Clark[22] concluded that T2DM not only increases the prevalence of NAFLD but is also associated with more severe forms of NAFLD, including NASH and fibrosis. In a study by Leite and colleagues,[35] patients with T2DM with ultrasonographic and biopsy evidence of NAFLD were examined. The prevalence of NASH was 78%. The prevalence of advanced fibrosis (stage $\geq$2) was 38% and 55%, the results of which depended on which of the 2 independent pathologists performed the histologic examination. NAFLD can occur in nonobese individuals with T2DM. Seto and colleagues[36] described the clinical entity of lean NAFLD, which is NAFLD occurring in nonobese individuals. Found in 20% of the Asian population based on prevalence studies in Asia, it is closely associated with insulin resistance, T2DM, and other metabolic complications.

All these findings highlight the impact of the metabolic risk factors on NAFLD and the need for awareness and lifestyle modification to treat this entity.

GENETIC POLYMORPHISM

Family studies and interethnic differences in susceptibility suggest that genetic factors play an important role in modulating the prevalence, severity, and progression of disease. Polymorphisms in genes affecting lipid metabolism, oxidative stress, and inflammatory cytokines may be directly linked to the development and progression of steatohepatitis and fibrosis. Recent whole genome–wide association studies (**Table 1**) have enabled researchers to identify genes contributing to inherited

Table 1
Genes and their variants

Gene Name	Genetic Variant	Amino Acid Change	Effect of Variant
PNPLA3	rs738409 rs6006460	I148M S453I	Increased intrahepatic TG content and insulin resistance Lower intrahepatic TG content
TM6SF2	rs58542926	E167K	Increased AST/ALT, GGT levels, increased intrahepatic TG content, lower serum TG level
MBOAT7	rs641738	TMC4	Increased intrahepatic TG content and inflammation
KLF6	rs3750861	IVS1	Increased hepatic clearance of insulin and hepatic insulin sensitivity, milder NAFLD
IRS1	rs9251008	G972R	Increased insulin resistance and apoptosis, accelerated fibrogenesis

Abbreviations: ALT, alanine transaminase; AST, aspartate transaminase; GGT, gamma-glutamyl transpeptidase.

susceptibility to hepatic steatosis and have provided important insights into the genetic contribution leading to NAFLD.

Patatinlike Phospholipase 3

Genome-wide association scanning has shown that a single nucleotide polymorphism (SNP) characterized by a C-to-G change encoding an isoleucine-to-methionine substitution at amino acid position 148 in the human patatinlike phospholipase 3 (PNPLA3) gene (rs738409) has been associated with an increased TG accumulation and fibrosis.[37,38] Subsequent studies not only confirmed the results but also showed its effect in different ethnic groups, especially in Asian and Hispanic cohorts, including Chinese, Japanese, Korean, Indian, and Mexican Americans populations.[39–44] Specifically, in the Hispanic population, PNPLA3 genetic variant not only affects liver fat content but was also associated with increased levels of serum aminotransferase.[45,46] The association with steatosis has been independently replicated in numerous candidate-gene studies, whereas its link to liver scarring stemmed from a meta-analysis in patients with chronic hepatitis C virus infection and alcoholic liver diseases.[47,48] Krawczyk and colleagues[49] evaluated patients with NAFLD diagnosed by imaging or liver biopsy and found that the PNPL3 genetic variant was significantly associated with the risk of developing steatosis grades S2 and S3 and fibrosis stage F2 to F4. More importantly, the PNPL3 genetic variant has been associated with increased risk for the development of HCC (**Fig. 2**).[50,51] In a European study of 100 white people with NAFLD-related HCC, carriers of each copy of the rs738409 minor G allele conferred an additive risk for HCC, with GG homozygotes having 5-fold increased risk of HCC compared with CC carriers. In addition, compared with the general UK population, GG homozygotes are 12 times more likely to develop HCC compared with CC homozygotes.[52]

It is proposed that PNPLA3 protein (also known as adiponutrin) expression serves as a reliable signal to the body's response to high fat intake.[53] PNPLA3 shows lipase activity against TG and acylglycerol transacetylase activity, and is involved in triacylglycerol hydrolysis in adipocytes.[54,55] The genetic variant eliminates its enzymatic activity, altering the enzymatic hydrolysis of emulsified TG, resulting in impaired secretion of very low-density lipoprotein and the development of hepatic insulin resistance.[56–58] It also decreases levels of circulating adiponectin, which functions to

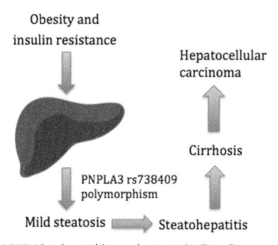

Fig. 2. The I148M PNPLA3 polymorphism and progressive liver disease.

modulate glucose levels and FA oxidation.[59–61] In contrast, the rs6006460, c.1531G>T mutation of PNPLA3, most commonly seen in the African American population, was shown to decrease hepatic fat content regardless of BMI.[62] Romeo and colleagues[62] performed a genome-wide association scan of nonsynonymous sequence variation in a multiethnic population–based probability sample of Dallas County residents the Dallas Heart Study and reported that the rs6006460 variant was more common in the African American cohort (10.4%) compared with white people (0.3%) and Hispanic Americans (0.8%). Moreover, the median hepatic fat content in African Americans who carry this genetic variant was 18% lower than that of the wild-type allele, suggesting that this genetic variation may protect against the development of NAFLD.[62]

TRANSMEMBRANE 6 SUPERFAMILY 2

Transmembrane 6 superfamily 2 (TM6SF2) or KIAA1926 is a protein of unknown function encoded by the gene on chromosome 19.[63] TM6SF2 is a regulator of liver fat metabolism with opposing effects on the secretion of TG-rich lipoproteins and hepatic lipid droplet content. Its inhibition is associated with the reduction of secretion of TG-rich lipoproteins into the serum and an increase in hepatic fat content, whereas its overexpression leads to a reduction in hepatic steatosis and an increase in serum TG level.[64] Similar results were replicated in a study in mice performed by Holmen and colleagues,[65] in which transient overexpression of the human TM6SF2 resulted in increased total cholesterol, low-density lipoprotein (LDL), and TG levels, and lower HDL-cholesterol levels. The knockdown of TM6SF2 produced the opposite effect.

One genetic variant in TM6SF2 SNP (rs58542926, c.499G>A) changes glutamic acid to lysine amino acid at protein residue 167 (p. E167K), inhibiting the expression of TM6SF2 protein. This inhibition was associated with a concomitant increase in hepatic TG levels and the development of NAFLD.[63,65,66] The frequency of the TM6SF2 genetic variant was higher in individuals of European ancestry (7.2%) than in Africans (3.4%) or Hispanic Americans (4.7%) in a study using samples from the Dallas Heart Study.[63] The modifier role of the TM6SF2 genetic variant on NAFLD and its spectrum of disease have been well shown in many large independent studies; however, its influence on liver histology remains controversial. A study by Sookoian and colleagues[67] evaluated 135 control subjects and 226 patients with histologically proven NAFLD. It showed that the TM6SF2 genetic variant is a low-frequency variant with a modest effect on NAFLD, and that carriers of the risk alleles are more likely to accumulate fat in the liver and develop NASH. The genetic variant was associated with increased histologic degree of hepatic steatosis but not lobular inflammation or fibrosis. It also has no major effects on serum liver chemistries. Krawczyk and colleagues[49] evaluated 361 patients with NAFLD diagnosed either by imaging or liver biopsy and showed that the TM6SF2 genetic variant was associated with increased serum aspartate transaminase, alanine transaminase, and gamma-glutamyl transpeptidase levels. This study supported the association of the TM6SF2 genetic variant with steatosis but not fibrosis. Liu and colleagues[68] performed a quantitative analysis within a well-characterized white European discovery cohort with histologically characterized NAFLD and replicated their findings in their larger validation cohort. They determined that the genetic variant was significantly associated with NAFLD and histologic fibrosis but not with histologic steatosis in the 2 explored cohorts after adopting an additive model, results of which directly conflict with the 2 studies mentioned earlier (Sookoian and colleagues,[67] Krawczyk and colleagues[49]). It can be concluded that the prevalence of fibrosis and steatosis in patients with this genetic variant are independent of one another.

Individuals carrying the TM6SF2 genetic variant are more prone to developing NAFLD with advanced fibrosis but have a lower risk for cardiovascular disease because the inhibition of liver fat secretion to serum results in increased hepatic fat content and decreased serum fat content. In a study by Dongiovanni and colleagues[66] evaluating the effects of the TM6SF2 genetic variant on cardiovascular risk and liver damage, subjects who carried the variant had more severe steatosis, necroinflammation, ballooning, and fibrosis, but were at lower risk of developing carotid atherosclerosis and had lower serum lipid levels. This phenomenon is called the Catch-22: protecting the heart at the expense of an increased risk of NAFLD progression.[69]

Membrane-Bound O-Acyltransferase Domain–Containing Protein 7

Lysophospholipid acyltransferase 7, also known as membrane-bound O-acyltransferase domain–containing protein 7 (MBOAT7) is an enzyme encoded by the MBOAT7 gene, and is involved in phospholipid acyl-chain remodeling, known as the Lands cycle. It transfers arachidonic acid (AA) to lysophosphatidylinositol and other lysophospholipids, reducing AA levels. AA acts to induce apoptosis and is a potent trigger for inflammation and fibrosis.[70,71]

The MBOAT7 rs641739 genetic variant has recently emerged as a new genetic risk factor for liver disease. The variant was associated with lower MBOAT7 protein expression in the liver, affecting the acyl remodeling of phosphatidylinositol, resulting in increased AA levels and an increase in the inflammatory response in the liver.[71,72] It has been shown to increase histologic liver damage in alcoholic cirrhosis; hepatitis C; and, most recently, chronic hepatitis B and NAFLD.[72–75] In a study of individuals of European descent, the MBOAT7 genetic variant was associated with increased hepatic fat content and more severe hepatic inflammation and fibrosis compared with controls without the variant.[72] Krawczyk and colleagues[49] showed that fibrosis stages were affected by the MBOAT7 genetic variant and were likely associated with the risk of hepatic fibrosis. More longitudinal studies are warranted to fully understand its role in the development of NAFLD.

Kruppel-Like Factor 6

Kruppel-like factor 6 (KLF6) belongs to the Kruppel-like family of transcription factors, has been identified as an early gene expressed in activated hepatic stellate cells in liver injury, and has been thought to be play a role in liver fibrogenesis.[76–78] A functional intron 1 SNP, *KLF6-IVS1-27G>A* (rs3750861) promotes KLF6 alternative splicing into antagonistic, truncated isoforms, thus decreasing KLF6's transactivation of factors involved in the development of liver fibrosis, such as collagen 1, transforming growth factor (TGF)-β1, and types I and II TGF-β receptors in hepatic stellate cells.[77–79] Miele and colleagues[78] recruited patients with biopsy-proven NAFLD in the United Kingdom and Italy to study the effect of this genetic variant, which promotes in vivo alternative splicing of KLF6. The study showed that the KLF6 genetic variant was associated with a milder NAFLD, with 25% compared with 45% of individuals without the variant having advanced fibrosis. In the same study, a linear regression analysis adjusting for age, sex, BMI, and blood glucose level identified wild-type KLF6 as an independent predictor of moderate/advanced fibrosis. In another study, Bechmann and colleagues[80] proposed that KLG6 genetic variant expression in steatotic hepatocytes is associated with a decrease in levels of glucose kinase regulator (GCKR), a negative regulator of glucokinase (GCK) activity, resulting in increased expression of GCK. GCK catalyzed the production of glucose-6-phosphate produced by the phosphorylation of glucose in the liver. Increased GCK activity also increases hepatic clearance of insulin and increased hepatic insulin sensitivity.

Insulin Receptor Substrate-1

Insulin receptor substrate-1 (IRS-1) is a signaling adapter protein critical in the insulin-signaling pathway. Insulin binds to high-affinity insulin receptors in hepatocytes, leading to insulin receptor phosphorylation, activation of IRS-1 and IRS-2 via tyrosine phosphorylation, and decreased glucose production and apoptosis via the activation of the downstream intracellular protein kinase B (Akt) pathway, a signal transduction pathway that promotes cell survival, growth, and glucose metabolism.[81,82] A glycine-to-arginine change at codon 972 in IRS-1 reduces insulin receptor autophosphorylation by acting as a competitive inhibitor of the insulin receptor, thus increasing the risk of insulin resistance and diabetes. IRS-1 genetic variant causes hepatocellular damage by decreasing cell survival, leading to accelerated fibrogenesis.[83] A combined study from Italy and the United Kingdom showed that the IRS-1 genetic variant was associated with an increased prevalence of advanced fibrosis and a marked reduction of approximately 70% in AKT activation status, leading to reduced insulin-signaling activity and insulin resistance. This effect was independent of the ethnic background.[84] Another study of transgenic mice expressing this variant evaluated the action of insulin in the liver, skeletal muscle, and adipose tissue. Glucose use and insulin signaling were impaired in all target tissues in the mice carrying the allele, confirming the findings of increased insulin resistance and decreased beta-cell function leading to hyperglycemia.[85]

RACE AND ETHNICITY

NAFLD has become a global health issue given its increasing prevalence in the United States and in many other countries owing to the dramatic change in lifestyle and the desire to be sedentary, resulting in increasing rates of obesity and diabetes across the world. Two ethnic groups that particularly stand out for their high risk for the development of NAFLD are those of Asian and Hispanic descent.

Asian

Although the prevalence of NAFLD in Western countries ranges from 24% to 46%, the prevalence in Asia varies across the continent, with numbers ranging from 7.9% in Indonesia to 54% of elderly female population in Taiwan.[2,36,86] The rate of NAFLD has doubled over the past 7 to 10 years in China, and the prevalence of NAFLD in Japan has increased by 18%, reflecting the severity of this global epidemic.[87,88]

Urbanization and economic prosperity leading to a more sedentary lifestyle in major cities in Asia, including Beijing, Shanghai, and Hong Kong, have been shown to be factors leading to an increase in the prevalence of NAFLD.[89–92]

Asian populations show a greater risk of fat-related disorders such as NAFLD, heart disease, and diabetes compared with their counterparts in Western countries of the same anthropometric measurements (weight and height).[93,94] Weston and colleagues[95] compared the demographic and clinical features of NAFLD in a racially diverse representative region of the US population (Alemeda County, CA) and showed that Asians with NAFLD have lower BMIs compared with Hispanic Americans, African Americans, white people, and other races. Chang and colleagues[96] examined 15,347 Korean men aged 30 to 59 years and found that Korean men who had a BMI between 18.5 and 22.9 had a significantly increased risk for ultrasonographically detected fatty liver if they had a weight gain of 2.3 kg or more. In Iran, a study by Bahrami and colleagues[97] evaluated 53 patients with biopsy-proven NAFLD. The Langevin Institute for food quality control with NAFLD had an average BMI of 29.3, and of these only 5.7% had diabetes, 54.7% had insulin resistance, and 75.5% had some form of dyslipidemia. More importantly, 13.2% of the subjects without the standard risk factors for NASH showed evidence of NASH on liver biopsy. In a retrospective analysis of liver biopsy data in 238 adults with NAFLD in Chicago, Mohanty and colleagues[98] showed that Asians showed higher grades of ballooning and increased prevalence of Mallory bodies compared with white people and other ethnicities combined (except Hispanic Americans). Asian patients also had a lower BMI (29.3) compared with other groups.

It is unclear why Asians seem to be a greater risk to develop NAFLD. Asians have been shown to have lower adiponectin levels and higher TNF-alpha levels than other races and these factors may be contributing to the development of NAFLD.[99] Besides the common risk factors shared among all ethnicities, there are emerging data that risk factors such as hypothyroidism and obstructive sleep apnea may be contributing to NAFLD in Asia.[100,101] Genetic variation of PNPLA3 is another factor contributing to NAFLD development, as shown by studies in China, Japan, and India, and among the different ethnic groups in Malaysia.[40,102–104] The PNPLA-3 rs738409 gene mutation, particularly the CG and GG genotypes, increases the risk of progression to HCC, even in people with cirrhosis of causes other than NAFLD.[51,105] Visceral adiposity reflected by increased waist circumference (instead of increased BMI) results in an increased production of proinflammatory cytokines, which accelerates the progression from simple steatosis to more advanced forms of NAFLD and worsening of insulin resistance.[106] A recent study showed that patients with lean NAFLD have a distinct metabolomic profile that is different from that of obese patients with NAFLD, specifically with regard to the types of amino acids and cholines found in the lean NAFLD group.[107] This finding suggests the need for emphasis on therapeutic intervention rather than weight loss alone in these high-risk patients. Future studies are needed to investigate this pathophysiologic distinctiveness.

Hispanic Americans/African Americans/Non-Hispanic White People

Obesity and diabetes have been reported to be more prevalent in the African American and Hispanic populations compared with non-Hispanic white people.[108–110] In the United States, 70% of African Americans, 73% of Mexican Americans, and 63% of non-Hispanic white people identified themselves as being either overweight or obese.[111] Mean hemoglobin A1c levels were higher among African Americans compared with white people (8.14% vs 7.40%).[112] Despite the increased prevalence of MetS in both the African American and the Hispanic populations, African Americans showed a lower risk for developing NAFLD/NASH compared with other patient groups. Browning and colleagues[54] examined and compared the distribution of hepatic TG content in multiethnic groups using proton magnetic resonance spectroscopy. This study revealed significant differences in the frequency of hepatic steatosis, with a rate of 45% in Hispanic Americans, 33% in non-Hispanic white people, and 24% in African Americans. The higher prevalence of obesity and insulin resistance could explain the higher prevalence of NAFLD in Hispanic Americans, but the same cannot be said for African Americans. In the study by Mohanty and colleagues,[98] Hispanic Americans showed higher grades of ballooning and increased Mallory bodies than all other ethnicities combined except for Asians. To date, there have been multiple other studies showing similar observations via radiologic, laboratory, and liver biopsy assessment.[113–116]

The difference in the prevalence of NAFLD by race may be explained by the distribution of adipose tissue in the body, with Hispanic Americans having more visceral fat compared with African Americans, a phenomenon called the insulin resistance paradox.[117] Diet may play a role because Hispanic Americans consume a higher amount of carbohydrates than non-Hispanic white people and African Americans, which affects lipid metabolism.[44] The greater propensity for a more prominent inflammatory status and more advanced fibrosis progression caused by higher levels of liver enzymes such as aminotransferases among the Hispanic population can lead to greater severity of chronic liver disease.[118] Significantly increased alanine transaminase level has been observed with the PNPLA-3 rs738409 gene mutation, and this observation was limited to individuals of Hispanic descent.[62,119] It has been shown that Hispanic Americans are twice as likely to carry the PNPLA-3 genetic variant compared with African Americans (40% vs 19%), leading to greater prevalence of NAFLD among Hispanic Americans compared with African Americans (24% vs 9%).[62] This risk allele has been shown to increase susceptibility to higher hepatic fat content from high dietary fat consumption in Hispanic children.[120] In contrast, the PNPLA3 variant at position S453I is associated with lower hepatic fat content, and can be found more in African Americans, with lower frequencies in European Americans and Hispanic Americans. Thus, African Americans with the same demographics as Hispanic Americans may show a lower risk of NAFLD development and progression purely because of differences in gene expression.[62]

Taken altogether, distribution of adipose tissue and variants with gene expression within the Asian and Hispanic cohorts may play a role in the degree of hepatic injury, identifying them as high-risk groups for the development of NAFLD/NASH.

GENDER

There are conflicting data on the influence of gender on NAFLD. Although early studies suggested that NAFLD was more common in women, recent studies have shown that NAFLD may be evenly distributed between women and men, or may even have a higher prevalence in men.[121,122] Using the NHANES data, NAFLD was significantly more prevalent in men.[2,4,123] Using the same data, Younossi and colleagues[124] stratified cohorts into lean and overweight-obese groups and reported that lean NAFLD was more common in women than in men. In the Nonalcoholic Steatohepatitis Clinical Research Network database, patients with NASH were more likely to be female than male in a 2:1 distribution, reflecting a higher disease burden in women and gender differences among those pursuing health care.[125] In a study by Stepanova and colleagues[126] of 289 patients with NAFLD, approximately 60% of the cohort was women even though there was no significant difference in age or race. Ayonrinde and colleagues[127] showed a higher prevalence of female NAFLD compared with male NAFLD (16.3% vs 10.1%) in an adolescent age group, although male individuals with NAFLD had greater visceral adiposity and adverse metabolic features. In contrast, in a study of 13,768 Korean adults, men had a 2.5-times greater risk of having NAFLD compared with women, and the association between metabolic risk factor and NAFLD was 1.5-fold to 2.0-fold stronger in men than in women, a finding that was attributed to gender differences in fat distribution. In addition, women who were of normal weight and had no risk factors were 40% less likely to develop NAFLD than men of the same group.[128] In another study of nearly 2500 patients in Hong Kong, male gender constituted 53% of the NAFLD cohort and 40% in subjects without NAFLD.[90] In addition, Williams and colleagues[2] evaluated NAFLD among a largely middle-aged population and showed a male gender predominance in NAFLD, with 58.9% being male and 41.1% being female. Lifestyle factors, including alcohol use, propensity for increased waist/circumference ratio, and perhaps different levels of female hormones may further explain the gender difference in the prevalence of NAFLD.[123,129–131]

POLYCYSTIC OVARIAN SYNDROME

Polycystic ovarian syndrome (PCOS) in the most common endocrine disorder in women of reproductive age, and the prevalence of NAFLD, is markedly increased in patients with PCOS. Data extrapolated from more than a dozen studies reveal that the prevalence of women with PCOS and NAFLD ranges from 35% to 70% compared with 20% to 30% in healthy women without PCOS who were matched for age, BMI, and waist circumference.[132] A recent study of 600 white women diagnosed with PCOS showed that NAFLD was more prevalent in cohorts with PCOS who had increased waist circumference, increased lipid accumulation product (LAP; an index of central lipid accumulation calculated from waist circumference and plasma TG level), increased insulin resistance, and increased total serum cholesterol and TG levels. Compared with an age-matched control with a similar prevalence of T2DM and MetS, patients with PCOS had a higher incidence of NAFLD.[133] This finding was replicated in a study by Ayonrinde and colleagues,[134] who showed that NAFLD was more prevalent in adolescent girls with PCOS than in controls (37.5% vs 15.1% of 244 individuals), and the former had greater adiposity, higher LAP levels, increased C-reactive protein levels, increased ferritin levels, increased insulin resistance, and lower sex hormone–binding globulin levels. In China, a study conducted on 602 lean young Chinese women with and without PCOS showed a greater prevalence of NAFLD in women with PCOS than in matched controls (33% vs 19%), and that metabolic risk factors were more prevalent in women with PCOS.[135] Insulin resistance is the key factor linking PCOS to NAFLD, because it is associated with impaired suppression of lipolysis in adipose tissue leading to increased influx of FFA into the liver.[136] Visceral adiposity and hypertriglyceridemia play a role in the pathogenesis of NAFLD in women with PCOS, as shown by the reduction of hepatic steatosis after weight loss and serum TG level reduction with the use of omega-3 FAs.[137,138] Studies on the role of hyperandrogenemia in NAFLD prevalence in PCOS phenotypes yield conflicting results. Theoretically, insulin resistance increases ovarian androgen synthesis and downregulates hepatic sex hormone–binding globulin, causing an increased in circulating free androgen levels, hence it is plausible that insulin resistance is the common factor that ties both NAFLD and high androgen levels (**Fig. 3**).[134]

FUTURE PROSPECTS

NAFLD is a burgeoning health epidemic owing largely to its modifiable risk factors, such as obesity and insulin resistance, and innate factors affecting visceral adiposity and genetic polymorphisms. Despite improved understanding of NAFLD pathophysiology and risk factors, there is still a lack of highly effective long-term therapy. Continuous clinical studies are warranted to improve primary prevention strategies and early diagnostic work-up, perhaps targeting high-risk population based on the aforementioned risk factors to improve outcomes for this disease.

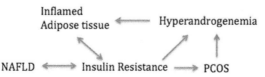

Fig. 3. Insulin resistance–mediated pathogenesis in NAFLD and PCOS.

REFERENCES

1. Younossi ZM, Stepanova M, Afendy M, et al. Changes in the prevalence of the most common causes of chronic liver diseases in the United States from 1988 to 2008. Clin Gastroenterol Hepatol 2011;9:524–30.e1 [quiz: e60].

2. Williams CD, Stengel J, Asike MI, et al. Prevalence of nonalcoholic fatty liver disease and nonalcoholic steatohepatitis among a largely middle-aged population utilizing ultrasound and liver biopsy: a prospective study. Gastroenterology 2011;140:124–31.

3. Vernon G, Baranova A, Younossi ZM. Systematic review: the epidemiology and natural history of non-alcoholic fatty liver disease and non-alcoholic steatohepatitis in adults. Aliment Pharmacol Ther 2011;34:274–85.

4. Lazo M, Hernaez R, Eberhardt MS, et al. Prevalence of nonalcoholic fatty liver disease in the United States: the Third National Health and Nutrition Examination Survey, 1988-1994. Am J Epidemiol 2013;178:38–45.

5. Brunt EM. Nonalcoholic steatohepatitis. Semin Liver Dis 2004;24:3–20.

6. Ludwig J, Viggiano TR, McGill DB, et al. Nonalcoholic steatohepatitis: Mayo Clinic experiences with a hitherto unnamed disease. Mayo Clin Proc 1980;55: 434–8.

7. Fleischman MW, Budoff M, Zeb I, et al. NAFLD prevalence differs among Hispanic subgroups: the Multi-Ethnic Study of Atherosclerosis. World J Gastroenterol 2014;20:4987–93.

8. Farrell GC, Wong VW, Chitturi S. NAFLD in Asia–as common and important as in the West. Nat Rev Gastroenterol Hepatol 2013;10:307–18.

9. Speliotes EK, Yerges-Armstrong LM, Wu J, et al. Genome-wide association analysis identifies variants associated with nonalcoholic fatty liver disease that have distinct effects on metabolic traits. PLoS Genet 2011;7:e1001324.

10. Alberti KG, Eckel RH, Grundy SM, et al. Harmonizing the metabolic syndrome: a joint interim statement of the International Diabetes Federation Task Force on Epidemiology and Prevention; National Heart, Lung, and Blood Institute; American Heart Association; World Heart Federation; International Atherosclerosis Society; and International Association for the Study of Obesity. Circulation 2009;120:1640–5.

11. Smits MM, Ioannou GN, Boyko EJ, et al. Non-alcoholic fatty liver disease as an independent manifestation of the metabolic syndrome: results of a US national survey in three ethnic groups. J Gastroenterol Hepatol 2013;28:664–70.

12. Marchesini G, Bugianesi E, Forlani G, et al. Nonalcoholic fatty liver, steatohepatitis, and the metabolic syndrome. Hepatology 2003;37:917–23.

13. Hamaguchi M, Kojima T, Takeda N, et al. The metabolic syndrome as a predictor of nonalcoholic fatty liver disease. Ann Intern Med 2005;143:722–8.

14. Bugianesi E, Gastaldelli A, Vanni E, et al. Insulin resistance in non-diabetic patients with non-alcoholic fatty liver disease: sites and mechanisms. Diabetologia 2005;48:634–42.

15. Reaven GM. Insulin resistance, the insulin resistance syndrome, and cardiovascular disease. Panminerva Med 2005;47:201–10.

16. Gallagher EJ, Leroith D, Karnieli E. The metabolic syndrome–from insulin resistance to obesity and diabetes. Med Clin North Am 2011;95:855–73.

17. Feldstein AE, Werneburg NW, Canbay A, et al. Free fatty acids promote hepatic lipotoxicity by stimulating TNF-alpha expression via a lysosomal pathway. Hepatology 2004;40:185–94.

18. Kelley DE, Mokan M, Simoneau JA, et al. Interaction between glucose and free fatty acid metabolism in human skeletal muscle. J Clin Invest 1993;92:91–8.
19. Cohen DH, LeRoith D. Obesity, type 2 diabetes, and cancer: the insulin and IGF connection. Endocr Relat Cancer 2012;19:F27–45.
20. Zarember KA, Godowski PJ. Tissue expression of human Toll-like receptors and differential regulation of Toll-like receptor mRNAs in leukocytes in response to microbes, their products, and cytokines. J Immunol 2002;168:554–61.
21. Bhargava P, Lee CH. Role and function of macrophages in the metabolic syndrome. Biochem J 2012;442:253–62.
22. Lazo M, Clark JM. The epidemiology of nonalcoholic fatty liver disease: a global perspective. Semin Liver Dis 2008;28:339–50.
23. Lee CJ, Clark JM, Asamoah V, et al. Prevalence and characteristics of individuals without diabetes and hypertension who underwent bariatric surgery: lessons learned about metabolically healthy obese. Surg Obes Relat Dis 2015; 11:142–6.
24. Inge TH, Zeller M, Harmon C, et al. Teen-longitudinal assessment of bariatric surgery: methodological features of the first prospective multicenter study of adolescent bariatric surgery. J Pediatr Surg 2007;42:1969–71.
25. Doycheva I, Watt KD, Alkhouri N. Nonalcoholic fatty liver disease in adolescents and young adults: the next frontier in the epidemic. Hepatology 2017;65(6): 2100–9.
26. Li L, Liu DW, Yan HY, et al. Obesity is an independent risk factor for nonalcoholic fatty liver disease: evidence from a meta-analysis of 21 cohort studies. Obes Rev 2016;17:510–9.
27. Fabbrini E, Sullivan S, Klein S. Obesity and nonalcoholic fatty liver disease: biochemical, metabolic, and clinical implications. Hepatology 2010;51:679–89.
28. Mittendorfer B, Magkos F, Fabbrini E, et al. Relationship between body fat mass and free fatty acid kinetics in men and women. Obesity (Silver Spring) 2009;17: 1872–7.
29. Pardina E, Baena-Fustegueras JA, Catalan R, et al. Increased expression and activity of hepatic lipase in the liver of morbidly obese adult patients in relation to lipid content. Obes Surg 2009;19:894–904.
30. Westerbacka J, Kolak M, Kiviluoto T, et al. Genes involved in fatty acid partitioning and binding, lipolysis, monocyte/macrophage recruitment, and inflammation are overexpressed in the human fatty liver of insulin-resistant subjects. Diabetes 2007;56:2759–65.
31. Shimomura I, Bashmakov Y, Horton JD. Increased levels of nuclear SREBP-1c associated with fatty livers in two mouse models of diabetes mellitus. J Biol Chem 1999;274:30028–32.
32. Sanyal AJ, Campbell-Sargent C, Mirshahi F, et al. Nonalcoholic steatohepatitis: association of insulin resistance and mitochondrial abnormalities. Gastroenterology 2001;120:1183–92.
33. Angelico F, Del Ben M, Conti R, et al. Insulin resistance, the metabolic syndrome, and nonalcoholic fatty liver disease. J Clin Endocrinol Metab 2005;90: 1578–82.
34. Kelley DE, McKolanis TM, Hegazi RA, et al. Fatty liver in type 2 diabetes mellitus: relation to regional adiposity, fatty acids, and insulin resistance. Am J Physiol Endocrinol Metab 2003;285:E906–16.
35. Leite NC, Villela-Nogueira CA, Pannain VL, et al. Histopathological stages of nonalcoholic fatty liver disease in type 2 diabetes: prevalences and correlated factors. Liver Int 2011;31:700–6.

36. Seto WK, Yuen MF. Nonalcoholic fatty liver disease in Asia: emerging perspectives. J Gastroenterol 2017;52:164–74.
37. Krawczyk M, Portincasa P, Lammert F. PNPLA3-associated steatohepatitis: toward a gene-based classification of fatty liver disease. Semin Liver Dis 2013; 33:369–79.
38. Sookoian S, Pirola CJ. Meta-analysis of the influence of I148M variant of patatin-like phospholipase domain containing 3 gene (PNPLA3) on the susceptibility and histological severity of nonalcoholic fatty liver disease. Hepatology 2011; 53:1883–94.
39. Peng XE, Wu YL, Lin SW, et al. Genetic variants in PNPLA3 and risk of nonalcoholic fatty liver disease in a Han Chinese population. PLoS One 2012;7: e50256.
40. Li Y, Xing C, Tian Z, et al. Genetic variant I148M in PNPLA3 is associated with the ultrasonography-determined steatosis degree in a Chinese population. BMC Med Genet 2012;13:113.
41. Kitamoto T, Kitamoto A, Yoneda M, et al. Genome-wide scan revealed that polymorphisms in the PNPLA3, SAMM50, and PARVB genes are associated with development and progression of nonalcoholic fatty liver disease in Japan. Hum Genet 2013;132:783–92.
42. Lee SS, Byoun YS, Jeong SH, et al. Role of the PNPLA3 I148M polymorphism in nonalcoholic fatty liver disease and fibrosis in Korea. Dig Dis Sci 2014;59: 2967–74.
43. Kanth VV, Sasikala M, Rao PN, et al. Pooled genetic analysis in ultrasound measured non-alcoholic fatty liver disease in Indian subjects: a pilot study. World J Hepatol 2014;6:435–42.
44. Kallwitz ER, Daviglus ML, Allison MA, et al. Prevalence of suspected nonalcoholic fatty liver disease in Hispanic/Latino individuals differs by heritage. Clin Gastroenterol Hepatol 2015;13:569–76.
45. Palmer ND, Musani SK, Yerges-Armstrong LM, et al. Characterization of European ancestry nonalcoholic fatty liver disease-associated variants in individuals of African and Hispanic descent. Hepatology 2013;58:966–75.
46. Qu HQ, Li Q, Grove ML, et al. Population-based risk factors for elevated alanine aminotransferase in a South Texas Mexican-American population. Arch Med Res 2012;43:482–8.
47. Fan JH, Xiang MQ, Li QL, et al. PNPLA3 rs738409 polymorphism associated with hepatic steatosis and advanced fibrosis in patients with chronic hepatitis C virus: a meta-analysis. Gut Liver 2016;10:456–63.
48. Salameh H, Raff E, Erwin A, et al. PNPLA3 gene polymorphism is associated with predisposition to and severity of alcoholic liver disease. Am J Gastroenterol 2015;110:846–56.
49. Krawczyk M, Rau M, Schattenberg JM, et al. Combined effects of the PNPLA3 rs738409, TM6SF2 rs58542926, and MBOAT7 rs641738 variants on NAFLD severity: a multicenter biopsy-based study. J Lipid Res 2017;58:247–55.
50. Hassan MM, Kaseb A, Etzel CJ, et al. Genetic variation in the PNPLA3 gene and hepatocellular carcinoma in USA: risk and prognosis prediction. Mol Carcinog 2013;52(Suppl 1):E139–47.
51. Guyot E, Sutton A, Rufat P, et al. PNPLA3 rs738409, hepatocellular carcinoma occurrence and risk model prediction in patients with cirrhosis. J Hepatol 2013;58:312–8.

52. Liu YL, Patman GL, Leathart JB, et al. Carriage of the PNPLA3 rs738409 C >G polymorphism confers an increased risk of non-alcoholic fatty liver disease associated hepatocellular carcinoma. J Hepatol 2014;61:75–81.

53. Hao L, Ito K, Huang KH, et al. Shifts in dietary carbohydrate-lipid exposure regulate expression of the non-alcoholic fatty liver disease-associated gene PNPLA3/adiponutrin in mouse liver and HepG2 human liver cells. Metabolism 2014;63:1352–62.

54. Browning JD. Common genetic variants and nonalcoholic fatty liver disease. Clin Gastroenterol Hepatol 2013;11:1191–3.

55. Naik A, Kosir R, Rozman D. Genomic aspects of NAFLD pathogenesis. Genomics 2013;102:84–95.

56. Perttila J, Huaman-Samanez C, Caron S, et al. PNPLA3 is regulated by glucose in human hepatocytes, and its I148M mutant slows down triglyceride hydrolysis. Am J Physiol Endocrinol Metab 2012;302:E1063–9.

57. Pirazzi C, Adiels M, Burza MA, et al. Patatin-like phospholipase domain-containing 3 (PNPLA3) I148M (rs738409) affects hepatic VLDL secretion in humans and in vitro. J Hepatol 2012;57:1276–82.

58. Kumashiro N, Yoshimura T, Cantley JL, et al. Role of patatin-like phospholipase domain-containing 3 on lipid-induced hepatic steatosis and insulin resistance in rats. Hepatology 2013;57:1763–72.

59. Valenti L, Rametta R, Ruscica M, et al. The I148M PNPLA3 polymorphism influences serum adiponectin in patients with fatty liver and healthy controls. BMC Gastroenterol 2012;12:111.

60. Bianchi G, Bugianesi E, Frystyk J, et al. Adiponectin isoforms, insulin resistance and liver histology in nonalcoholic fatty liver disease. Dig Liver Dis 2011;43:73–7.

61. Polyzos SA, Toulis KA, Goulis DG, et al. Serum total adiponectin in nonalcoholic fatty liver disease: a systematic review and meta-analysis. Metabolism 2011;60:313–26.

62. Romeo S, Kozlitina J, Xing C, et al. Genetic variation in PNPLA3 confers susceptibility to nonalcoholic fatty liver disease. Nat Genet 2008;40:1461–5.

63. Kozlitina J, Smagris E, Stender S, et al. Exome-wide association study identifies a TM6SF2 variant that confers susceptibility to nonalcoholic fatty liver disease. Nat Genet 2014;46:352–6.

64. Mahdessian H, Taxiarchis A, Popov S, et al. TM6SF2 is a regulator of liver fat metabolism influencing triglyceride secretion and hepatic lipid droplet content. Proc Natl Acad Sci U S A 2014;111:8913–8.

65. Holmen OL, Zhang H, Fan Y, et al. Systematic evaluation of coding variation identifies a candidate causal variant in TM6SF2 influencing total cholesterol and myocardial infarction risk. Nat Genet 2014;46:345–51.

66. Dongiovanni P, Petta S, Maglio C, et al. Transmembrane 6 superfamily member 2 gene variant disentangles nonalcoholic steatohepatitis from cardiovascular disease. Hepatology 2015;61:506–14.

67. Sookoian S, Castano GO, Scian R, et al. Genetic variation in transmembrane 6 superfamily member 2 and the risk of nonalcoholic fatty liver disease and histological disease severity. Hepatology 2015;61:515–25.

68. Liu YL, Reeves HL, Burt AD, et al. TM6SF2 rs58542926 influences hepatic fibrosis progression in patients with non-alcoholic fatty liver disease. Nat Commun 2014;5:4309.

69. Kahali B, Liu YL, Daly AK, et al. TM6SF2: catch-22 in the fight against nonalcoholic fatty liver disease and cardiovascular disease? Gastroenterology 2015; 148:679–84.

70. Serini S, Piccioni E, Merendino N, et al. Dietary polyunsaturated fatty acids as inducers of apoptosis: implications for cancer. Apoptosis 2009;14:135–52.

71. Guicciardi ME, Gores GJ. Apoptosis: a mechanism of acute and chronic liver injury. Gut 2005;54:1024–33.

72. Mancina RM, Dongiovanni P, Petta S, et al. The MBOAT7-TMC4 variant rs641738 increases risk of nonalcoholic fatty liver disease in individuals of European descent. Gastroenterology 2016;150:1219–30.e6.

73. Buch S, Stickel F, Trepo E, et al. A genome-wide association study confirms PNPLA3 and identifies TM6SF2 and MBOAT7 as risk loci for alcohol-related cirrhosis. Nat Genet 2015;47:1443–8.

74. Thabet K, Asimakopoulos A, Shojaei M, et al. MBOAT7 rs641738 increases risk of liver inflammation and transition to fibrosis in chronic hepatitis C. Nat Commun 2016;7:12757.

75. Thabet K, Chan HL, Petta S, et al. The MBOAT7 variant rs641738 increases inflammation and fibrosis in chronic hepatitis B. Hepatology 2017;65(6): 1840–50.

76. Lalazar A, Wong L, Yamasaki G, et al. Early genes induced in hepatic stellate cells during wound healing. Gene 1997;195:235–43.

77. Ratziu V, Lalazar A, Wong L, et al. Zf9, a Kruppel-like transcription factor upregulated in vivo during early hepatic fibrosis. Proc Natl Acad Sci U S A 1998;95:9500–5.

78. Miele L, Beale G, Patman G, et al. The Kruppel-like factor 6 genotype is associated with fibrosis in nonalcoholic fatty liver disease. Gastroenterology 2008; 135:282–91.e1.

79. Kim Y, Ratziu V, Choi SG, et al. Transcriptional activation of transforming growth factor beta1 and its receptors by the Kruppel-like factor Zf9/core promoter-binding protein and Sp1. Potential mechanisms for autocrine fibrogenesis in response to injury. J Biol Chem 1998;273:33750–8.

80. Bechmann LP, Gastaldelli A, Vetter D, et al. Glucokinase links Kruppel-like factor 6 to the regulation of hepatic insulin sensitivity in nonalcoholic fatty liver disease. Hepatology 2012;55:1083–93.

81. Copps KD, White MF. Regulation of insulin sensitivity by serine/threonine phosphorylation of insulin receptor substrate proteins IRS1 and IRS2. Diabetologia 2012;55:2565–82.

82. Ramocki NM, Wilkins HR, Magness ST, et al. Insulin receptor substrate-1 deficiency promotes apoptosis in the putative intestinal crypt stem cell region, limits Apcmin/+ tumors, and regulates Sox9. Endocrinology 2008;149:261–7.

83. McGettrick AJ, Feener EP, Kahn CR. Human insulin receptor substrate-1 (IRS-1) polymorphism G972R causes IRS-1 to associate with the insulin receptor and inhibit receptor autophosphorylation. J Biol Chem 2005;280:6441–6.

84. Dongiovanni P, Valenti L, Rametta R, et al. Genetic variants regulating insulin receptor signalling are associated with the severity of liver damage in patients with non-alcoholic fatty liver disease. Gut 2010;59:267–73.

85. Hribal ML, Tornei F, Pujol A, et al. Transgenic mice overexpressing human G972R IRS-1 show impaired insulin action and insulin secretion. J Cell Mol Med 2008;12:2096–106.

86. Caballeria L, Pera G, Auladell MA, et al. Prevalence and factors associated with the presence of nonalcoholic fatty liver disease in an adult population in Spain. Eur J Gastroenterol Hepatol 2010;22:24–32.

87. Fan JG, Farrell GC. Epidemiology of non-alcoholic fatty liver disease in China. J Hepatol 2009;50:204–10.

88. Kojima S, Watanabe N, Numata M, et al. Increase in the prevalence of fatty liver in Japan over the past 12 years: analysis of clinical background. J Gastroenterol 2003;38:954–61.

89. Zhu JZ, Zhou QY, Wang YM, et al. Prevalence of fatty liver disease and the economy in China: a systematic review. World J Gastroenterol 2015;21:5695–706.

90. Fung J, Lee CK, Chan M, et al. High prevalence of non-alcoholic fatty liver disease in the Chinese - results from the Hong Kong liver health census. Liver Int 2015;35:542–9.

91. Yan J, Xie W, Ou WN, et al. Epidemiological survey and risk factor analysis of fatty liver disease of adult residents, Beijing, China. J Gastroenterol Hepatol 2013;28:1654–9.

92. Li Z, Xue J, Chen P, et al. Prevalence of nonalcoholic fatty liver disease in mainland of China: a meta-analysis of published studies. J Gastroenterol Hepatol 2014;29:42–51.

93. Das K, Das K, Mukherjee PS, et al. Nonobese population in a developing country has a high prevalence of nonalcoholic fatty liver and significant liver disease. Hepatology 2010;51:1593–602.

94. Liu CJ. Prevalence and risk factors for non-alcoholic fatty liver disease in Asian people who are not obese. J Gastroenterol Hepatol 2012;27:1555–60.

95. Weston SR, Leyden W, Murphy R, et al. Racial and ethnic distribution of nonalcoholic fatty liver in persons with newly diagnosed chronic liver disease. Hepatology 2005;41:372–9.

96. Chang Y, Ryu S, Sung E, et al. Weight gain within the normal weight range predicts ultrasonographically detected fatty liver in healthy Korean men. Gut 2009;58:1419–25.

97. Bahrami H, Daryani NE, Mirmomen S, et al. Clinical and histological features of nonalcoholic steatohepatitis in Iranian patients. BMC Gastroenterol 2003;3:27.

98. Mohanty SR, Troy TN, Huo D, et al. Influence of ethnicity on histological differences in non-alcoholic fatty liver disease. J Hepatol 2009;50:797–804.

99. Wong VW, Hui AY, Tsang SW, et al. Metabolic and adipokine profile of Chinese patients with nonalcoholic fatty liver disease. Clin Gastroenterol Hepatol 2006;4:1154–61.

100. Tao Y, Gu H, Wu J, et al. Thyroid function is associated with non-alcoholic fatty liver disease in euthyroid subjects. Endocr Res 2015;40:74–8.

101. Chou TC, Liang WM, Wang CB, et al. Obstructive sleep apnea is associated with liver disease: a population-based cohort study. Sleep Med 2015;16:955–60.

102. Kawaguchi T, Sumida Y, Umemura A, et al. Genetic polymorphisms of the human PNPLA3 gene are strongly associated with severity of non-alcoholic fatty liver disease in Japanese. PLoS One 2012;7:e38322.

103. Bhatt SP, Nigam P, Misra A, et al. Genetic variation in the patatin-like phospholipase domain-containing protein-3 (PNPLA-3) gene in Asian Indians with nonalcoholic fatty liver disease. Metab Syndr Relat Disord 2013;11:329–35.

104. Zain SM, Mohamed R, Mahadeva S, et al. A multi-ethnic study of a PNPLA3 gene variant and its association with disease severity in non-alcoholic fatty liver disease. Hum Genet 2012;131:1145–52.

105. Singal AG, Manjunath H, Yopp AC, et al. The effect of PNPLA3 on fibrosis progression and development of hepatocellular carcinoma: a meta-analysis. Am J Gastroenterol 2014;109:325–34.
106. van der Poorten D, Milner KL, Hui J, et al. Visceral fat: a key mediator of steatohepatitis in metabolic liver disease. Hepatology 2008;48:449–57.
107. Feldman A, Eder SK, Felder TK, et al. Clinical and metabolic characterization of lean Caucasian subjects with non-alcoholic fatty liver. Am J Gastroenterol 2017; 112:102–10.
108. Brancati FL, Kao WH, Folsom AR, et al. Incident type 2 diabetes mellitus in African American and white adults: the Atherosclerosis Risk in Communities study. JAMA 2000;283:2253–9.
109. Hedley AA, Ogden CL, Johnson CL, et al. Prevalence of overweight and obesity among US children, adolescents, and adults, 1999-2002. JAMA 2004;291: 2847–50.
110. Crespo CJ, Loria CM, Burt VL. Hypertension and other cardiovascular disease risk factors among Mexican Americans, Cuban Americans, and Puerto Ricans from the Hispanic Health and Nutrition Examination Survey. Public Health Rep 1996;111(Suppl 2):7–10.
111. Flegal KM, Carroll MD, Ogden CL, et al. Prevalence and trends in obesity among US adults, 1999-2008. JAMA 2010;303:235–41.
112. Hausmann LR, Ren D, Sevick MA. Racial differences in diabetes-related psychosocial factors and glycemic control in patients with type 2 diabetes. Patient Prefer Adherence 2010;4:291–9.
113. Louthan MV, Theriot JA, Zimmerman E, et al. Decreased prevalence of nonalcoholic fatty liver disease in black obese children. J Pediatr Gastroenterol Nutr 2005;41:426–9.
114. Wagenknecht LE, Scherzinger AL, Stamm ER, et al. Correlates and heritability of nonalcoholic fatty liver disease in a minority cohort. Obesity (Silver Spring) 2009; 17:1240–6.
115. Pan JJ, Fisher-Hoch SP, Chen C, et al. Burden of nonalcoholic fatty liver disease and advanced fibrosis in a Texas Hispanic community cohort. World J Hepatol 2015;7:1586–94.
116. Kallwitz ER, Guzman G, TenCate V, et al. The histologic spectrum of liver disease in African-American, non-Hispanic white, and Hispanic obesity surgery patients. Am J Gastroenterol 2009;104:64–9.
117. Pan JJ, Fallon MB. Gender and racial differences in nonalcoholic fatty liver disease. World J Hepatol 2014;6:274–83.
118. Guerrero R, Vega GL, Grundy SM, et al. Ethnic differences in hepatic steatosis: an insulin resistance paradox? Hepatology 2009;49:791–801.
119. Wagenknecht LE, Palmer ND, Bowden DW, et al. Association of PNPLA3 with non-alcoholic fatty liver disease in a minority cohort: the Insulin Resistance Atherosclerosis Family Study. Liver Int 2011;31:412–6.
120. Davis JN, Le KA, Walker RW, et al. Increased hepatic fat in overweight Hispanic youth influenced by interaction between genetic variation in PNPLA3 and high dietary carbohydrate and sugar consumption. Am J Clin Nutr 2010;92:1522–7.
121. Sheth SG, Gordon FD, Chopra S. Nonalcoholic steatohepatitis. Ann Intern Med 1997;126:137–45.
122. Hashimoto E, Yatsuji S, Kaneda H, et al. The characteristics and natural history of Japanese patients with nonalcoholic fatty liver disease. Hepatol Res 2005;33: 72–6.

123. Schneider AL, Lazo M, Selvin E, et al. Racial differences in nonalcoholic fatty liver disease in the U.S. population. Obesity (Silver Spring) 2014;22:292–9.
124. Younossi ZM, Stepanova M, Negro F, et al. Nonalcoholic fatty liver disease in lean individuals in the United States. Medicine (Baltimore) 2012;91:319–27.
125. Neuschwander-Tetri BA, Clark JM, Bass NM, et al. Clinical, laboratory and histological associations in adults with nonalcoholic fatty liver disease. Hepatology 2010;52:913–24.
126. Stepanova M, Rafiq N, Makhlouf H, et al. Predictors of all-cause mortality and liver-related mortality in patients with non-alcoholic fatty liver disease (NAFLD). Dig Dis Sci 2013;58:3017–23.
127. Ayonrinde OT, Olynyk JK, Beilin LJ, et al. Gender-specific differences in adipose distribution and adipocytokines influence adolescent nonalcoholic fatty liver disease. Hepatology 2011;53:800–9.
128. Lee K, Sung JA, Kim JS, et al. The roles of obesity and gender on the relationship between metabolic risk factors and non-alcoholic fatty liver disease in Koreans. Diabetes Metab Res Rev 2009;25:150–5.
129. Schaffler A, Scholmerich J, Buchler C. Mechanisms of disease: adipocytokines and visceral adipose tissue–emerging role in intestinal and mesenteric diseases. Nat Clin Pract Gastroenterol Hepatol 2005;2:103–11.
130. Ishibashi E, Eguchi Y, Eguchi T, et al. Waist circumference correlates with hepatic fat accumulation in male Japanese patients with non-alcoholic fatty liver disease, but not in females. J Gastroenterol Hepatol 2008;23:908–13.
131. McKenzie J, Fisher BM, Jaap AJ, et al. Effects of HRT on liver enzyme levels in women with type 2 diabetes: a randomized placebo-controlled trial. Clin Endocrinol (Oxf) 2006;65:40–4.
132. Targher G, Rossini M, Lonardo A. Evidence that non-alcoholic fatty liver disease and polycystic ovary syndrome are associated by necessity rather than chance: a novel hepato-ovarian axis? Endocrine 2016;51:211–21.
133. Macut D, Tziomalos K, Bozic-Antic I, et al. Non-alcoholic fatty liver disease is associated with insulin resistance and lipid accumulation product in women with polycystic ovary syndrome. Hum Reprod 2016;31:1347–53.
134. Ayonrinde OT, Adams LA, Doherty DA, et al. Adverse metabolic phenotype of adolescent girls with non-alcoholic fatty liver disease plus polycystic ovary syndrome compared with other girls and boys. J Gastroenterol Hepatol 2016;31:980–7.
135. Qu Z, Zhu Y, Jiang J, et al. The clinical characteristics and etiological study of nonalcoholic fatty liver disease in Chinese women with PCOS. Iran J Reprod Med 2013;11:725–32.
136. Tziomalos K, Athyros VG, Karagiannis A. Non-alcoholic fatty liver disease in type 2 diabetes: pathogenesis and treatment options. Curr Vasc Pharmacol 2012;10:162–72.
137. Cussons AJ, Watts GF, Mori TA, et al. Omega-3 fatty acid supplementation decreases liver fat content in polycystic ovary syndrome: a randomized controlled trial employing proton magnetic resonance spectroscopy. J Clin Endocrinol Metab 2009;94:3842–8.
138. Gomez-Meade CA, Lopez-Mitnik G, Messiah SE, et al. Cardiometabolic health among gastric bypass surgery patients with polycystic ovarian syndrome. World J Diabetes 2013;4:64–9.

The Genetics of Pediatric Nonalcoholic Fatty Liver Disease

Nidhi P. Goyal, MD, MPH[a,b], Jeffrey B. Schwimmer, MD[a,b],*

KEYWORDS

- Nonalcoholic steatohepatitis • Children • Liver • Steatosis • *PNPLA3* • *TM6SF2*
- Obesity • Alanine aminotransferase

KEY POINTS

- Genetic polymorphisms play a role in the pathogenesis and severity of pediatric nonalcoholic fatty liver disease (NAFLD).
- The *PNPLA3* I148 M variant is associated with higher alanine aminotransferase in children with obesity.
- The *TM6SF2* (rs58542926 c.449 C > T, p.Glu167Lys) variant allele is associated with hepatic steatosis in children.
- Future studies of the genetics of pediatric NAFLD should focus on histologic severity and/or clinical outcomes.
- Replication studies will be important due to the heterogeneity in pediatric NAFLD by age, gender, race, and ethnicity.

INTRODUCTION

Nonalcoholic fatty liver disease (NAFLD) is the leading cause of chronic liver disease in children. The prevalence of fatty liver, after adjusting for age, race, gender, and ethnicity, is estimated at 9.6%.[1] Pediatric nonalcoholic steatohepatitis (NASH) can be distinct from adult NASH and denotes hepatic steatosis with inflammation, with or without ballooning injury to hepatocytes.[2] This can include zone 3 (venule)–centered injury pattern or confluent pattern typically with ballooning or portal predominant (zone 1)–centered injury pattern often without ballooning.[3] Children with zone 1 steatosis are more likely to present with fibrosis, including advanced fibrosis, compared with

The authors have nothing to disclose.

[a] Division of Gastroenterology, Hepatology, and Nutrition, Department of Pediatrics, University of California, San Diego, Gilman Drive, La Jolla, CA 92993, USA; [b] Department of Gastroenterology, Rady Children's Hospital, San Diego, Children's Way, San Diego, CA 92123, USA
* Corresponding author. Division of Gastroenterology, Hepatology, and Nutrition, Department of Pediatrics, University of California, San Diego, 3030 Children's Way, San Diego, CA 92123.
E-mail address: jschwimmer@ucsd.edu

children with zone 3 steatosis.[4] Severe fibrosis and cirrhosis are observed in some children with NAFLD and can occur within a few years of diagnosis in the most severe cases.[5] Children with NASH are at higher risk of serious comorbidities, such as type 2 diabetes and hypertension.[6,7] Knowledge of the genetics of pediatric NAFLD may someday improve both diagnosis and treatment. NAFLD is now the leading cause of liver transplantation in young adults, yet a treatment remains to be discovered. Tailoring therapeutics to genetic predispositions is an avenue yet to be explored for this disease.

It is likely that NAFLD has a strong genetic component based on 2 key observations. First is the racial and ethnic difference in the prevalence of NAFLD and second is the evidence that NAFLD tends to cluster in families. Hispanic children have the highest prevalence of NAFLD and black children have the lowest. In the Study of Child and Adolescent Liver Epidemiology, in which diagnosis was based on liver histopathology, NAFLD was present in 11.8% of Hispanic children, 10.2% of Asian children, 8.6% of white children, and 1.5% of black children.[1] These differences have also been seen in adulthood.[8]

The clustering of NAFLD within families was evaluated by a heritability study by Schwimmer and colleagues.[9] In this study, 33 obese children with biopsy-proved NAFLD, 11 obese children without NAFLD, and 152 of their family members (parents, siblings, second-degree relatives, or third-degree relatives) were studied. Presence of NAFLD in family members was evaluated by MRI proton density fat fraction. In children without NAFLD, 17% of siblings and 37% of parents had NAFLD compared with 59% of siblings and 78% of parents of children with biopsy-proved NAFLD. The heritability estimates (with 0 no heritability and 1 representing a trait that is completely heritable) were 0.85 for the unadjusted dichotomous variable for NAFLD and 1.0 after adjusting for age, gender, race, and BMI. For the continuous measurement of hepatic steatosis, the adjusted heritability estimate was 0.39 or 39%.

Many aspects of the pathogenesis of NAFLD, such as the mechanism for the progression from steatosis to steatohepatitis, remain unclear. Additionally, it is not known why NAFLD occurs in some obese individuals and not others. Although less common, NAFLD also exists in 5% of children with a normal BMI.[1] With respect to treatment, there is wide variability in the response of children with NAFLD to lifestyle interventions,[10] and the underlying genetics of NAFLD may play a part in the differential response to dietary and/or exercise interventions. These observations suggest that genetics are a modifying factor and that there is an interplay of genetics and environment in the pathogenesis of this disease. Understanding how genes influence the development and progression of pediatric NAFLD will help to address critical gaps in knowledge in the field.

In this review, the existing data on the genetics of pediatric NAFLD are summarized. The articles cited were identified based on a search of PubMed done in February 2017 using the criteria "NAFLD and genetic and children" with the results limited to studies in humans.

PNPLA3

PNPLA3 belongs to the patatin-like phospholipase domain-containing family of proteins and it encodes a 481–amino acid protein called adiponutrin, which is involved in lipid metabolism. Although the exact role of this protein in the liver is unclear, there is a large body of evidence that PNPLA3 is associated with NAFLD.

In the landmark study for this field, a genome-wide association study (GWAS) resulted in the discovery of a single nucleotide polymorphism (SNP) in the gene

PNPLA3 that confers susceptibility to NAFLD. The Dallas Heart Study was a multi-ethnic, population-based study in adults (n = 1032 African American, 696 European Americans, and 383 Hispanics) that evaluated hepatic fat content via proton magnetic resonance spectroscopy and performed a GWAS to search for sequence variations. A single variant in *PNPLA3* (rs739409), a cytosine (C) to guanine (G) substitution of codon 148 resulting in a nonsynonymous change to methionine from isoleucine, was highly associated with hepatic fat content independent of body mass index (BMI), diabetes, or alcohol use.[11] The highest frequency of this allele was present in Hispanics (0.49) followed by European Americans (0.23) and African-Americans (0.17), consistent with differing rates of NAFLD by ethnicity and race. Studies in adults have demonstrated an association with *PNPLA3* and histologic severity, with the minor allele associated with increased steatosis, NASH, and fibrosis.[12] These results indicate that the *PNPLA3* gene locus is not only associated with steatosis but likely also with steatohepatitis or NASH.

Data from pediatric studies have also demonstrated the importance of this gene in children with NAFLD. Several pediatric studies have evaluated the association of *PNPLA3* with alanine aminotransferase (ALT), imaging evidence of NAFLD, and histology (**Table 1**). In a study of 475 overweight or obese children, children who were homozygous for the variant I148 M allele had higher serum ALT activity compared with those with homozygous wild-type allele, ALT 32 U/L compared to 21 U/L, respectively.[13] When stratified by genotype, of those subjects with homozygous minor alleles for *PNPLA3*, 32% had ALT greater than 30 U/L versus 10% in those with homozygous wild-type alleles. Similarly, in another Italian cohort of 1048 children with obesity, the mean ALT was 25 U/L for those with the homozygous wild-type and 38 U/L in those with the homozygous variant genotype.[14] In a study of 520 Taiwanese children with obesity, ALT value was also associated with the *PNPLA3* genotype in an additive effect. In this study, the mean serum ALT was higher by 4.8 IU/L in carriers and 10.9 IU/L in those with the homozygous variant genotype compared with children with the wild-type genotype. The variant allele was also associated with ultrasound evidence of hepatic steatosis.[15] In a study of more than 1000 children from Mexico, the percentage of children with ALT greater than 35 U/L was 8.6% for wild-type, 30.5% for carriers of the variant allele, and 61% for the homozygous variant *PNPLA3*.[16] The percentage of children with elevated ALT who had the homozygous variant was 32% to 33% in the 2 studies of Italian children compared with 61% in the study of children from Mexico. This could be due to the varying cutoffs used to define an elevated ALT as well as differences due to ethnicity. The relationship of an elevated ALT in children carrying the risk allele of *PNPLA3* has subsequently also been observed in children from Finland and Austria.[17,18]

Two pediatric studies have evaluated the association of *PNPLA3* with liver steatosis, as measured by MRI. Santoro and colleagues[19] evaluated 85 children with obesity and found a positive association of MRI signal fat fraction (SFF) with presence of at least 1 G allele in white and African American children. This association, however, was not statistically significant in Hispanic children and there was no association with *PNPLA3* and ALT in any racial group. In the second study, the liver fat fraction was evaluated in 188 Hispanic children, and the mean SFF was 11% for those children with homozygous variant alleles compared with 4.7% with the wild-type alleles.[20] One study evaluated *PNPLA3* association with ultrasound evidence of hepatic steatosis. This study was conducted in 1093 overweight or obese children in China and reported that for each variant allele present the odds ratio (OR) for hepatic steatosis was 1.57 (95% CI, 1.15–2.16).[21]

Table 1
Association of *PNPLA3* with pediatric nonalcoholic fatty liver disease

Study, Year	Population	Location	N	Age (Years)	Nonalcoholic Fatty Liver Disease Criteria	Results
ALT						
Romeo et al,[13] 2010	Obesity clinic	Italy	475	Mean 10	ALT	• ALT >30 U/L in 32% with GG and 10% with CC • Mean ALT 32 U/L with GG and 21 U/L with CC
Giudice et al,[14] 2011	Childhood obesity service	Italy	1048	2–16	ALT	• ALT >40 U/L: GG 33%, CG 17%, CC 13%, elevated ALT GG vs CC: OR 2.97 • Mean ALT 38 U/L with GG and 25 U/L with CC
Lin et al,[15] 2011	Obese children recruited from school	Taiwan	520	6–18	Ultrasound	• Mean ALT 31 U/L with GG and 22 U/L with CC • The frequency of the GG genotype was significantly higher in the hepatic steatosis group (25% vs 14%)
Larrieta-Carrasco et al,[16] 2013	Summer camp	Mexico	1037	6–12	ALT	• GG genotype with higher ALT in normal weight, overweight and obese children compared to CC in each weight category; overall GG with 3.7 OR for elevated ALT • Percentage of children with ALT >35 U/L was 9% CC, 31% CG, and 61% GG
Viitasalo et al,[17] 2015	Children enrolled in school	Finland	481	6–8	ALT	• G allele carriers with higher ALT at baseline and higher ALT increase at 2 y follow-up if overweight
Mangge et al,[18] 2015	Overweight/obese whites	Austria	169	10–20	ALT	• Mean ALT 37.5 U/L with GG and 23.5 U/L with CC

Imaging

Study	Setting	Country	N	Age	Method	Findings
Santoro et al,[19] 2010	Pediatric obesity clinic	US	85	8–18	MRI SFF	• Carriers of G allele with higher SFF (*P* = .04) • Results not significant in Hispanic population, only white and Asian • No association with ALT
Goran et al,[20] 2010	Hispanic children in general clinical research center	US	188	8–18	MRI SFF	• Mean SFF was 11% for GG genotype and was 5% for CC genotype
Wang et al,[21] 2016	Overweight and obese children from school	China	1093	7–18	Ultrasound	• For each G allele present the OR for hepatic steatosis was 1.57 (95% CI, 1.15–2.16) • In inactive children (physical activity <1 h/d or sedentary behavior ≥2 h/d), the percentage of children with steatosis increased for each G allele (CC 13%, CG 18%, GG 28%)

Histology

Study	Setting	Country	N	Age	Method	Findings
Rotman et al,[22] 2010	NASH Clinical Research Network	US	223	Mean 12.4	Histology	• No association was found
Valenti et al,[23] 2010	NAFLD clinic	Italy	149	6–13	Histology	• *PNPLA3* G allele had 1.9 times the odds for presence of fibrosis (95% CI, 1.14–3.45 per number of G alleles) • Perivenular fibrosis or higher-grade fibrosis in 31% (20/65) of CC, 48% (29/61) of CG, and 74% (17/23) of GG
Rossi et al,[24] 2012	NAFLD clinic	Italy	118	Mean 10.2	Histology	• NASH was present in 0% of CC, 73% of CG, and 100% of GG

Studies of the relationship between *PNPLA3* and liver histology have had inconsistent findings. A study by Rotman and colleagues[22] in 2010 included 223 pediatric patients from the NASH Clinical Research Network and reported that there was no association of the *PNPLA3* locus with the histologic severity of NAFLD. In a somewhat smaller study, Valenti and colleagues[23] evaluated liver histology in 149 Italian pediatric patients with NAFLD. They reported that the *PNPLA3* variant allele was associated with the severity of steatosis, lobular inflammation, hepatocellular ballooning, and fibrosis. The prevalence of grade 2 and grade 3 steatosis was greater in children with homozygous variant alleles compared with heterozygotes. Lobular necroinflammation was observed in 3% of the children with wild-type homozygous alleles (2/65), 30% in carriers of the allele (18/61), and 70% in children with homozygous variant alleles (16/23). The prevalence of histologic NASH was 3% (2/65) in those with homozygous wild-type alleles (2/65) versus 74% (46/61) for the heterozygotes (45/61) and 100% (23/23) in those with homozygous variant alleles. A similar pattern was reported for hepatocellular ballooning. The variant genotype was associated with perivenular fibrosis or higher-grade fibrosis in 31% (20/65) of those with homozygous wild-type, 48% (29/61) of those heterozygous, and 74% (17/23) of those homozygous variants. There was no association with periportal fibrosis, which is a more common pattern in pediatric NAFLD. Similarly, in another study of 118 Italian children at the same medical center, 100% of children with *PNPLA3* homozygous risk variant had NASH, 73% of heterozygous patients had NASH, and no homozygous wild-type patients had NASH.[24]

OTHER GENES

A majority of data that exist for genetic associations with pediatric NAFLD are for the *PNPLA3* polymorphism. After the initial discovery of the association of *PNPLA3* and NAFLD in 2008, many other genes and their relation to pediatric NAFLD have been evaluated. For any 1 genetic polymorphism, however, most have only been evaluated in single studies thus far (**Table 2**). The field of genetics and how it relates to NAFLD is still young; however, there is increasing interest in determining at risk populations based on genetics in the hope of finding genotypes that correlate to NAFLD phenotype. The following subsections divide these pediatric studies based on the outcome variable evaluated: ALT, imaging measure of hepatic steatosis, or liver histology.

ALANINE AMINOTRANSFERASE

The association with ALT was evaluated for 2 genes: hypoxia-inducible factor 3 alpha subunit (*HIF3A*) and membrane-bound O-acyltransferase domain-containing protein 7 (*MBOAT7*). Based on prior studies postulating a possible relationship with epigenetic modifications, such as DNA methylation, and obesity, Wang and colleagues[25] evaluated methylation at the first intron of the *HIF3A* gene and its relation to obesity and ALT. To date, this is the only epigenetic study for pediatric NAFLD. In this study of 110 children with obesity and 110 normal-weight and age-matched controls from China, ALT was found associated with DNA methylation of *HIF3A* at the CpG11 methylation site after adjusting for BMI ($r = 0.226$; $P = .007$). The other methylation sites evaluated were not significantly associated with ALT once adjusted for BMI.

MBOAT7 is a gene encoding proteins involved in phospholipid remodeling. This gene has been associated with NAFLD in several adult studies. The first and only pediatric study was conducted in 2016.[26] In this study, the association between the minor T allele and ALT was evaluated in 467 children ages 6 years to 9 years. Carriers of this polymorphism had an ALT that was 7% higher than noncarriers (17.8 U/L vs 19.1 U/L). At 2-year follow-up, the ALT was 10% higher than noncarriers (18.0 U/L vs 19.7 U/L). In addition, this study also looked at 2 other genes, *PNPLA3* and transmembrane 6 superfamily 2 human (*TM6SF2*). Children who were carriers of the minor allele for all 3 of these genes had an ALT of 32 U/L compared with 19 U/L if they were carriers of *MBOAT* alone, suggesting that multiple risk genotypes potentially have an additive effect.

IMAGING

The *TM6SF2* gene polymorphism and its association with pediatric NAFLD has been evaluated in 2 studies. This SNP was initially found associated with NAFLD in an adult study. It has been postulated that the variant form of the protein is misfolded, thereby leading to accelerated degradation, which leads to increased intrahepatic fat accumulation and decreased secretion of VLDL from the hepatocyte.[27] After *PNPLA3*, the *TM6SF2* SNP is the most studied in NAFLD patients. In a study of 454 children at a pediatric obesity clinic in the United States, Goffredo and colleagues[28] looked at the association between the *TM6SF2* SNP and MRI hepatic fat fraction (HFF). The variant allele frequency was 0.061 in whites, 0.033 in African Americans, and 0.089 in Hispanics, which is similar to prior studies. Children carrying the minor allele (n = 92) had a mean HFF of 11.1%, whereas children with the wild-type had a mean HFF of 6.7%. When stratified by race and ethnicity, this effect was significant for white and African American children but not Hispanic children. Although MRI HFF was not associated with genotype in the Hispanic population, ALT was 26 U/L for wild-type genotype compared with 47 U/L for those carrying the variant allele in Hispanic children. There was no association with ALT in white or African American children. Additionally, in whites and Hispanics, lower low-density lipoprotein, small dense low-density lipoprotein, and very small low-density lipoprotein were observed. In a study of 531 Italian children with obesity and ultrasound evidence of hepatic steatosis, 8.9% were carriers of the variant allele (1 child was homozygous), and 89% of children carrying the *TM6SF2* variant allele demonstrated ultrasound evidence of steatosis compared with approximately 47% with the homozygous wild-type allele.[29] There was also an association with ALT, where ALT was greater than or equal to 40 in 29% of children who were heterozygous or homozygous for the *TM6SF2* variant allele compared with 16% of children with wild-type allele. In terms of lipids, carriers of the polymorphism had lower total cholesterol (144 mg/dL vs 160 mg/dL), low-density lipoprotein cholesterol (85 mg/dL vs 95 mg/dL), triglycerides (90 mg/dL vs 99 mg/dL), and non–high-density lipoprotein cholesterol levels (102 mg/dL vs 116 mg/dL). In addition, the investigators assessed the additive effect of the *PNPLA3* and the *TM6SF2* SNPs. For those patients that were homozygous variant at the *PNPLA3* locus and carriers of the variant *TM6SF2* allele (n = 14), the OR of having an elevated ALT was 12.2 (CI, 3.8–39.6).

Association with ultrasound evidence of hepatic steatosis in Taiwanese children has been evaluated for the genes uridine-5-diphosphoglucuronosyltransferase 1A1 (*UGT1A1*), peroxisome proliferator-activated receptor gamma coactivator 1-alpha (*PPARGC1A*), and heme oxygenase-1 (*HO-1*). *UGT1A1* is responsible for the conjugation of bilirubin in the liver, and defects in this gene are known to cause neonatal hyperbilirubinemia and Gilbert syndrome. Two polymorphisms of this gene are common and these polymorphisms were studied in children with obesity from Taiwan. In this population of 234 children, 12% had ultrasound evidence of hepatic steatosis, and the *UGT1A1*6* genotype was a protective factor for hepatic steatosis, with an estimated adjusted OR of 0.31 (95% CI, 0.11–0.91). The other polymorphism, *UGT1A1*28*, was not associated with hepatic steatosis.[30]

Table 2
Genetic polymorphisms and their association with pediatric nonalcoholic fatty liver disease

Study	Gene	Population	Location	N	Age (Years)	Nonalcoholic Fatty Liver Disease Criteria	Results
Lin et al,[30] 2009	UGT1A1	Obese elementary school children	Taiwan	234	6–13	Ultrasound	• UGT1A1*28 genotypes not significantly associated with hepatic steatosis • UGT1A1*6 genotypes associated with lower odds of hepatic steatosis, OR 0.31 (95% CI, 0.11–0.91)
El-Koofy et al,[35] 2011	MTP and MnSOD	Pediatric obesity clinic	Egypt	33	2–15	Histology	• 7 patients with NASH, 8 with steatosis, 18 normal • Of those with both the MTP and MnSOD risk genotypes 6/7 had NASH compared with 2/20 controls
Rossi et al,[24] 2012	CB2	NAFLD clinic	Italy	118	Mean 10.2	Histology	• CB2 Q63 R variant associated with grade 2 inflammation: 0/13 children with the wild-type genotype, 10/46 heterozygous genotype (22%), and 13/59 with the homozygous variant genotype (22%) • No association with ALT
Valenti et al,[33] 2012	LPIN1	NAFLD clinic	Italy	142	Mean 10.2	Histology	• Homozygosity for the LPIN1 T allele was a predictor of the absence of histologic fibrosis independent of PNPLA3 genotype: homozygous variant fibrosis rate 30% (3/10) compared with 70% (92/132) in those who were carriers or homozygous wild-type
Lin et al,[31] 2013	PPARGC1A	Obese children	Taiwan	781	7–18	Ultrasound	• Mean ALT 28.2 U/L in carriers of A allele vs 22.8 U/L in noncarriers • Overall carrier rate 68% with 59.3% in those with hepatic steatosis and 49% in those without hepatic steatosis.

Study	Gene	Population	Country	N	Age	Method	Findings
Chang et al,[32] 2015	HO-1 promoter	Pediatric obesity clinic	Taiwan	101	6–17	Ultrasound	• Higher GT repeat length in promoter of HO-1 polymorphism was associated with hepatic steatosis: 10/27 with long repeat with NAFLD and 1/27 with short repeat with NAFLD. • Mean ALT 30 U/mL in short repeat and 46 U/mL in long repeat
Wang et al,[25] 2015	HIF3A methylation	Obese and overweight children and normal weight controls	China	212	7–17	ALT	• ALT associated with DNA methylation – correlation coefficient 0.263
Goffredo et al,[28] 2016	TM6SF2	Pediatric obesity clinic	US	454	Mean 13	MRI SFF	• Subjects carrying minor allele showed a higher SFF in children of black or white race but not Hispanic ethnicity • Overall, those carrying the minor allele (n = 92) had a mean SFF of 11.1%; children with wild-type SFF 6.7% • Mean ALT was 26 U/L for wild-type genotype and 47 U/L for those carrying the variant allele in Hispanics
Grandone et al,[29] 2016	TM6SF2	Pediatric obesity clinic	Italy	531	4–16	Ultrasound	• 8.9% were carriers of allele, only 1 patient was homozygous • Hepatic steatosis was present in 40/45 children with the variant allele vs 227/486 children homozygous for the wild-type allele • ALT ≥40 U/L in 29% of children with the variant allele and in 16% of children with wild-type allele
Viitasalo et al,[26] 2016	MBOAT7	School children in first grade	Finland	467	6–9	ALT	• Carriers had an ALT that was 7% higher than noncarriers (17.8 U/L vs 19.1 U/L) • Carriers of MBOAT, TM6SF2, and PNPLA3 – ALT 32 U/L compared with 19 U/L if carrier of MBOAT alone

Abbreviations: MnSOD, manganese superoxide dismutase; MTP, microsomal triacylglycerol transfer protein.

The *PPARGC1A* gene encodes a protein that regulates oxidative stress, lipogenesis, and gluconeogenesis. The most common polymorphism of this gene has also been associated with diseases in adults, including type 2 diabetes mellitus, hypertension, obesity, and NAFLD. In the lone pediatric study, this polymorphism was evaluated in 781 Taiwanese children with obesity.[31] There was a high carrier rate of 68% (532/781). Among the 23% of children with liver ultrasonography consistent with hepatic steatosis, 59% were carriers of the risk allele, which was higher than those with normal liver ultrasound (49% carriers). Carriers of the risk allele also had higher mean ALT, 28.2 U/L, compared with children with the wild-type allele, 22.8 U/L. The association between the *PPARGC1A* polymorphism and ALT level remained significant after controlling for *PNPLA3* genotype.

HO-1 plays a role in the oxidative process and its promoter has a GT dinucleotide repeat that modulates transcription in that longer GT repeats decrease gene transcription. In a study of 101 children with obesity from Taiwan, 27% had ultrasound evidence of hepatic steatosis and a higher repeat length was associated with NAFLD where 10/27 with long repeat had NAFLD compared with 1/27 with short repeat with NAFLD. The mean ALT was 30 IU/mL in short repeat and 46 IU/mL in long repeat.[32]

HISTOLOGY

There have been 3 studies thus far evaluating the association between liver histology in children with NAFLD and genetic polymorphisms other than *PNPLA3*. In aggregate, these 3 studies comprise fewer than 300 children.

The next 2 histology-based studies were conducted in children from Italy; genes evaluated included cannabinoid receptor 2 (*CB2*) and lipin 1 (*LPIN1*). CB2 is found predominantly outside of the central nervous system and data from murine models suggest that it may have a hepatoprotective role. In a study of 118 Italian children with NAFLD, the *CB2* polymorphism was significantly associated with inflammation but not with steatosis grade or fibrosis stage.[24] Grade 2 inflammation was seen 22% of those that were carriers or homozygous for the risk allele but not in children with homozygous wild-type alleles. There was no association with ALT. Another Italian study looked at the association between *LPIN1* and pediatric NAFLD.[33] *LPIN1* is a phosphatidate phosphatase that is highly expressed in adipose tissue and is involved in the flux of phospholipids between the liver and adipose tissue. In children homozygous for the variant allele, the prevalence of fibrosis was 30% (3/10) compared with 70% (92/132) in those who were carriers or homozygous wild-type. Also, the frequency distribution of the variant allele was lower in those with NAFLD (7%) compared with controls (14%). Controls were defined as children with ALT less than 35 IU/mL in boys and ALT less than 30 IU/mL in girls.

DISCUSSION

To date, there have been 22 original research articles on the topic of the genetics of pediatric NAFLD. Based on these studies, the best validated finding is an association of *PNPLA3* rs738409 genotype with higher ALT, which has been observed in multiple populations of children. There have been 3730 children studied from Asia (Taiwan), Europe (Austria, Finland, and Italy), and North America (Mexico). Taken in aggregate, mean ALT activity is 9 U/L higher in children with the GG genotype compared with the CC genotype. Although the effect size on ALT seems small in a clinical context, in a population study, it is often the difference between having normal or elevated ALT. The association of *PNPLA3* with imaging evidence of NAFLD is less well developed. Although there have been 1366 children studied to date, MRI SFF was measured in approximately 20%, with most studies relying on ultrasound. Because ultrasound performs poorly for the diagnosis or grading of hepatic steatosis in children, the resulting association data are likely to have large errors in their estimates of effect size.[34] The data regarding liver histology in children are inconsistent. There have been 490 children evaluated in 3 studies with positive findings between *PNPLA3* and histologic severity in Italian children and negative findings in American children. Thus substantial gaps remain regarding the role of *PNPLA3* in pediatric NAFLD.

The second most studied gene in the context of pediatric NAFLD is *TM6SF2*, because it is the only gene with more than one study. Because the c.449 C > T, p.Glu167Lys variant allele has a much lower frequency, large studies are needed. Although the existing studies include approximately 2000 children, the number of children actually carrying the variant allele was fewer than 200. The allele frequency of the *TM6SF2* SNP is much lower than that of *PNPLA3*. For example, for the Hispanic population the allele frequency for *PNPLA3* is approximately 0.49 and for *TM6SF2* is approximately 0.09. Thus far, these 2 studies demonstrate a positive association with *TM6SF2* and NAFLD. Additionally, these 2 studies have also demonstrated an association with lower lipid levels, such as low-density lipoprotein. Additional large studies are needed, however, to be able to make generalizable conclusions about its association with NAFLD. In particular, data are needed on the effect size of this genetic association, especially with the severity of liver histology. Studies evaluating cardiovascular outcomes are also necessary given the association with lipid levels.

The genetics of pediatric NAFLD is a relatively new field and as such there is growing need for future studies. Major challenges in study design include adequately powered sample sizes, liver histology, and appropriate control groups. Additionally, replication within a diverse pediatric population is required given the key differences in disease histology by age, race and ethnicity, and gender. Studies that included data on clinical outcomes are also a major need.

More recent studies have been evaluating multiple genetic polymorphisms in the same patients and trying to determine the potential risk of NAFLD. Studying multiple genes within the same patient population is likely the best approach, because different races and ethnicities may have different risk genes. Future studies of the genetics of pediatric NAFLD should look at multiple genes in a diverse patient population with NAFLD diagnosed histologically. With this information, the field can help determine if certain genotypes carry higher risk of NASH and fibrosis, because these are the histologic outcomes that are associated with the largest risk of patient morbidity. These types of studies could help delineate higher-risk populations that require closer follow-up and potential therapeutic management. Future clinical trials can then stratify effectiveness of therapy per patient genotype, because one therapy may not be universally efficacious. Only with such studies will we be able to take advantage of the growing field of genetics and make progress in understanding how to best care for and develop treatments for children with NAFLD.

REFERENCES

1. Schwimmer JB, Deutsch R, Kahen T, et al. Prevalence of fatty liver in children and adolescents. Pediatrics 2006;118(4):1388–93.

2. Schwimmer JB, Behling C, Newbury R, et al. Histopathology of pediatric nonalcoholic fatty liver disease. Hepatology 2005;42(3):641–9.

3. Vos MB, Abrams SH, Barlow SE, et al. NASPGHAN clinical practice guideline for the diagnosis and treatment of nonalcoholic fatty liver disease in children: recommendations from the Expert Committee on NAFLD (ECON) and the North

American Society of Pediatric Gastroenterology, Hepatology and Nu. J Pediatr Gastroenterol Nutr 2017;64(2):319–34.

4. Africa JA, Behling CA, Brunt EM, et al. Children with nonalcoholic fatty liver disease, zone 1 steatosis is associated with advanced fibrosis. Clin Gastroenterol Hepatol 2017. http://dx.doi.org/10.1016/j.cgh.2017.02.030.

5. Goyal NP, Schwimmer JB. The progression and natural history of pediatric nonalcoholic fatty liver disease. Clin Liver Dis 2016;20(2):325–38.

6. Newton KP, Hou J, Crimmins NA, et al. Prevalence of prediabetes and type 2 diabetes in children with nonalcoholic fatty liver disease. JAMA Pediatr 2016; 170(10):e161971.

7. Schwimmer JB, Zepeda A, Newton KP, et al. Longitudinal assessment of high blood pressure in children with nonalcoholic fatty liver disease. PLoS One 2014;9(11):e112569.

8. Lazo M, Hernaez R, Eberhardt MS, et al. Prevalence of nonalcoholic fatty liver disease in the United States: the third national health and nutrition examination survey, 1988-1994. Am J Epidemiol 2013;178(1):38–45.

9. Schwimmer JB, Celedon MA, Lavine JE, et al. Heritability of nonalcoholic fatty liver disease. Gastroenterology 2009;136(5):1585–92.

10. Africa JA, Newton KP, Schwimmer JB. Lifestyle interventions including nutrition, exercise, and supplements for nonalcoholic fatty liver disease in children. Dig Dis Sci 2016;61(5):1375–86.

11. Romeo S, Kozlitina J, Xing C, et al. Genetic variation in PNPLA3 confers susceptibility to nonalcoholic fatty liver disease. Nat Genet 2008;40(12):1461–5.

12. Valenti L, Al-Serri A, Daly AK, et al. Homozygosity for the patatin-like phospholipase-3/adiponutrin I148M polymorphism influences liver fibrosis in patients with nonalcoholic fatty liver disease. Hepatology 2010;51(4):1209–17.

13. Romeo S, Sentinelli F, Cambuli VM, et al. The 148M allele of the PNPLA3 gene is associated with indices of liver damage early in life. J Hepatol 2010;53(2):335–8.

14. Giudice EM, Grandone A, Cirillo G, et al. The association of PNPLA3 variants with liver enzymes in childhood obesity is driven by the interaction with abdominal fat. PLoS One 2011;6(11):e27933.

15. Lin YC, Chang PF, Hu FC, et al. A common variant in the PNPLA3 gene is a risk factor for non-alcoholic fatty liver disease in obese Taiwanese children. J Pediatr 2011;158(5):740–4.

16. Larrieta-Carrasco E, León-Mimila P, Villarreal-Molina T, et al. Association of the I148M/PNPLA3 variant with elevated alanine transaminase levels in normal-weight and overweight/obese Mexican children. Gene 2013;520(2):185–8.

17. Viitasalo A, Pihlajamaki J, Lindi V, et al. Associations of I148M variant in PNPLA3 gene with plasma ALT levels during 2-year follow-up in normal weight and overweight children: the PANIC study. Pediatr Obes 2015;10(2):84–90.

18. Mangge H, Baumgartner BG, Zelzer S, et al. Patatin-like phospholipase 3 (rs738409) gene polymorphism is associated with increased liver enzymes in obese adolescents and metabolic syndrome in all ages. Aliment Pharmacol Ther 2015;42(1):99–105.

19. Santoro N, Kursawe R, D'Adamo E, et al. A common variant in the patatin-like phospholipase 3 gene (PNPLA3) is associated with fatty liver disease in obese children and adolescents. Hepatology 2010;52(4):1281–90.

20. Goran MI, Walker R, Le K-A, et al. Effects of PNPLA3 on liver fat and metabolic profile in hispanic children and adolescents. Diabetes 2010;59(12):3127–30.

21. Wang S, Song J, Shang X, et al. Physical activity and sedentary behavior can modulate the effect of the PNPLA3 variant on childhood NAFLD: a case-control study in a Chinese population. BMC Med Genet 2016;17(1):90.
22. Rotman Y, Koh C, Zmuda JM, et al. The association of genetic variability in patatin-like phospholipase domain-containing protein 3 (PNPLA3) with histological severity of nonalcoholic fatty liver disease. Hepatology 2010;52(3):894–903.
23. Valenti L, Alisi A, Galmozzi E, et al. I148M patatin-like phospholipase domain-containing 3 gene variant and severity of pediatric nonalcoholic fatty liver disease. Hepatology 2010;52(4):1274–80.
24. Rossi F, Bellini G, Alisi A, et al. Cannabinoid receptor type 2 functional variant influences liver damage in children with non-alcoholic fatty liver disease. Lafrenie R, ed. PLoS One 2012;7(8):e42259.
25. Wang S, Song J, Yang Y, et al. HIF3A DNA methylation is associated with childhood obesity and ALT. PLoS One 2015;10(12):e0145944.
26. Viitasalo A, Eloranta A-M, Atalay M, et al. Association of MBOAT7 gene variant with plasma ALT levels in children: the PANIC study. Pediatr Res 2016;80(5): 651–5.
27. Kozlitina J, Smagris E, Stender S, et al. Exome-wide association study identifies a TM6SF2 variant that confers susceptibility to nonalcoholic fatty liver disease. Nat Genet 2014;46(4):352–6.
28. Goffredo M, Caprio S, Feldstein AE, et al. Role of *TM6SF2* rs58542926 in the pathogenesis of nonalcoholic pediatric fatty liver disease: a multiethnic study. Hepatology 2016;63(1):117–25.
29. Grandone A, Cozzolino D, Marzuillo P, et al. *TM6SF2* Glu167Lys polymorphism is associated with low levels of LDL-cholesterol and increased liver injury in obese children. Pediatr Obes 2016;11(2):115–9.
30. Lin Y-C, Chang P-F, Hu F-C, et al. Variants in the UGT1A1 gene and the risk of pediatric nonalcoholic fatty liver disease. Pediatrics 2009;124(6):e1221–7.
31. Lin Y-C, Chang P-F, Chang M-H, et al. A common variant in the peroxisome proliferator-activated receptor- coactivator-1 gene is associated with nonalcoholic fatty liver disease in obese children. Am J Clin Nutr 2013;97(2):326–31.
32. Chang P-F, Lin Y-C, Liu K, et al. Heme oxygenase-1 gene promoter polymorphism and the risk of pediatric nonalcoholic fatty liver disease. Int J Obes 2015;39(8): 1236–40.
33. Valenti L, Motta BM, Alisi A, et al. LPIN1 rs13412852 polymorphism in pediatric nonalcoholic fatty liver disease. J Pediatr Gastroenterol Nutr 2012;54(5):588–93.
34. Awai HI, Newton KP, Sirlin CBB, et al. Evidence and recommendations for imaging liver fat in children, based on systematic review. Clin Gastroenterol Hepatol 2014;12(5):765–73.
35. El-Koofy N, El-Karaksy H, Mandour I, et al. Genetic polymorphisms in non-alcoholic fatty liver disease in obese Egyptian children. Saudi J Gastroenterol 2011;17(4):265.

Diagnosis and Evaluation of Nonalcoholic Fatty Liver Disease/Nonalcoholic Steatohepatitis, Including Noninvasive Biomarkers and Transient Elastography

Eugenia Tsai, MD[a], Tai-Ping Lee, MD[b],*

KEYWORDS

- Nonalcoholic fatty liver disease • Steatohepatitis • Noninvasive biomarker
- Transient elastography

KEY POINTS

- Liver biopsy, the current gold standard for diagnosis of nonalcoholic fatty liver disease (NAFLD)/nonalcoholic steatohepatitis (NASH), is not perfect.
- Noninvasive biomarkers are useful in assessing NAFLD/NASH.
- FibroMeter, FIB-4 (Fibrosis-4), and NAFLD fibrosis score have high diagnostic yields in evaluating advanced fibrosis and cirrhosis.
- Transient elastography is very effective and has high accuracy in staging advanced fibrosis and cirrhosis.
- The combination of noninvasive biomarkers and transient elastography improves diagnostic accuracy of NAFLD/NASH.

Nonalcoholic fatty liver disease (NAFLD) is the most common cause of abnormal liver tests in industrial countries. It encompasses the spectrum of liver damage from simple steatosis to nonalcoholic steatohepatitis (NASH) and cirrhosis.[1] NAFLD is associated with insulin resistance and is considered a hepatic manifestation of metabolic syndrome (MetS).[2,3]

Disclosures: The authors have nothing to disclose.
[a] Department of Internal Medicine, Division of Gastroenterology and Hepatology, Tulane Medical Center, 1430 Tulane Avenue, SL 35, New Orleans, LA 70119, USA; [b] Department of Internal Medicine, Division of Hepatology, Sandra A. Bass Center of Liver Diseases Northwell Health, 400 Community Drive, Manhasset, NY 11030, USA
* Corresponding author.
E-mail address: Tlee@northwell.edu

The incidence and prevalence of NAFLD are increasing worldwide in parallel with the obesity and diabetes epidemics.[3,4] In the United States, NAFLD is estimated to affect one-third of the general adult population.[3–5] Persons with only hepatic steatosis are thought to have a benign long-term prognosis. However, 20% to 30% of those with simple steatosis develop NASH (1.5%–6.45% of the general population), which may further progress to cirrhosis.[2,3]

NAFLD with advanced fibrosis or cirrhosis increases the risk of development of hepatocellular carcinoma (HCC), which has poor outcomes and limited therapeutic options.[6,7] NASH is a rapidly growing indication for liver transplant in the United States.[8,9] In data of adults listed for liver transplant extracted from the UNOS (United Network for Organ Sharing) registry in 2015, NASH surpassed chronic hepatitis C as the leading indication for liver transplant among adults.[10]

Screening for NAFLD is not currently recommended in clinical practice because of unclear cost-effectiveness and uncertainties with diagnostic testing and treatments.[11,12] Most patients are asymptomatic until there is significant liver dysfunction. However, because of significant NASH-associated morbidity and mortality, early diagnosis is prudent.[11] Patients with older age, type 2 diabetes mellitus (T2DM), obesity, and MetS are at high risk of developing NAFLD.[13,14] In this subset of high-risk patients, clinicians should maintain high clinical suspicion for the diagnosis of NAFLD, even if liver enzyme levels are normal.

DIAGNOSIS OF NONALCOHOLIC FATTY LIVER DISEASE AND NONALCOHOLIC STEATOHEPATITIS

The initial diagnosis of NAFLD is based on clinical history, biochemical data, and radiographic features. Clinical history requires excluding secondary causes of fatty liver, such as[12]:

- Viral hepatitis (hepatitis C, genotype 3)
- Alcoholic fatty liver disease (>3 drinks/d for men, >2 drinks/d for women)
- Drugs (eg, amiodarone, corticosteroids, methotrexate, tamoxifen, synthetic estrogens, valproic acid, intravenous tetracycline, and highly active antiretroviral drugs)
- Medical conditions (eg, Wilson disease, hemochromatosis, and celiac disease)
- Metabolic abnormalities (eg, inborn errors of metabolism, cholesterol ester storage disease, glycogen storage diseases, abetalipoproteinemia, lysosomal acid lipase deficiency, and Reye syndrome)
- Nutritional status (eg, starvation and parenteral nutrition)

It also includes obtaining clinical history regarding certain risk factors for NAFLD (**Box 1**).

The current gold standard for the diagnosis and staging of NAFLD is liver biopsy. It can determine necroinflammatory activity, degree of steatosis, and extent of fibrosis.[15–18] Liver biopsy has inherent limitations because of sample size and sampling variability. The intraobserver and interobserver variability may also decrease diagnostic accuracy.[18–21] Risks and life-threatening complications render liver biopsy a less-than-ideal gold standard. Potential complications include[22–26]:

- Mortality after percutaneous liver biopsy reported at 0.009% to 0.14%
- Pain
- Intraperitoneal bleeding
- Hemobilia
- Hypotension

Box 1
Risk factors for nonalcoholic fatty liver disease

Age $\geq$50 y

Hispanic ethnicity

T2DM

Hypertension

BMI $\geq$30 kg/m^2

Postmenopausal women

Increased fasting insulin level

Abbreviation: BMI, body mass index.
  Data from Chalasani N, Younossi Z, Lavine JE, et al. The diagnosis and management of non-alcoholic fatty liver disease: practice guideline by the American Association for the Study of Liver Diseases, American College of Gastroenterology, and the American Gastroenterological Association. Hepatology 2012;55:2005–23.

With the increasing prevalence of NAFLD, liver biopsy to diagnose NASH or fibrosis would be an enormous task and impractical for routine use. Regular monitoring for NAFLD progression or response to intervention by repeat or serial liver biopsies may not be favorable to patients either. This situation has led to the focus on alternative less invasive or noninvasive tests to assess nonalcoholic fatty liver.[25]

A major advantage of noninvasive methods is easy reproducibility over time. It allows longitudinal assessment and the monitoring of disease progression.[27] This article discusses the noninvasive diagnosis of NAFLD and NASH via biomarkers and elastography.

NONINVASIVE DIAGNOSTIC TESTS

Although a good screening test should have high sensitivity to identify disease, a good diagnostic test should have high specificity to exclude disease. Important characteristics of diagnostic tests include cost-effectiveness, ease, and reproducibility.[28]

There are 2 main noninvasive approaches to diagnose NAFLD/NASH.

Biological-Based Diagnosis

Biological markers of disease presence and progression are not strictly liver specific but they have been associated with pathophysiologic disease processes.[29] Several biomarkers have been studied and proposed for the noninvasive evaluation of hepatic steatosis, NASH, and significant/advanced fibrosis.

Physical-Based Diagnosis

This method relies on the physical measurement of liver stiffness (liver stiffness measurement [LSM]), which corresponds with the intrinsic physical property of liver parenchyma. Current validated modalities used in clinical practice include transient elastography (TE), acoustic radiation force impulse imaging, and magnetic resonance elastography (MRE).

BIOMARKERS
Biomarkers and Steatosis

In simple hepatic steatosis, aminotransferase levels are often normal. When NAFLD progresses, liver tests may become mildly increased and fluctuate. Identifying NAFLD in its early stages could prevent possible disease progression to cirrhosis and decrease the risk of HCC by early intervention. In the evaluation of liver transplant donors, assessment for steatosis would reduce the risk for potential postoperative morbidity and mortality. Thus, several panels have been proposed to diagnose hepatic steatosis (**Table 1**).

- SteatoTest (2005) has been evaluated by several groups. In a meta-analysis with morbidly obese subjects, SteatoTest showed reasonable accuracy for evaluating moderate to severe steatosis.[30] The formula is currently undisclosed.
- Fatty Liver Index (2006) grades steatosis on a scale from 0 to 100. It showed good accuracy in detecting steatosis compared with routine ultrasonography.[31] Results must be interpreted carefully because a gold standard was not used.
- NAFLD Liver Fat Score (LFS; 2009) has been compared with magnetic resonance spectroscopy. Results were favorable for determining hepatic steatosis.[32]
- Lipid accumulation product (2010) still needs additional external validation for clinical use.[33]

Table 1
Current available diagnostic panels used for predicting steatosis

Diagnostic Panel	Study	Biomarkers Evaluated	Sensitivity (%)	Specificity (%)
SteatoTest	Poynard et al,[30] 2005	α-MG, haptoglobin, apolipoprotein A1, total bilirubin, GGT, fasting glucose, triglycerides, cholesterol, ALT, age, gender, and BMI	90	70
FLI	Bedogni et al,[31] 2006	Triglycerides, BMI, GGT, waist circumference	87	86
NAFLD-LFS	Kotronen et al,[32] 2009	MetS, T2DM, fasting insulin, AST, ALT	95	95
LAP	Bedogni et al,[33] 2010	Waist circumference, triglycerides	NA	NA

Abbreviations: α-MG, alpha-2 macroglobulin; ALT, alanine aminotransferase; AST, aspartate aminotransferase; FLI, fatty liver index; GGT, gamma-glutamyl transpeptidase; LAP, lipid accumulation product; LFS, liver fat score; NA, not applicable.

Data from Machado MV, Cortez-Pinto H. Non-invasive diagnosis of non-alcoholic fatty liver disease. A critical appraisal. J Hepatol 2013;58(5):1007–19.

Biomarkers and Nonalcoholic Steatohepatitis

Although there are no current recommended treatment options for NASH, differentiating NASH from simple steatosis confers prognostic value. There are no clinical signs and symptoms that differentiate steatosis from NASH, and aminotransferases are unreliable for identifying NASH. Thus, several biomarkers have been proposed for the prediction of NASH. Biomarkers focus on the specific pathways involved in the progression of disease; namely, hepatocyte death or apoptosis, oxidative stress, and inflammation (**Fig. 1**).[34–36]

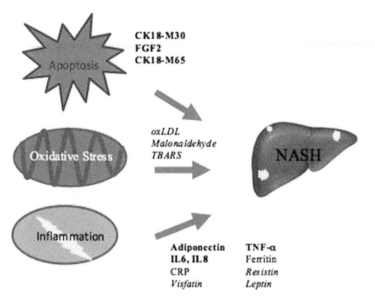

Fig. 1. Serum biomarkers for predicting NASH. CK18-M30, cytokeratin 18 cleaved with cas-pase 3; CK18-M65, cytokeratin 18, uncleaved; CRP, C-reactive protein; FGF2, fibroblast growth factor 2; IL6, interleukin-6; IL8, interleukin-8; oxLDL, oxidized low density lipopro-tein; TBARS, thiobarbituric acid reactive substance. (*Adapted from* Fitzpatrick E, Dhawan A. Noninvasive biomarkers in nonalcoholic fatty liver disease: current status and a glimpse of the future. World J Gastroenterol 2014;20(31):10851–63; with permission.)

Markers of inflammation

Ferritin and high-sensitivity C-reactive protein (CRP) are nonspecific markers of inflammation that have been shown to be associated with NASH.[37–39] Although adipo-kines, adipocytokines, and other cytokines are reported to be strongly associated with presence and severity of disease,[40] overall circulating levels of adipokines have been inconsistent in predicting the disease. Studies have shown that low levels of adipo-nectin and high levels of tumor necrosis factor-α (TNF-α) are associated with higher levels of liver damage.[41] A limited number of studies have shown that interleukin-6 and interleukin-8 are strongly correlated with NASH.[42–44] Leptin, resistin, and visfatin have also been studied but data for these markers are variable.[45–49]

Markers of oxidative stress

Oxidative stress contributes to the pathogenesis of NASH. Oxidized low-density lipo-protein, malonaldehyde, and thiobarbituric acid reactive substances have been eval-uated in predicting NASH but results have been conflicting.[50,51] Measurements of serum markers of oxidative stress are difficult because of their volatile nature.[52]

Markers of apoptosis

Cytokeratin 18 (CK18) fragments are major intermediate filaments of hepatocytes. Serum CK18 levels correlate with histologic changes and reflect severity of NASH.[53–58] Studies have shown its high specificity for NAFLD and fibrosis.[59] Combi-nation with other biomarkers, such as fibroblast growth factor 21 (FGF21), showed greater association with disease progression.[60] Another marker of cell death that has been studied is CK18-M65 (uncleaved CK18), with strong accuracy in predicting NASH.[61]

Complex models have been developed to predict NASH. The few models that have been externally validated are included in **Table 2**. Most of these scoring systems were only tested in morbidly obese populations and require further validation.

Table 2				
Validated diagnostic panels for predicting nonalcoholic steatohepatitis				
Diagnostic Panel	**Study**	**Biomarkers Evaluated**	**Sensitivity (%)**	**Specificity (%)**
NASH test	Poynard et al,[62] 2006	Undisclosed formula using α-MG, haptoglobin, apolipoprotein A1, total bilirubin, GGT, ALT, AST, triglycerides, cholesterol, age, gender, height, weight	33	94
NASH diagnostics	Younossi et al,[61] 2008	Undisclosed formula using CK18-M30, CK18-M65, adiponectin, and resistin	72	91
Apoptosis panel	Tamimi et al,[63] 2011	CK18 fragments, soluble Fas, and Fas ligand	88	89

Data from Machado MV, Cortez-Pinto H. Non-invasive diagnosis of non-alcoholic fatty liver disease. A critical appraisal. J Hepatol 2013;58(5):1007–19.

Other complex models have also been proposed still need external validation. These include:

- HAIR (evaluation of hypertension, increased alanine aminotransferase [ALT] level, and insulin resistance).[64]
- Palekar score: model using combination of age greater than or equal to 50 years, female sex, increased aspartate transaminase (AS) level, body mass index (BMI) greater than or equal to 30 kg/m², AST/ALT ratio greater than or equal to 0.8, hyaluronic acid level greater than or equal to 55 μg/L.[65]
- Gholam model: uses ALT level and presence of T2DM.[66]
- NASH diagnostic panel: undisclosed formula using T2DM, sex, BMI, triglyceride level, and M30 and M35 antigens.[67]
- Nice model: formula using ALT levels, CK 18 fragments, presence of MetS.[68]

Biomarkers and Fibrosis

The Metavir scoring system is most widely used for staging fibrosis.[69] Stages are defined as:

- F0: no fibrosis
- F1: portal fibrosis without septa
- F2: portal fibrosis with few septa, extending outside of portal areas
- F3: bridging fibrosis or numerous septa without cirrhosis
- F4: cirrhosis

Significant fibrosis is characterized as greater than or equal to F2 disease. Serum aminotransferases are not useful in diagnosing fibrosis and levels often decrease when fibrosis worsens. An AST/ALT ratio greater than 1 has been shown to be predictive of fibrosis because of impaired AST clearance.[70]

Hyaluronic acid (HA) production increases in fibrosis and its clearance decreases in advanced liver disease.[71,72] Studies have reported good correlation of high HA levels with advanced fibrosis. However, different cutoff values were used, rendering interpretation difficult.[73,74] Type IV collagen and pentraxin-3 were shown to correlate with advanced fibrosis but further studies are required to validate these biomarkers.[75–77]

Complex models for predicting advanced fibrosis have been studied:

- FibroTest (2006), known as FibroSure in the United States, has been compared with other scoring systems and externally validated. The formula is currently undisclosed.
- NAFLD fibrosis score (2007) has been externally validated by 13 studies. The score is based on the formula ($-1.675 + 0.037 \times$ age in years $+ 0.094 \times$ BMI $[kg/m^2] + 1.13 \times$ IFG/diabetes [yes $= 1$, no $= 0$] $+ 0.99 \times$ AST/ALT ratio $- 0.013 \times$ platelet count $[\times 109/L] - 0.66 \times$ albumin [g/dL]) (Easy-access online calculator: http://nafldscore.com/.)[78]
- BARD (BMI, AST/ALT Ratio, Diabetes, 2008) has also been compared with other scores by several groups and showed strong accuracy in excluding advanced fibrosis (negative predictive value, 96%) with lower accuracy in confirming disease (positive predictive value, 43%).[80]
- FibroMeter (2009) was originally developed for staging fibrosis in hepatitis C virus but its use in NAFLD has shown good diagnostic accuracy.[81]
- FIB-4 (Fibrosis-4; 2010) has been externally validated in viral hepatitis as well as NAFLD (**Table 3**).[82]

Table 3
Validated diagnostic panels for predicting fibrosis in nonalcoholic fatty liver disease

Diagnostic Panel	Study	Biomarkers Evaluated	Sensitivity (%)	Specificity (%)
NAFLD fibrosis score	Angulo et al,[78] 2007	Age, glucose level, BMI, platelet count, albumin, and AST/ALT ratio	82	98
FibroTest	Ratziu et al,[79] 2006	Age, α2-macroglobulin, total bilirubin, GGT, and apolipoprotein A1	77	98
BARD	Harrison et al,[80] 2008	BMI ≥ 28 kg/m², AST/ALT ratio ≥ 0.8, presence of T2DM	NA	NA
FibroMeter	Cales et al,[81] 2009	Glucose, AST, ferritin, platelet count, ALT, body weight, age	79	96
FIB-4	McPherson et al,[82] 2011	Age, AST/platelet count, ALT	85	65

Data from Machado MV, Cortez-Pinto H. Non-invasive diagnosis of non-alcoholic fatty liver disease. A critical appraisal. J Hepatol 2013;58(5):1007–19.

Other models include:

BAAT ([BMI, Age, ALT, Triglyceride], 2000): score calculated based on age, BMI (≥ 28 kg/m²), triglycerides, ALT. Sensitivity, 14%; specificity, 100%.[83]

ELF ([enhanced liver fibrosis], 2004): original European liver fibrosis score calculates a score based on age, HA, type III collagen, and TIMP-1 (tissue inhibitor of metalloproteinase-1).[84]

NAFLD diagnostic panel (2011): undisclosed formula using T2DM, triglycerides, TIMP-1, and AST. Sensitivity, 93%; specificity, 91%.[67]

Emerging Biomarkers in Nonalcoholic Fatty Liver Disease/Nonalcoholic Steatohepatitis

Emerging technology in proteomics, glycomics, and microRNAs (miRNAs) provide insight into the pathophysiology of NAFLD/NASH.

- Proteomics is the identification of putative markers expressed in certain diseases. Proteins peaks with significant differential expression have been seen in NAFLD/NASH and fibrosis.[85–87] Studies have suggested increased expression of lumican (involved in collagen cross-linking), calreticulin, and endoplasmin, in patients with NASH.[88,89] In addition, it was reported that a higher baseline hemoglobin level is associated with development of NAFLD.[90] This current technology has mainly been studied with the use of liver tissue, restricting its applicability to the clinical setting. The use of proteomics in is still in its early stages.[91]
- Glycomics is the study of posttranslational modification of proteins with glycosylation (carbohydrate moieties). This modification provides structural diversity and can alter cell-cell interactions. N-glycan–based biomarker specifically recognizes liver inflammation for the development of steatohepatitis and can differentiate between steatosis and NASH.[92,93]
- Circulating miRNAs are noncoding RNAs that regulate posttranscriptional biological processes such as cell growth, tissue differentiation, cell proliferation, and apoptosis.[94] These circulating, cell-free miRNAs have been proposed as potential diagnostic and prognostic biomarkers for liver injury. miRNA-21(miR-21), miR-34a, miR-122, and miR-451 were associated with NAFLD and steatosis severity.[95,96] However, available data are insufficient to confirm a role as diagnostic markers for inflammation or apoptosis in NAFLD.

TRANSIENT ELASTOGRAPHY (FibroScan)

TE is a unidimensional, noninvasive method that has been shown to be useful for the detection of liver fibrosis.[97,98] Initially designed at the Langevin Institute for food quality control in 1995, its application in medical practice started in 2001 under the name FibroScan (**Fig. 2**).[99]

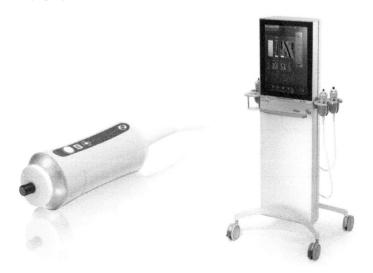

Fig. 2. FibroScan. (© Copyright Echosens; Paris, France. All rights reserved.)

FibroScan Technology

Both ultrasonography (5 MHz) and low-frequency (50 Hz) elastic waves are used in TE.[99] The measured propagation velocity is directly related to liver stiffness, based on Hook's law, which states that the velocity of shear waves that travel through an elastic object is proportional to the object's stiffness. Thus, the stiffer the medium, the faster the wave transmits.[100]

In practice, the low-frequency vibrations are transmitted to the skin by placement of the probe at the intercostal space where a liver biopsy would be performed. A shear wave is induced that subsequently propagates in a spherical manner, through the liver. The wave passes through tissue 2.5 to 6.5 cm below the skin surface and a pulse echo acquisition is then used to measure the propagating wave's velocity in meters per second.

Results correspond with the median value of 10 validated measurements to improve test reliability. Machine-based software determines the success and validity of each measurement and unsuccessful measurements are automatically excluded by the device. The manufacturer's criteria for acceptable LSM interpretation[97,101,102] requires:

1. Greater than or equal to 10 shots
2. Success rate greater than or equal to 60%
3. Interquartile range (IQR) less than or equal to 30%

Stricter parameters, such as IQR less than or equal to 25%, have been proposed for a more reproducible LSM.[103]

LSM values range from 1.5 to 75 kPa, with lower values indicating a more elastic liver. Compared with liver biopsy for diagnosing fibrosis and cirrhosis, TE confers many advantages[104]:

1. Evaluates a larger region of interest: volume greater than 100 times that of liver biopsy
2. Painless
3. Reproducible
4. Noninvasive: safe, with no risk of bleeding
5. Fast: less than 5-minute evaluation
6. Applicable as a screening tool and for monitoring disease progression

This user-friendly, noninvasive test is often more desirable to patients than an invasive liver biopsy. TE for the evaluation of cirrhosis has shown validity and excellent diagnostic accuracy in chronic hepatitis C, chronic hepatitis B, alcoholic liver disease, primary biliary cholangitis, primary sclerosing cholangitis, and after liver transplant.[105–108] It has high sensitivity and specificity in evaluating significant fibrosis but lower sensitivity and specificity in mild and moderate fibrosis.[109–113] TE is a better tool for excluding cirrhosis than it is for confirming cirrhosis.[114]

Transient Elastography Limitations

Overestimation of liver fibrosis can occur in various clinical settings, which include[115–118]:

- Active hepatitis or acute inflammation (ALT level >5× upper limit of normal)
- Extrahepatic cholestasis
- Congestive heart failure

In a subset of patients, unreliable readings may be more frequently seen because of technical limitations such as[119,120]:

- Obesity (BMI $\geq$30 kg/m^2)
- Presence of ascites: elastic waves do not travel through liquids
- Features of MetS: T2DM, hypertension, increased waist circumference
- Narrow intercostal spaces

Operator inexperience (<500 examinations) and waist circumference (>80 cm in women, >94 cm in men) have been found to be the most important determinants of TE failure and unreliable results. Other limitations include age, presence of T2DM, female sex, hypertension, recent food intake, and alcohol consumption.[121]

Transient Elastography in Nonalcoholic Fatty Liver Disease

The validity of TE in the identification of fibrosis in patients with NAFLD has been extensively studied. A 2016 meta-analysis assessing TE for the diagnosis of fibrosis in NAFLD showed that as fibrosis increases, the sensitivity and specificity also improve (**Table 4**).[122]

Table 4 Fibrosis stages and proposed transient elastography cutoffs			
Fibrosis Stage	Cutoff (kPa)	Sensitivity (%)	Specificity (%)
F $\geq$2	5.35–7.4	87.5	78.4
F $\geq$3	8.0–12.85	93.7	91.1
F $\geq$4	10.3–17.5	96.2	92.2

Data from Hashemi SA, Alavian SM, Gholami-Fesharaki M. Assessment of transient elastography (FibroScan) for diagnosis of fibrosis in non-alcoholic fatty liver disease: a systematic review and meta-analysis. Caspian J Intern Med 2016;7(4):242–52.

In 2016, a head-to-head comparison of 9 fibrosis tests (BARD, NAFLD fibrosis score, FibroMeter[NAFLD], APRI (AST to platelet ratio index), FIB-4, FibroTest, Hepascore, FibroMeter[V2G], and LSM) identified TE as the most accurate method for the noninvasive diagnosis of fibrosis in patients with NAFLD. The investigators developed new fibrosis classifications for FibroScan, specific to NAFLD: F0/1, F1 $\pm$ 1, F1/F2, F2/3, F3 $\pm$ 1, F3/4, F4, based on the NASH-CRN (Nonalcoholic Steatohepatitis Clinical Research Network) scoring system. Baseline liver stiffness thresholds for the prognostic groups were also set at notably higher levels to maximize sensitivity and specificity, at 8.8, 12.0, and 38.6 kPa.[123]

Transient Elastography Limitations in Nonalcoholic Fatty Liver Disease

Liver stiffness as measured by the M probe is not always successful in obese patients. An improved FibroScan probe, the XL probe, has been shown to achieve better diagnostic accuracy. Cutoff values, compared with M probe values, are approximately 1.5 to 2 kPa lower.[104] The advantages of FibroScan XL probe are listed in **Box 2**.[104,121,122]

Box 2
Advantages of FibroScan XL probe
More sensitive ultrasound transducer (lower frequency of 2.5 MHz)
Larger vibration amplitude
Deeper focal length
Deeper signal penetration (through tissues >35–75 mm in depth)

In conclusion, TE can be considered a strong alternative to liver biopsy in patients with NAFLD for diagnosing fibrosis and cirrhosis.

Controlled Attenuation Parameter

On histology, steatosis has greater than or equal to 5% fatty deposit in hepatocytes.[124] Conventional ultrasonography, commonly used in the clinical setting for diagnosis of fatty liver, has limited sensitivity for detection of mild steatosis (<30% fat in the liver).[125,126]

Controlled attenuation parameter (CAP) is a fairly new method that uses the FibroScan technology to measure liver attenuation.[127] Fat affects ultrasound propagation and thus measurements of liver attenuation are directly related to the amount of steatosis. Studies have shown strong correlation of CAP with steatosis in the liver compared with liver biopsy for many chronic liver diseases.[128] The measurements range from 100 to 400 dB/m. Generally accepted CAP staging and proposed cutoff values are listed in **Table 5**.[129,130]

Table 5		
Controlled attenuation parameter staging and proposed values		
Steatosis Stage	**Steatosis (% Fat in Liver)**	**Proposed Median CAP Values in dB/m (Range)**
S0 = no steatosis	<5	205 (180–227)
S1 = mild steatosis	5–33	245 (231–268)
S2 = moderate steatosis	34–66	299 (268–323)
S3 = severe steatosis	>67%	321 (301–346)

Data from Petta S, Wong VW, Cammà C, et al. Improved noninvasive prediction of liver fibrosis by liver stiffness measurement in patients with nonalcoholic fatty liver disease accounting for controlled attenuation parameter values. Hepatology 2017;65(4):1145–55.

LSM can overestimate fibrosis in patients with lower stages of NAFLD because of altered attenuation by fat. A recent study on patients with biopsy-confirmed NAFLD showed increased CAP values leading to overestimation of fibrosis by TE.[131] Higher rates of false-positive LSM were found in both greater than or equal to F2 and greater than or equal to F3 diseases if CAP measurements were higher. The differences in LSM with higher CAP measurements and proposed adjusted cutoffs are summarized in **Table 6**.[131]

Table 6
Fibrosis stages with liver stiffness measurement cutoffs and proposed adjusted cutoffs values

Fibrosis Stage	LSM (kPa) Cutoff; Middle CAP (300–339 dB/m)	Proposed Adjusted Cutoff (kPa)	LSM (kPa) Cutoff; Higher CAP (>340 dB/m)	Proposed Adjusted Cutoff (kPa)
≥F2	9.5–10.5	≥10.5	8.5–10.5	≥11.6
≥F3	10.1–12.5	≥12.5	10.1–13.6	≥13.6

Data from Petta S, Wong VW, Cammà C, et al. Improved noninvasive prediction of liver fibrosis by liver stiffness measurement in patients with nonalcoholic fatty liver disease accounting for controlled attenuation parameter values. Hepatology 2017;65(4):1145–55.

The advantages of CAP include easy use, operator independency, simultaneous measurement of liver stiffness, and no sampling error.[132] CAP is good at detecting significant hepatic steatosis, but its accuracy decreases in patients with high BMI.[133] TE with CAP is an excellent diagnostic tool for assessing and following patients with NAFLD/NASH.[134] Its ability to exclude patients with advanced fibrosis may be used to identify patients with low-risk NAFLD in whom liver biopsy is not needed, therefore reducing the risk of complications and the financial costs.

SEQUENTIAL ALGORITHMS

There has been a shift in focus to the sequential use of 2 or more noninvasive methods for evaluating suspected NAFLD/NASH. The combination of TE with noninvasive biomarkers can increase overall diagnostic accuracy and decrease the need for liver biopsy.[135,136] Limitations include increased costs and need for more sophisticated testing, such as MRE[137,138] or invasive liver biopsy, if there is any discrepancy among the tests.

SUMMARY

The incidence and prevalence of NAFLD are increasing. Identification of people at risk of disease progression to NASH, fibrosis, and cirrhosis is extremely important because most are asymptomatic. The current gold standard for the diagnosis of NAFLD/NASH is liver biopsy, which is not perfect. Noninvasive tests, such as biomarkers and TE to assess NAFLD/NASH, are promising. The most validated diagnostic panels include NAFLD fibrosis score, FIB-4, and FibroMeter. TE is very useful in evaluating advanced fibrosis and cirrhosis. Biomarkers and TE may improve the ability to assess NAFLD/NASH by a sequential approach in near future.

REFERENCES

1. Bedongni G, Miglioli L, Masutti F, et al. Prevalence of and risk factors for nonalcoholic fatty liver disease: the Dionysos Nutrition and Liver Study. Hepatology 2005;42:44–52.
2. Bugianesi E, Moscatiello S, Ciaravella MF, et al. Insulin resistance in nonalcoholic fatty liver disease. Curr Pharm Des 2010;16(17):1941–51.
3. Loomba R, Sanyal A. The global NAFLD epidemic. Nat Rev Gastroenterol Hepatol 2013;10:686–90.
4. Michelotti GA, Machado MV, Diehl AM. NAFLD, NASH and liver cancer. Nat Rev Gastroenterol Hepatol 2013;10:656–65.

5. Do A, Lim JK. Epidemiology of nonalcoholic fatty liver disease: a primer. Clin Liver Dis 2016;7(5):106–8.

6. Baffy G, Brunt E, Caldwell SH. Hepatocellular carcinoma in non-alcoholic fatty liver disease: an emerging menace. J Hepatol 2012;56(6):1384–91.

7. D'Avola D, Labgaa I, Villanueva A. Natural history of nonalcoholic steatohepatitis/nonalcoholic fatty liver disease-hepatocellular carcinoma: magnitude of the problem from a hepatology clinic perspective. Clin Liver Dis 2016;8(4):100–4.

8. Zezos P, Renner EL. Liver transplantation and non-alcoholic fatty liver disease. World J Gastroenterol 2014;20(42):15532–8.

9. Malik SM, deVera ME, Fontes P, et al. Outcome after liver transplantation for NASH cirrhosis. Am J Transplant 2009;9:782–93.

10. Banini BA, et al. Abstract #46. Presented at: American College of Gastroenterology Annual Scientific Meeting. Las Vegas (NV), October 14–19, 2016.

11. Fazel Y, Koenig AB, Sayiner M, et al. Epidemiology and natural history of non-alcoholic fatty liver disease. Metab Clin Exp 2016;65(8):1017–25.

12. Chalasani N, Younossi Z, Lavine JE, et al. The diagnosis and management of non-alcoholic fatty liver disease: practice guideline by the American Association for the Study of Liver Diseases, American College of Gastroenterology, and the American Gastroenterological Association. Hepatology 2012;55:2005–23.

13. Cusi K. Role of insulin resistance and lipotoxicity in non-alcoholic steatohepatitis. Clin Liver Dis 2009;13:545–63.

14. Adams LA, Feldstein AE. Nonalcoholic steatohepatitis: risk factors and diagnosis. Expert Rev Gastroenterol Hepatol 2010;4(5):623–35.

15. Nalbantoglu I, Brunt EM. Role of liver biopsy in nonalcoholic fatty liver disease. World J Gastroenterol 2014;20(27):9026–37.

16. Brunt EM. Nonalcoholic fatty liver disease: what the pathologist can tell the clinician. Dig Dis 2012;1(30 Suppl):61–8.

17. Gaidos JK, Hillner BE, Sanyal AJ. A decision analysis study of the value of a liver biopsy in nonalcoholic steatohepatitis. Liver Int 2008;28:650–8.

18. Bravo AA, Sheth SG, Chopra S. Liver biopsy. N Engl J Med 2001;341:495–500.

19. Ratziu V, Charlotte F, Heurtier A, et al. Sampling variability of liver biopsy in nonalcoholic fatty liver disease. Gastroenterology 2005;128(7):1898–906.

20. Regev A, Berho M, Jeffers LJ, et al. Sampling error and intraobserver variation in liver biopsy in patients with chronic HCV infection. Am J Gastroenterol 2002; 97(10):2614–8.

21. Merriman RB, Ferrell LD, Patti MG, et al. Correlation of paired liver biopsies in morbidly obese patients with suspected nonalcoholic fatty liver disease. Hepatology 2006;44:874–80.

22. Myers RP, Fong A, Shaheen AAM. Utilization rates, complications and costs of percutaneous liver biopsy: a population-based study including 4275 biopsies. Liver Int 2008;28(5):705–12.

23. Kose S, Ersan G, Tatar B, et al. Evaluation of percutaneous liver biopsy complications in patients with chronic viral hepatitis. Eur J Med 2015;47(3):161–4.

24. Fallatah HI. Noninvasive biomarkers of liver fibrosis: an overview. Adv Hepatol 2014;2014:1–15.

25. Machado MV, Cortez-Pinto H. Non-invasive diagnosis of non-alcoholic fatty liver disease. A critical appraisal. J Hepatol 2013;58(5):1007–19.

26. Ratziu V, Bellentani S, Cortez-Pinto H, et al. A position statement on NAFLD/ NASH based on the EASL 2009 special conference. J Hepatol 2010;53:372–84.

27. Wieckowska A, McCullough AJ, Felstein AE. Noninvasive diagnosis and moni-toring of nonalcoholic steatohepatitis: present and future. Hepatology 2007; 46(2):582–9.
28. Simundic AM. Measures of diagnostic accuracy: basic definitions. EJIFCC 2009;19(4):203–11.
29. Pepe MS, Etzioni R, Feng Z, et al. Phases of biomarker development for early detection of cancer. J Natl Cancer Inst 2001;93(14):1054–61.
30. Poynard T, Ratziu V, Naveau S, et al. The diagnostic value of biomarkers (Stea-toTest) for the prediction of liver steatosis. Comp Hepatol 2005;4(10):1–14.
31. Bedogni G, Bellentani S, Miglioli L, et al. The fatty liver index: a simple and ac-curate predictor of hepatic steatosis in the general populations. BMC Gastroen-terol 2006;6(33):1–7.
32. Kotronen A, Peltonen M, Hakkarainen A, et al. Prediction of non-alcoholic fatty liver disease and liver fat using metabolic and genetic factors. Gastroenterology 2009;137:865–72.
33. Bedogni G, Kahn HS, Bellentani S, et al. A simple index of lipid overaccumula-tion is a good marker of liver steatosis. BMC Gastroenterol 2010;10(98):1–8.
34. Sanal MG. Biomarkers in non-alcoholic fatty liver disease-the emperor has no clothes? World J Gastroenterol 2015;21(11):3223–31.
35. Shen J, Chan HL-Y, Wong GL, et al. Non-invasive diagnosis of non-alcoholic steatohepatiis by combined serum biomarkers. J Hepatol 2012;56:1363–70.
36. Fitzpatrick E, Dhawan A. Noninvasive biomarkers in nonalcoholic fatty liver dis-ease: current status and a glimpse of the future. World J Gastroenterol 2014; 20(31):10851–63.
37. Targher G. Relationship between high-sensitivity C-reactive protein levels and liver histology in subjects with nonalcoholic fatty liver disease. J Hepatol 2006;45:879–81.
38. Musso G, Gambino R, Cassader M, et al. Meta-analysis natural history of non-alcoholic fatty liver disease (NAFLD) and diagnostic accuracy of non-invasive tests for liver disease severity. Ann Med 2011;43:617–49.
39. Hui JM, Farrell GC, Kench JG, et al. High sensitivity C-reactive protein values do not reliably predict the severity of histological changes in NAFLD. Hepatology 2004;39:1458–9.
40. Jarrar MH, Baranova A, Collantes R, et al. Adipokines and cytokines in non-alcoholic fatty liver disease. Aliment Pharmacol Ther 2008;27:412–21.
41. Hui JM, Hodge A, Farrell GC, et al. Beyond insulin resistance in NASH: TNF-alpha or adiponectin? Hepatology 2004;40:46–54.
42. Abiru S, Migita K, Maeda Y, et al. Serum cytokine and soluble cytokine receptor levels in patients with nonalcoholic steatohepatitis. Liver Int 2006;26:39–45.
43. Wieckowska A, Papouchado BG, Li Z, et al. Increased hepatic and circulating interleukin-6 levels in human nonalcoholic steatohepatitis. Am J Gastroenterol 2008;103:1372–9.
44. Ajmera V, Perito ER, Bass NM, et al, NASH Clinical Research Network. Novel plasma biomarkers associated with liver disease severity in adults with nonalco-holic fatty liver disease. Hepatology 2017;65:65–77.
45. Pagano C, Soardo G, Pilon C, et al. Increased serum resistin in nonalcoholic fatty liver disease is related to liver disease severity and not to insulin resistance. J Clin Endocrinol Metab 2006;91(3):1081–6.
46. Lebensztejn DM, Wojtkowska M, Skiba E, et al. Serum concentration of adipo-nectin, leptin and resistin in obese children with non-alcoholic fatty liver disease. Adv Med Sci 2009;54(2):177–82.

47. Abenavoli L, Luigiano C, Guzzi PH, et al. Serum adipokine levels in overweight patients and their relationship with non-alcoholic fatty liver disease. Panminerva Med 2014;56(2):189–93.

48. Shen C, Zhao CY, Wang W, et al. The relationship between hepatic resistin over-expression and inflammation in patients with nonalcoholic steatohepatitis. BMC Gastroenterol 2014;14:39.

49. Le D, Marks D, Lyle E, et al. Serum leptin levels, hepatic leptin receptor tran-scription, and clinical predictors of non-alcoholic steatohepatitis in obese bariat-ric surgery patients. Surg Endosc 2007;21:1593–9.

50. Yesilova Z, Yaman H, Oktenli C, et al. Systemic markers of lipid peroxidation and antioxidants in patients with nonalcoholic fatty liver disease. Am J Gastroenterol 2005;100:850–5.

51. Chalasani N, Deeg MA, Crabb DW. Systemic levels of lipid peroxidation and its metabolic and dietary correlates in patients with nonalcoholic steatohepatitis. Am J Gastroenterol 2004;99:1497–502.

52. Sanyal AJ, Campbell-Sargent C, Mirshahi F, et al. Nonalcoholic steatohepatitis: association of insulin resistance and mitochondrial abnormalities. Gastroenter-ology 2001;120:1183–92.

53. Feldstein AE, Wieckowska A, Lopez AR, et al. Cytokeratin-18 fragment levels as noninvasive biomarkers for nonalcoholic steatohepatitis: a multicenter validation study. Hepatology 2009;50:1072–8.

54. Wieckowska A, Zein NN, Yerian LM, et al. In vivo assessment of liver cell apoptosis as a novel biomarker of disease severity in nonalcoholic fatty liver dis-ease. Hepatology 2006;44:27–33.

55. Yilmaz Y, Dolar E, Ulukaya E, et al. Soluble forms of extracellular cytokeratin 18 may differentiate simple steatosis from nonalcoholic steatohepatitis. World J Gastroenterol 2007;13:837–44.

56. Diab DL, Yerian L, Schauer P, et al. The clinical utility of biomarkers and the nonalcoholic steatohepatitis CRN liver biopsy scoring system in patients with nonalcoholic fatty liver disease. J Gastroenterol Hepatol 2009;24:564–8.

57. Joka D, Wahl K, Moeller S, et al. Prospective biopsy-controlled evaluation of cell death biomarkers for prediction of liver fibrosis and nonalcoholic steatohepatitis. Hepatology 2012;55:455–64.

58. Kawanaka M, Nishino K, Nakamura J, et al. Correlation between serum cytoker-atin -18 and the progression or regression of non-alcoholic fatty liver disease. Ann Hepatol 2015;14(6):837–44.

59. Cusi K, Chang Z, Harrison S, et al. Limited value of plasma cytokeratin-18 as a biomarker for NASH and fibrosis in patients with nonalcoholic fatty liver disease. J Hepatol 2014;60(1):167–74.

60. Shen J, Chan HL, Wong GL, et al. Non-invasive diagnosis of non-alcoholic stea-tohepatitis by combined serum biomarkers. J Hepatol 2012;56:1224–9.

61. Younossi ZM, Jarrar M, Nugent C, et al. A novel diagnostic biomarker panel for obesity-related nonalcoholic steatohepatitis (NASH). Obes Surg 2008;18:1430–7.

62. Poynard T, Ratziu V, Charlotte F, et al. Diagnostic value of biochemical markers (NASHTest) for the prediction of nonalcoholic steatohepatitis in patients with non-alcoholic fatty liver disease. BMC Gastroenterol 2006;6(34):1–16.

63. Tamimi TI, Elgouhari HM, Alkhouri N, et al. An apoptosis panel for nonalcoholic steatohepatitis diagnosis. J Hepatol 2011;54:1224–9.

64. Dixon JB, Bhathal PS, O'Brien PE. Nonalcoholic fatty liver disease: predictors of nonalcoholic steatohepatitis and liver fibrosis in the severely obese. Gastroenterology 2001;121:91–100.

65. Palekar NA, Naus R, Larson SP, et al. Clinical model for distinguishing nonalcoholic steatohepatitis from simple steatosis in patients with nonalcoholic fatty liver disease. Liver Int 2006;26:151–6.

66. Gholam PM, Flancbaum L, Machan JT, et al. Nonalcoholic fatty liver disease in severely obese patients. Am J Gastroenterol 2007;102:399–408.

67. Younossi ZM, Page S, Rafiq N, et al. A biomarker panel for non-alcoholic steatohepatitis (NASH) and NASH-related fibrosis. Obes Surg 2011;21:431–9.

68. Anty R, Iannelli A, Patouraux S, et al. A new composite model including metabolic syndrome, alanine aminotransferase and cytokeratin-18 for the diagnosis of non-alcoholic steatohepatitis in morbidly obese patients. Aliment Pharmacol Ther 2010;32:1315–22.

69. Goodman ZD. Grading and staging systems for inflammation and fibrosis in chronic liver diseases. J Hepatol 2007;47(4):598–607.

70. Williams AL, Hoofnagle JH. Ratio of serum aspartate to alanine aminotransferase in chronic hepatitis. Relationship to cirrhosis. Gastroenterology 1988;95:734–9.

71. Piperno A, Sampietro M, Pietrangelo A, et al. Heterogeneity of hemochromatosis in Italy. Gastroenterology 1998;144:996–1002.

72. Hartley JL, Brown RM, Tybulewicz A, et al. Hyaluronic acid predicts hepatic fibrosis in children with hepatic disease. J Pediatr Gastroenterol Nutr 2006;43:217–21.

73. Kaneda H, Hashimoto E, Yatsuji S, et al. Hyaluronic acid levels can predict severe fibrosis and platelet counts can predict cirrhosis in patients with nonalcoholic fatty liver disease. J Gastroenterol Hepatol 2006;21:1458–65.

74. Suzuki A, Angulo P, Lymp J, et al. Hyaluronic acid, an accurate serum marker for severe hepatic fibrosis in patients with non-alcoholic fatty liver disease. Liver Int 2005;25:779–86.

75. Yoneda M, Mawatari H, Fujita K, et al. Type IV collagen 7s domain is an independent clinical marker of the severity of fibrosis in patients with nonalcoholic steatohepatitis before the cirrhotic stage. J Gastroenterol 2007;42:375–81.

76. Sakugawa H, Nakayoshi T, Kobashigawa K, et al. Clinical usefulness of biochemical markers of liver fibrosis in patients with nonalcoholic fatty liver disease. World J Gastroenterol 2005;11:255–9.

77. Yoneda M, Uchiyama T, Kato S, et al. Plasma pentraxin 3 is a novel marker for nonalcoholic steatohepatitis (NASH). BMC Gastroenterol 2008;8(53):1–9.

78. Angulo P, Hui JM, Marchesini G, et al. The NAFLD fibrosis score: a noninvasive system that identifies liver fibrosis in patients with NAFLD. Hepatology 2007;45:846–54.

79. Ratziu V, Massard J, Charlotte F, et al. Diagnostic value of biochemical markers (FibroTest-FibroSURE) for the prediction of liver fibrosis in patients with non-alcoholic fatty liver disease. BMC Gastroenterol 2006;6(6):1–13.

80. Harrison SA, Oliver D, Arnold HL, et al. Development and validation of a simple NAFLD clinical scoring system for identifying patients without advanced disease. Gut 2008;57:1441–7.

81. Cales P, Laine F, Boursier J, et al. Comparison of blood tests for liver fibrosis specific or not to NAFLD. J Hepatol 2011;26:1536–43.

82. McPherson S, Stewart SF, Henderson E, et al. Simple non-invasive fibrosis scoring systems can reliably exclude advanced fibrosis in patients with non-alcoholic fatty liver disease. Gut 2010;59:1265–9.
83. Ratziu V, Giral P, Charlotte F. Liver fibrosis in overweight patients. Gastroenterology 2000;118:1117–23.
84. Rosenberg WM, Voelker M, Thiel R, et al. Serum markers detect the presence of liver fibrosis: a cohort study. Gastroenterology 2004;127:1704–13.
85. Younossi ZM, Baranova A, Ziegler K, et al. A genomic and proteomic study of the spectrum of nonalcoholic fatty liver disease. Hepatology 2005;42:665–74.
86. Bell LN, Theodorakis JL, Vuppalanchi R, et al. Serum proteomics and biomarker discovery across the spectrum of nonalcoholic fatty liver disease. Hepatology 2010;51(1):111–20.
87. Lim JW, Dillon J, Miller M. Proteomic and genomic studies of non-alcoholic fatty liver disease - clues in the pathogenesis. World J Gastroenterol 2014;20(26): 8325–40.
88. Charlton M, Viker K, Krishnan A, et al. Differential expression of lumican and fatty acid binding protein-1: new insights into the histologic spectrum of nonalcoholic fatty liver disease. Hepatology 2009;49(4):1375–84.
89. Rodriguez-Suarez E, Duce AM, Caballeria J, et al. Nonalcoholic fatty liver disease proteomics. Proteomics Clin Appl 2010;4(4):362–71.
90. Yu C, Xu C, Xu L, et al. Serum proteomic analysis revealed diagnostic value of hemoglobin for nonalcoholic fatty liver disease. J Hepatol 2012;56:241–7.
91. Ladaru A, Balanescu P, Stan M, et al. Candidate proteomic biomarkers for non-alcoholic fatty liver disease (steatosis and non-alcoholic steatohepatitis) discovered with mass-spectrometry: a systematic review. Proteomics Clin Appl 2010; 4(4):362–71.
92. Blomme B, Francque S, Trepo E, et al. N-glycan based biomarker distinguishing nonalcoholic steatohepatitis from steatosis independently of fibrosis. Dig Liver Dis 2012;44(4):315–22.
93. Yamasaki Y, Nouso K, Miyahara K, et al. Use of non-invasive serum glycan markers to distinguish nonalcoholic steatohepatitis from simple steatosis. J Gastroenterol Hepatol 2015;30(3):528–34.
94. Pirola CJ, Fernandez GT, Castano GO, et al. Circulating microRNA signature in non-alcoholic fatty liver disease: from serum non-coding RNAs to liver histology and disease pathogenesis. Gut 2015;64(5):800–12.
95. Mehta R, Otgonsuren M, Younoszai Z, et al. Circulating miRNA in patients with nonalcoholic fatty liver disease and coronary artery disease. BMJ Open Gastroenterol 2016;3(1–7):e000096.
96. Yamada H, Suzuki K, Ichino N, et al. Associations between circulating micro-RNAs (miR-21, miR-34a, miR-122 and miR-451) and non-alcoholic fatty liver. Clin Chim Acta 2013;424:99–103.
97. Castera L, Forns X, Alberti A. Non-invasive evaluation of liver fibrosis using transient elastography. J Hepatol 2008;48:835–47.
98. Afdhal NH. Fibroscan (transient elastography) for the measurement of liver fibrosis. Gastroenterol Hepatol (N Y) 2012;8(9):605–7.
99. Sandrin L, Fourquet B, Hasquenoph JM, et al. Transient elastography: a new noninvasive method for assessment of hepatic fibrosis. Ultrasound Med Biol 2003;29(12):1705–13.
100. Mueller S, Sandrin L. Liver stiffness: a novel parameter for the diagnosis of liver disease. Hepat Med 2010;2:49–67.

101. Fraquelli M, Rigamonti C, Casazza G, et al. Reproducibility of transient elastography in the evaluation of liver fibrosis in patients with chronic liver disease. Gut 2007;56:968–73.

102. Roulot D, Czernichow S, Le Clésiau H, et al. Liver stiffness values in apparently healthy subjects: influence of gender and metabolic syndrome. J Hepatol 2008; 48:606–13.

103. Boursier J, Konate A, Gorea G, et al. Reproducibility of liver stiffness measurement by ultrasonographic elastometry. Clin Gastroenterol Hepatol 2008;6: 1263–9.

104. Mikolasevic I, Orlic L, Franjic N, et al. Transient elastography (FibroScan®) with controlled attenuation parameter in the assessment of liver steatosis and fibrosis in patients with nonalcoholic fatty liver disease - where do we stand? World J Gastroenterol 2016;22(32):7236–51.

105. Wilder J, Patel K. The clinical utility of FibroScan as a noninvasive diagnostic tests for liver disease. Med Devices (Auckl) 2014;7:107–14.

106. Castera L. Noninvasive methods to assess liver disease in patients with hepatitis B or C. Gastroenterology 2012;142:1293–302.

107. de Ledinghen V, Douvin C, Kettaneh A, et al. Diagnosis of hepatic fibrosis and cirrhosis by transient elastography in HIV/hepatitis C virus–coinfected patients. J Acquir Immune Defic Syndr 2006;41(2):175–9.

108. Sanchez AG, Garcia PF, Vallecillo MA, et al. FibroScan evaluation of liver fibrosis in liver transplantation. Transplant Proc 2009;41(3):1044–6.

109. Friedrich-Rust M, Ong MF, Martens S, et al. Performance of transient elastography for the staging of liver fibrosis: a meta-analysis. Gastroenterology 2008;134: 960–74.

110. Talwalkar JA, Kurtz DM, Schoenleber SJ, et al. Ultrasound-based transient elastography for the detection of hepatic fibrosis: systemic review and meta-analysis. Clin Gastroenterol Hepatol 2007;5:1214–20.

111. Tsochatzis EA, Gurusamy KS, Ntaoula S, et al. Elastography for the diagnosis of severity of fibrosis in chronic liver disease: a meta-analysis of diagnostic accuracy. J Hepatol 2011;54:650–9.

112. Awad MD, Shiha GE, Sallam FA, et al. Evaluation of liver stiffness measurement by Fibroscan as compared to liver biopsy for assessment of hepatic fibrosis in children with chronic hepatitis C. J Egypt Soc Parasitol 2013;43(3):805–19.

113. Afdhal NH, Bacon BR, Patel K, et al. Accuracy of Fibroscan, compared with histology, in analysis of liver fibrosis in patients with hepatitis B or C: a United States multicenter study. Clin Gastroenterol Hepatol 2015;13(4):772–9.

114. Foucher J, Chanteloup E, Vergniol J, et al. Diagnosis of cirrhosis by transient elastography (FibroScan): a prospective study. Gut 2006;55(3):403–8.

115. Coco B, Oliveri F, Maina AM, et al. Transient elastography: a new surrogate marker of liver fibrosis influenced by major changes of transaminases. J Viral Hepat 2007;14:360–9.

116. Arena U, Vizzutti F, Corti G, et al. Acute viral hepatitis increases liver stiffness values measured by transient elastography. Hepatology 2008;47:380–4.

117. Hopper I, Kemp W, Porapakkham P, et al. Impact of heart failure and changes to volume status on liver stiffness: non-invasive assessment using transient elastography. Eur J Heart Fail 2012;14:621–7.

118. Yashima Y, Tsujino T, Masuzaki R, et al. Increased liver elasticity in patients with biliary obstruction. J Gastroenterol 2011;46:86–91.

119. Kettaneh A, Marcellin P, Douvin C, et al. Features associated with success rate and performance of FibroScan measurements for the diagnosis of cirrhosis in

HCV patients: a prospective study of 935 patients. J Hepatol 2007;46(4): 628–34.

120. Foucher J, Castera L, Bernard PH, et al. Prevalence and factors associated with failure of liver stiffness measurement using FibroScan in a prospective study of 2114 examinations. Eur J Gastroenterol Hepatol 2006;18(4):411–2.

121. Castera L, Foucher J, Bernard PH, et al. Pitfalls of liver stiffness measurement: a 5-year prospective study of 13,369 examinations. Hepatology 2010;51(3): 828–35.

122. Hashemi SA, Alavian SM, Gholami-Fesharaki M. Assessment of transient elastography (FibroScan) for diagnosis of fibrosis in non-alcoholic fatty liver disease: a systematic review and meta-analysis. Caspian J Intern Med 2016;7(4):242–52.

123. Boursier J, Vergniol J, Guillet A, et al. Diagnostic accuracy and prognostic significance of blood fibrosis tests and liver stiffness measurement by FibroScan in non-alcoholic fatty liver disease. J Hepatol 2016;65(3):570–8.

124. Kleiner DE, Brunt EM. Nonalcoholic fatty liver disease: pathologic patterns and biopsy evaluation in clinical research. Semin Liver Dis 2012;32:3–13.

125. Ryan CK, Johson LA, Germin BI, et al. One hundred consecutive hepatic biopsies in the workup of living donors for right lobe liver transplantation. Liver Transpl 2002;8:1114–22.

126. Palmentieri B, deSio I, La Mura V, et al. The role of bright liver echo pattern on ultrasound B-mode examination in the diagnosis of liver steatosis. Dig Liver Dis 2006;38:485–9.

127. Sasso M, Miette V, Sandrin L, et al. The controlled attenuation parameter (CAP): a novel tool for the non-invasive evaluation of steatosis using Fibroscan®. Clin Res Hepatol Gastroenterol 2012;36:13–20.

128. de Lédinghen V, Vergniol J, Foucher J, et al. Non-invasive diagnosis of liver steatosis using controlled attenuation parameter (CAP) and transient elastography. Liver Int 2012;32:911–8.

129. Karlas T, Petroff D, Garnov N, et al. Non-invasive assessment of hepatic steatosis in patients with NAFLD using controlled attenuation parameter and 1H-MR spectroscopy. PLoS One 2014;9(3):e91987.

130. Sasso M, Beaugrand M, de Ledinghen V, et al. Controlled attenuation parameter (CAP): a novel VCTE guided ultrasonic attenuation measurement for the evaluation of hepatic steatosis: preliminary study and validation in a cohort of patients with chronic liver disease from various causes. Ultrasound Med Biol 2010; 36(11):1825–35.

131. Petta S, Wong VW, Cammà C, et al. Improved noninvasive prediction of liver fibrosis by liver stiffness measurement in patients with nonalcoholic fatty liver disease accounting for controlled attenuation parameter values. Hepatology 2017;65(4):1145–55.

132. Myers RP, Pollett A, Kirsch R, et al. Controlled attenuation parameter (CAP): a noninvasive method for the detection of hepatic steatosis based on transient elastography. Liver Int 2012;32:902–10.

133. Chan WK, Mustapha N, Raihan N, et al. Controlled attenuation parameter for the detection and quantification of hepatic steatosis in nonalcoholic fatty liver disease. J Gastroenterol Hepatol 2014;29:1470–6.

134. de Ledinghen V, Wong GL, Vergniol J, et al. Controlled attenuation parameter for the diagnosis of steatosis in non-alcoholic fatty liver disease. J Gastroenterol Hepatol 2016;31(4):848–55.

135. Festi D, Schiumerini R, Marzi L, et al. The diagnosis of non-alcoholic fatty liver disease–availability and accuracy of non-invasive methods. Aliment Pharmacol Ther 2013;37:392–400.

136. Dyson JK, Anstee QM, McPherson S. Non-alcoholic fatty liver disease: a practical approach to diagnosis and staging. Liver 2013;5(3):211–8.

137. Singh S, Venkatesh SK, Loomba R, et al. Magnetic resonance elastography for staging liver fibrosis in non-alcoholic fatty liver disease: a diagnostic accuracy systematic review and individual participant data pooled analysis. Eur Radiol 2016;26(5):1431–40.

138. Imajo K, Kessoku T, Honda Y, et al. Magnetic resonance imaging more accurately classifies steatosis and fibrosis in patients with nonalcoholic fatty liver than transient elastography. Gastroenterology 2016;150(3):626–37.

Radiologic Imaging in Nonalcoholic Fatty Liver Disease and Nonalcoholic Steatohepatitis

Yonah B. Esterson, MD, MS*, Gregory M. Grimaldi, MD

KEYWORDS

- Steatosis • Nonalcoholic fatty liver disease • Nonalcoholic steatohepatitis
- Ultrasound • MRI • CT • Elastography • Imaging

KEY POINTS

- Imaging plays a role in the diagnosis and monitoring of patients with nonalcoholic fatty liver disease (NAFLD).
- MRI has the best sensitivity and specificity profile for diagnosing hepatic steatosis of any degree. MRI may be superior to biopsy in terms of estimating hepatic fat fraction and may be used to longitudinally follow patients with treatment.
- Image-based elastography is increasingly being used to evaluate for fibrosis in patients with NAFLD and may obviate biopsy.
- Up to 50% of patients with NAFLD with hepatocellular carcinoma have no morphologic evidence of cirrhosis, and special screening considerations may be needed in this population.

INTRODUCTION

Nonalcoholic fatty liver disease (NAFLD) encompasses a spectrum of liver pathologies defined by the presence of fat in the liver in the absence of alcohol consumption.[1] The disease spectrum ranges from simple steatosis to nonalcoholic steatohepatitis (NASH) to hepatic fibrosis and cirrhosis.[2,3] NAFLD is a frequently encountered entity in the Western world, with its prevalence estimated to be as high as 30%.[2,4]

Clinically, its recognition is vital, as the all-cause mortality rate of patients with NAFLD is at least 34% higher than that of the general population,[3] with the presence of NASH long considered to be a significant predictor of morbidity and mortality in

Disclosure Statement: The authors have nothing to disclose.
Department of Radiology, Northwell Health System, Hofstra Northwell School of Medicine, 300 Community Drive, Manhasset, NY 11030, USA
* Corresponding author.
E-mail address: YEsterson@northwell.edu

patients with NAFLD.[5,6] However, more recent studies have suggested that among patients with NAFLD, it is not NASH but rather advanced fibrosis that independently predicts liver-related mortality.[1] In fact, a study by Soderberg and colleagues[6] of patients with NAFLD demonstrated no difference in mortality between those with biopsy-proven NASH and those without NASH. In contrast, a study by Younossi and colleagues[7] demonstrated high-grade liver fibrosis to be an independent risk factor for liver-related mortality with a hazard ratio of 5.7. In this study, the presence of NASH was only associated with mortality when fibrosis was included in the analysis. Therefore, it is the identification of fibrosis in a patient with NAFLD that indicates that patient's mortality risk. The degree of fibrosis in patients with NASH may progress, regress, or remain stable over time.[3]

Liver biopsy remains the gold standard for diagnosis of NAFLD and fibrosis and is the only way to diagnose NASH, which has no imaging findings.[1] However, biopsy has considerable disadvantages. It is invasive, costly, and carries the risk of potential complications, such as hemorrhage. Furthermore, it is subject to sampling variability and may not paint an accurate picture of the true disease severity.[8] Biopsy is, therefore, inappropriate to use as a screening test in at-risk patients or to evaluate the progression of disease in the many patients with NAFLD. Newer technologies, such as elastography, are increasingly being used to evaluate the degree of fibrosis.

Imaging plays a role in the diagnosis of NAFLD when patients are referred with abnormal liver chemistries, referred for the clinical suspicion of NAFLD (perhaps by having obesity, hyperlipidemia, or type 2 diabetes), or when abnormal findings are present at imaging performed for other reasons.[1,9] Imaging also plays a role in monitoring patients with known NAFLD. In the following article, the authors review the multimodality (ultrasound, computed tomography [CT], and magnetic resonance [MR]) imaging appearance of NAFLD and discuss the radiologic diagnostic criteria as well as the sensitivity and specificity of these imaging methods. The authors review the role of both ultrasound and MR elastography (MRE) for the diagnosis of fibrosis and for the longitudinal evaluation of patients following therapeutic intervention. Lastly, the authors briefly discuss the screening and diagnosis of hepatocellular carcinoma (HCC) in patients with NAFLD as there are special considerations in this population.

IMAGING DIAGNOSIS OF STEATOSIS
Ultrasonography

The intracellular fat vacuoles present in hepatic steatosis alter the properties of the liver such that its reflection of sound waves is increased relative to normal hepatic parenchyma.[2] This characteristic of intracellular hepatic fat produces an echogenic, or bright, liver on sonographic imaging. Most commonly, fat deposition is diffuse; therefore, the liver will appear homogeneously echogenic.[10] The right kidney, situated just inferior to the right hepatic lobe, may be used as an internal reference. The liver is typically evaluated on sagittal view with the kidney and liver at the same focal zone depth. In normal patients, the liver will be similar or slightly more echogenic than the renal cortex. A starker contrast between the echogenicity of the liver and the adjacent renal cortex is suggestive of hepatic steatosis. Additionally, the increased reflection of sound waves by the fat-infiltrated liver may result in a coarser hepatic echotexture than normal liver, decreased depth of penetration by the ultrasound beam, and loss of right hemidiaphragm and portal triad visualization, structures which are normally readily apparent at ultrasound.[2,9,10]

In clinical practice, ultrasound is used to provide a qualitative rather than a quantitative assessment of hepatic fat infiltration. Mild steatosis is defined as increased hepatic parenchymal echogenicity without obscuration of the portal triads. Moderate steatosis is characterized by increased hepatic parenchymal echogenicity that obscures the portal triads. Finally, severe steatosis is present when the liver is sufficiently echogenic to obscure the diaphragm and limit the evaluation of the deep liver parenchyma by attenuating the ultrasound beam (**Fig. 1**).

Although ultrasound is easily accessible, relatively low in cost, and does not rely on ionizing radiation, reports on its accuracy have varied greatly. The sensitivity of ultrasound has been reported to range from 53% to 100% and its specificity from 77% to 98% with higher diagnostic sensitivities and specificities when evaluating only cases of moderate to severe hepatic steatosis (histologic grade $\geq$30%–33%) and lower values when all grades of hepatic steatosis, including mild steatosis (histologic grade $\geq$3%–5%), are considered.[2,11–16] Additionally, studies evaluating the use of ultrasonography for detecting hepatic steatosis versus other entities that can increase hepatic parenchymal echogenicity, such as fibrosis, hepatitis, or iron overload, found the specificity of ultrasonography for the diagnosis of steatosis to be on the lower end of the above range.[9,13]

Beyond the lower sensitivity and specificity for the diagnosis of mild steatosis, as well as its decreased specificity in patients with other infiltrative liver diseases, ultrasound is also an operator-dependent modality. Several studies have demonstrated only fair to moderate interobserver and intraobserver agreement with regard to both the diagnosis of hepatic steatosis and the severity of hepatic steatosis when present.[9,17,18]

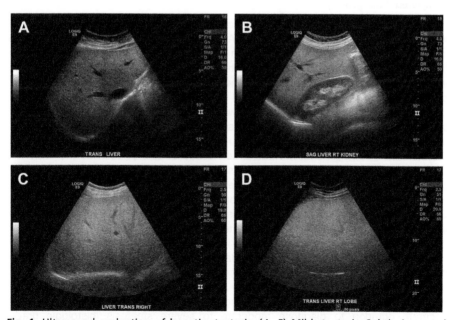

Fig. 1. Ultrasound evaluation of hepatic steatosis. (*A, B*) Mild steatosis. Subtle increased echogenicity of the liver parenchyma noted best when comparing the brightness of the liver with the adjacent renal cortex. (*C*) Moderate steatosis. Increased echogenicity of the liver parenchyma with obscuration of the portal triads. The echogenic diaphragm is still visualized. (*D*) Severe steatosis. Complete obscuration of the portal triads with obscuration of the diaphragm and decreased penetration with depth.

More recently, methods have been developed to make the ultrasound techniques currently used in clinical practice more quantitative and less operator dependent. The most promising thus far is the development of the hepatorenal index, which compares the brightness of the liver versus the kidney using a software program. Webb and colleagues[19] found that a hepatorenal index of at least 1.49 was 100% sensitive and 91% specific for diagnosing even mild steatosis. However, this study used proprietary software and only a single scanner, severely limiting its generalizability. Another study by Marshall and colleagues,[20] which used free software available through the National Institutes of Health and which touted the hepatorenal index as an "accurate, simple, and effective tool in screening for steatosis," found that a hepatorenal index of 1.28 was 100% sensitive for diagnosing even mild steatosis. However, the same study found the specificity of the hepatorenal index to be only 54%. The study also excluded patients with renal disease who typically have more echogenic kidneys and who may have altered the results of the study. Lastly, although the hepatorenal index software used by Marshall and colleagues[20] is available as freeware, the software is likely too time consuming and labor intensive to be used for screening the many patients at risk for hepatic steatosis seen in general practice.

In summary, ultrasound is commonly used to screen for hepatic steatosis and may detect steatosis in patients scanned for other indications; but its limitations include suboptimal sensitivity and specificity for the detection of mild steatosis, operator dependence, and, at the current time, that it is used only to make a qualitative assessment of the extent of disease. It is, therefore, not ideal for detecting the early stages of disease or for the longitudinal evaluation of patients carrying the diagnosis of NAFLD.

Computed Tomography

The brightness or darkness of a structure at unenhanced CT is based on the extent to which that structure attenuates radiation. At unenhanced CT, the normal liver will have slightly higher attenuation than the spleen (ie, the normal liver will be slightly brighter than the spleen). More quantitatively, each pixel in a CT image is assigned a numeric value in Hounsfield units (HU) based on the extent to which the tissue making up that pixel attenuates radiation. The Hounsfield unit scale is based on assigning a value of 0 to water. Fat, which is less dense than water, has Hounsfield unit values of approximately −50 to −100. On the other hand, soft tissue, which has slightly greater attenuation than water, has Hounsfield unit values ranging from +10 to +60. It follows that the infiltration of hypodense fat into a soft tissue structure, such as the liver, will decrease the attenuation of the liver, resulting in a darker appearance to the eye and a lower attenuation when its Hounsfield units are measured.

The spleen serves as a useful internal control when evaluating the liver for steatosis. Several studies have shown that decreased hepatic attenuation relative to splenic attenuation has good sensitivity of 88% to 95% and specificity of 90% to 99% for the diagnosis of hepatic steatosis.[9,21–24] In clinical practice, hepatic attenuation 10 HU less than splenic attenuation at unenhanced CT is one criterion used to diagnose hepatic steatosis (**Fig. 2**).[25] An absolute liver attenuation of less than 40 HU at unenhanced CT is another criterion commonly used in clinical practice to make the diagnosis[25,26] and has been shown by Kodama and colleagues[27] to be the most accurate criterion to diagnose moderate to severe steatosis (histologic grade ≥30%). Other more recent studies, such as one by Pickhardt and colleagues,[28] used an absolute liver attenuation cutoff of 48 HU, which was found to be 100% specific for the diagnosis but only 54% sensitive. Of note, iron deposition within the liver increases its attenuation; therefore, measurements of liver attenuation may be less accurate detecting steatosis in patients with hemochromatosis or hemosiderosis.[9]

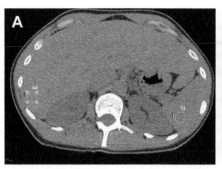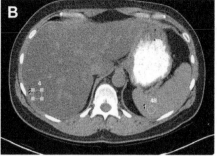

Fig. 2. Unenhanced CT evaluation of hepatic steatosis using hepatic-splenic attenuation difference. (*A*) No evidence of steatosis. The region-of-interest–measured hepatic attenuation is greater than the spleen (+13). (*B*) Diffuse hepatic steatosis. The hepatic to splenic attenuation difference is −44 HU.

In the case of contrast-enhanced CT, the attenuation characteristics of the liver and spleen will be altered based on a variety of factors, including iodine concentration, injection rate, injection volume, blood flow dynamics, and time delay between injection and scanning. The use of contrast-enhanced CT to evaluate for hepatic steatosis has yielded mixed results. Using comparison with splenic attenuation as the diagnostic criterion, Panicek and colleagues[29] found a sensitivity of 88% and a specificity of only 30% using a liver-spleen attenuation difference of less than 0 HU on noncontrast imaging as the reference standard. A different study with a 5-fold larger sample size by Lawrence and colleagues[26] found a sensitivity of 60.5% but a specificity of 100% when using a liver-spleen attenuation difference of less than 10 HU on noncontrast imaging as the reference standard. Lawrence and colleagues[26] also found that using absolute liver attenuation of less than 40 HU as the diagnostic criterion, even in the presence of intravenous contrast, yielded a sensitivity of 53% and a specificity of 100%.

In summary, several CT criteria have been shown to be highly specific for the diagnosis of hepatic steatosis. However, most studies have been performed in cases of moderate to severe steatosis and have been performed without longitudinal follow-up. Little is known regarding the value of CT in cases of mild steatosis or regarding the ability of CT to detect minor changes in the severity of hepatic steatosis over time.

Magnetic Resonance

MRI has become the gold standard imaging modality for quantification of hepatic fat. The detection of hepatic steatosis at MRI is based on chemical shift imaging. Protons in water and fat oscillate at regular frequencies. At certain known echo times related to the magnetic field strength, the protons in water and fat will be in phase (ie, they will be aligned in the same direction) and their signal will be summed resulting in a brighter signal on imaging. At other known echo times, the protons in water and fat will be out of phase (ie, they will be aligned in opposite directions) and their signals will cancel each other out resulting in a darker signal on imaging. Therefore, tissue that contains both fat and water will be relatively bright on in-phase imaging and relatively dark on out-of-phase imaging. Standard liver protocol MRI studies typically include dual-echo chemical shift imaging, meaning that both in-phase and out-of-phase images are produced. The normal, nonsteatotic liver will appear similar on in-phase compared with out-of-phase images. However, in patients with hepatic steatosis, the increased fat content of the liver will result in diminished signal intensity of the liver on out-of-phase compared with in-phase images (**Fig. 3**). Several studies have assessed the ability of dual-echo chemical shift MRI to detect hepatic steatosis. These studies reported sensitivities of 77% to 100% and specificities of 87% to 91% for detection of any degree of hepatic steatosis (histologic grade ≥5%) by dual-echo chemical shift imaging.[14,16,17,30] Using the knowledge that the signal intensity of the liver on out-of-phase images represents the difference between water and fat signals and that the signal intensity of the liver on in-phase images represents the sum of water and fat signals, fat signal percentage can be calculated using the following simple formula: fat signal percentage = $(signal_{in\text{-}phase} - signal_{out\text{-}of\text{-}phase})/2(signal_{in\text{-}phase})$.[9]

Multi-echo chemical shift imaging takes these principles one step further and allows calculation of a more accurate proton density fat fraction (PDFF), which is the fraction of protons bound to fat in the liver divided by the total number of protons in the liver, including those bound to water or fat.[31,32] As mentioned earlier, fat and water protons resonate at different frequencies. At a magnetic strength of 1.5 T, water and fat protons will alternately be aligned in and out of phase with each other every 2.2 ms. Dual-echo chemical shift imaging captures images at the first time point that fat and water protons are in phase and at the first time point that fat and water protons are out of phase. Multi-echo chemical shift imaging captures at least 3 consecutive pairs of in-phase and out-of-phase imaging sequences to optimize the separation of fat and water signals and to address confounding factors of T1 bias and T2* decay, which are beyond the scope of this review.[2,9,33] These multi-echo T1-independent and T2*-corrected chemical shift imaging sequences have proven to provide more accurate estimates of hepatic fat compared with dual-echo chemical shift imaging sequences.[34–36] For example, a study by Lee and colleagues[34] found that fat fraction calculated by multi-echo chemical shift MR to have a correlation coefficient of 0.99 to the reference standard of MR spectroscopy (a technology explained later) compared with the correlation coefficient of 0.86 for the fat fraction calculated by dual-echo chemical shift imaging to the same reference standard. In contrast to other imaging methods whereby hepatic iron deposition limits the reader's ability to detect steatosis, multi-echo chemical shift imaging has proven to be accurate even in the presence of iron deposition disease.[2,9,34] Several studies have even suggested that PDFF may be superior to pathologic evaluation of a biopsy specimen in terms of estimating the total fat content of the liver.[37,38] Although fat accumulation tends to be diffuse, the distribution is often

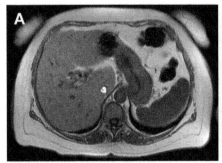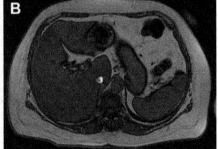

Fig. 3. MRI evaluation of hepatic steatosis using chemical shift imaging. (*A*) In-phase image. (*B*) Out-of-phase image. Out-of-phase image demonstrates diminished signal intensity of liver parenchyma consistent with hepatic steatosis. Note relative stability of signal in the spleen, which can be used as an internal reference.

nonuniform, which may lend to spatial variability in sampling at liver biopsy.[31] PDFF has been proven to be accurate in quantifying hepatic steatosis with a high degree of precision and reproducibility (**Fig. 4**).

Furthermore, PDFF shows promise that it may be used to follow patients longitudinally. In one study by Noureddin and colleagues,[39] changes in PDFF over the 24-week study period correlated with changes in body weight and liver enzymes. Le and colleagues[40] demonstrated a 5.6% increase in hepatic fat following 24 weeks of bile sequestrant administration compared with placebo administration in patients with NASH. In both studies, the small changes in hepatic fat content seen on MR were not appreciated on biopsy.

MR spectroscopy is based on a similar principle to that of chemical shift imaging; however, it measures the water and fat content of the liver more directly than chemical shift imaging and is, therefore, considered to be more accurate.[31] Even though all

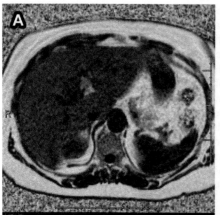
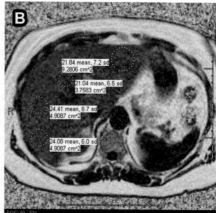
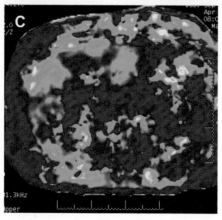

Fig. 4. PDFF/MR elastogram images of a patient with moderate hepatic steatosis, however, no evidence of fibrosis. (*A*) PDFF image without measurements demonstrates the liver signal to be moderately hyperintense compared with the spleen, compatible with steatosis. Note bright signal from subcutaneous fat used as a reference standard. (*B*) PDFF image with 4 region-of-interest measurements representing the hepatic fat fraction. Mean fat fraction is 23%. (*C*) Elastogram image in the same patient with average stiffness of 2.5 kPa, in the range of normal or inflammation. (*Courtesy of* Sandeep Deshmukh, MD, Department of Radiology, Thomas Jefferson University Hospital, Philadelphia, PA.)

protons are in essence identical hydrogen atoms, their resonant frequencies will differ based on the chemical group to which they are bound. The hydrogen atoms in a hydroxyl group, methylene group, and methyl group, for example, will each resonate at a distinct characteristic frequency. In MR spectroscopy, resonant frequencies of a substance are collected and the data are displayed in the form of a set of peaks on a graph, rather than as differing signal intensities on an anatomic image. On MR spectroscopy of the liver, water appears as a single characteristic peak at 4.7 ppm and fat appears as several smaller characteristic peaks at 0.8 to 2.3 ppm because fat is made up of multiple different hydrocarbon components.[9] MR spectroscopy is considered to be the most sensitive imaging modality for the evaluation of hepatic steatosis and has been shown in a direct comparison study by van Werven and colleagues to have a slightly higher sensitivity of 91% than the sensitivity of dual-echo chemical shift MR imaging calculated to be 90%. The same study by van Werven and colleagues found MR spectroscopy to have a slightly stronger correlation with histopathologic steatosis assessment (r = 0.86) compared with that for dual-echo chemical shift MRI (r = 0.85).[16] However, MR spectroscopy has several notable limitations. In contrast to chemical shift imaging, which evaluates the entirety of the liver, MR spectroscopy evaluates data collected from a single region or voxel selected by the operator. In this way, MR spectroscopy is similar to biopsy in that the small sample size evaluated may provide incomplete information regarding the true extent of disease. Additionally, MR spectroscopy is complex to acquire and analyze and is not available on all MR scanners, limiting its clinical use,[31] whereas chemical shift MRI is widely available and has been shown to have sensitivity and accuracy similar to that of MR spectroscopy.[35,36]

Although MRI is more expensive and somewhat less accessible relative to ultrasound and CT, it is a noninvasive and accurate way to assess hepatic fat content quantitatively; in the studies thus far, chemical shift MRI has proven superior to biopsy in detecting small changes in hepatic fat content following therapeutic intervention (**Table 1**).

IMAGING DIAGNOSIS OF FIBROSIS

To this point, the authors have discussed the role of ultrasound, CT, and MRI in evaluating hepatic steatosis. However, the clinical importance of NAFLD is that a

Table 1
Comparison of ultrasound, computed tomography, and MRI for detection and evaluation of hepatic steatosis

Imaging Modality	Strengths	Limitations
US	• Widely accessible • Inexpensive	• Suboptimal sensitivity/specificity for mild steatosis • Operator dependent • Qualitative
CT	• High sensitivity for moderate to severe steatosis	• Suboptimal sensitivity/specificity for mild steatosis • Radiation risks
MRI	• Best sensitivity and sensitivity for steatosis (even mild steatosis) • May be superior to biopsy specimen in terms of estimating total hepatic fat • Can be used to follow patients longitudinally with treatment	• Expensive • Limited availability as a screening tool

Abbreviation: US, ultrasound.

percentage of those carrying the diagnosis can progress to NASH and subsequently to hepatic fibrosis. Hepatic fibrosis, which is associated with an increased risk of esophageal varices and HCC, cannot be detected with conventional ultrasound, CT, or MRI, yet its early detection is critical to facilitate closer monitoring.[41] In recent years, ultrasound and MRE methods have been refined to evaluate liver stiffness as a proxy for fibrosis. In elastography, an external force is applied to the liver. The force temporarily distorts the hepatic parenchyma and produces shear waves, which travel through the liver perpendicular to the direction of the force (think of ripples radiating perpendicularly from the spot where a stone is dropped into a pond). The velocity of these shear waves, which can be identified with ultrasound or MR, is itself associated with the degree of fibrosis.[42,43] Transient elastography (TE), a non–image-based modality, has been used to detect advanced fibrosis and cirrhosis in patients with liver disease. In the following paragraphs, the authors discuss image-based ultrasound elastography, specifically acoustic radiation force impulse (ARFI) elastography, as well as MRE (**Table 2**).

Acoustic Radiation Force Impulse Elastography

Patients are placed in the supine or slight left lateral decubitus position, and an intercostal window is used to image segments VII and VIII of the right hepatic lobe with real-time B-mode (gray-scale ultrasound) imaging. While visualizing the right hepatic lobe, ARFI elastography uses rapid acoustic pulses delivered by the ultrasound probe to generate shear waves in a small region of interest that the operator places within the images of the liver being obtained in real time (**Fig. 5**). The velocity of the shear waves generated by ARFI elastography, measured as the waves propagate through the region of interest placed by the operator, is directly related to liver tissue stiffness. In order to optimize these stiffness measurements, the ARFI pulse should be delivered perpendicular to the liver capsule during a breath hold. Additionally, it is recommended that 10 stiffness measurements be obtained over the same area in segments

Table 2
Comparison of acoustic radiation force impulse and magnetic resonance elastography for detection and evaluation of hepatic fibrosis in patients with nonalcoholic fatty liver disease

Imaging Modality	Strengths	Limitations
ARFI	• Widely accessible • Inexpensive • Good sensitivity for detection of fibrosis, especially advanced fibrosis or cirrhosis • Can be combined with imaging for HCC screening • Less likely to fail in obese patients compared with TE	• Suboptimal sensitivity/specificity for mild fibrosis • Failure in patients with high degrees of steatosis and inflammation • Small sample size compared with MRE • No validated mean stiffness cutoff values for different stages of fibrosis
MRE	• Higher sensitivity and accuracy for detection of fibrosis compared with ARFI and TE • Excellent interobserver agreement • Large sample size • Less likely to fail in obese patients compared with ultrasound-based elastography methods • Can be combined with imaging for HCC diagnosis	• Expensive • Limited availability • Failure in patients with iron deposition • Patients may have contraindications to MRI

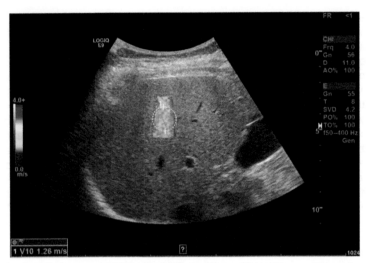

Fig. 5. Ultrasound elastogram (GE Logiq E9 Shear Wave, GE Healthcare, Wauwatosa, WI) in patient with hepatic steatosis. Elastogram image demonstrates one of the 10 measurements obtained in the same location of the right lobe. The median stiffness measure of 1.28 m/s is within normal liver stiffness range; no evidence of fibrosis.

VII and VIII with only the mean value of these measurements reported. A good-quality examination is suggested when the interquartile range of these 10 measurements is less than 30% of the calculated median liver stiffness value.[44]

A 2015 meta-analysis by Liu and colleagues[45] found ARFI to have a pooled sensitivity of 80% and a pooled specificity of 85% for detecting significant fibrosis in patients with NAFLD. A study included in this meta-analysis by Yoneda and colleagues[46] found the median shear wave velocity measured with ARFI to be significantly correlated with that measured with TE (r = 0.75). Yoneda and colleagues[46] also found ARFI to have excellent sensitivity and specificity of greater than 90% for diagnosing the two most advanced stages of hepatic fibrosis as well as a negative predictive value of 100%. In contrast to TE, which has a failure rate of 3% to 16% when it is attempted in obese patients,[47] ARFI measurements in this study were not significantly correlated with weight or height.[46] A study by Palmeri and colleagues,[48] also included in the aforementioned meta-analysis, found ARFI to be able to successfully distinguish low-grade from high-grade fibrosis with a sensitivity and specificity of 90% and, importantly, found that ARFI was not affected by body mass index. A smaller study of 57 patients by Friedrich-Rust and colleagues[49] demonstrated no difference in the results obtained by TE and ARFI.

Although incompletely studied in NAFLD, these studies suggest that ARFI has similar diagnostic accuracy to TE but that, in contrast to transient elastography, its use is not limited in obese patients. However, both TE and ARFI may be complicated by the degree of steatosis, which decreases shear wave velocity, and inflammation, which increases shear wave velocity.[45] Additionally, specific ARFI-based mean stiffness cutoff values have not yet been validated for the different stages of fibrosis in large-scale trials of patients with NAFLD.

Magnetic Resonance Elastography

MRE uses an active driver, located outside the magnet room, and a passive driver, placed directly against patients' lower right chest/upper right abdominal wall. The active generator generates continuous low-frequency vibrations that are transmitted to the passive driver via tubing connecting the two drivers.[47] The vibrations generate shear waves in the liver that are imaged with a 2-dimensional gradient-recalled echo MRE sequence with oscillating motion-sensitizing gradients synchronized to the frequency of the generated shear waves. This sequence and its motion encoding gradients allow imaging of both magnitude and phase data that are displayed as a wave image; a color coded cross sectional map demonstrating the propagation of shear waves through the tissues within a given axial MR slice, and as an elastogram/stiffness map; a color coded cross sectional map indicating the degree of stiffness of the tissues within a given axial MR slice.[47,50,51] Importantly, these maps are superimposed on images of the liver, meaning that the entirety of the cross-sectional area of the liver is sampled, a much larger sample than what may be achieved with biopsy or with the ultrasound-based elastography methods, which use only a small region of interest placed by the operator over real-time ultrasound images of the liver (see **Fig. 4C**; **Fig. 6**).

In 2015, Singh and colleagues performed a systematic review of nine studies comparing MRE to the gold standard of liver biopsy. The study showed MRE to have high accuracies for diagnosing any degree of fibrosis (F$\geq$stage 1 fibrosis), significant fibrosis (F$\geq$stage 2 fibrosis), advanced fibrosis (F$\geq$stage 3 fibrosis), or cirrhosis (F = stage 4 fibrosis), with areas under the receiver operator curve ranging from 0.86 to 0.91. Furthermore, the pooled sensitivities of MRE for diagnosing these 4 stages of liver fibrosis were 75% to 88%. Importantly, MRE was not affected by obesity, with similar accuracies reported in obese and nonobese patients; MRE was not affected by the presence of severe hepatic inflammation.[52] Much has been learned about MRE from studies performed in patients with the viral hepatitis, which may also lead to hepatic fibrosis. A study evaluating the interobserver agreement between radiologists interpreting MRE examinations and separately between pathologists interpreting liver biopsies performed in patients with viral hepatitis found that the intraclass correlation coefficient (ICC) was excellent for both radiologic and pathologic interpretations. However, the ICC among radiologists interpreting MRE examinations was significantly higher than that among pathologists staging hepatic biopsies (ICC of 0.99 for MRE vs 0.91 for pathologic fibrosis staging).[53]

Several more recent studies have been performed comparing MRE with TE and ARFI. Imajo and colleagues[54] compared MRE and TE in patients with biopsy-proven NAFLD and found MRE to have greater accuracy for diagnosing advanced fibrosis (area under the receiver operator curve of 0.91 for MRE vs 0.82 for TE). However, no significant difference was found between the accuracy of MRE and TE for detecting any degree of fibrosis or for detecting significant fibrosis. Similarly, Park and colleagues[55] performed a prospective cross-sectional study on patients undergoing biopsy for NAFLD evaluation and found that MRE was significantly more accurate for detecting the presence of fibrosis than TE (area under the receiver operator curve of 0.82 for MRE vs 0.67 for TE). Park and colleagues[55] also found that MRE trends toward greater accuracy for detecting the 3 more advanced grades of fibrosis than does TE. Cui and colleagues[50] compared MRE and ARFI in patients with biopsy-proven NAFLD and found MRE to be more accurate overall (area under the receiver operator curve of 0.80 for MRE vs 0.66 for ARFI) as well as more accurate for diagnosing the 3 most advanced stages of fibrosis. This study also showed MRE to be superior to ARFI for the diagnosis of any degree of fibrosis in obese patients.

Although the data on MRE are limited at the current time, the available results are promising, demonstrating good accuracy and sensitivity of MRE for the detection of fibrosis in patients with NAFLD as well as the superior accuracy of MRE compared

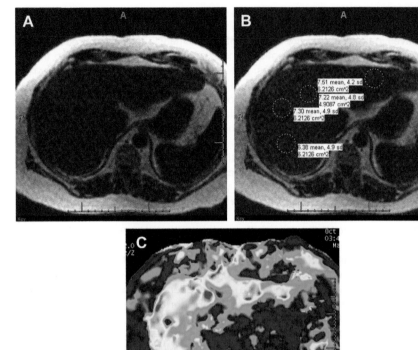

Fig. 6. PDFF/MR elastogram of a patient with mild hepatic steatosis and stage 3 to 4 fibrosis. (*A*) PDFF image without measurements demonstrates the liver signal to be similar to minimally increased compared with the spleen, compatible with steatosis. Note bright signal from subcutaneous fat used as a reference standard. (*B*) PDFF image with 4 region-of-interest (ROI) measurements representing the hepatic fat fraction. Mean fat fraction is 7%. (*C*) Elastogram image in the same patient, average stiffness of 4.7 kPa, in the range of stage 3 to 4 fibrosis. (*Courtesy of* Sandeep Deshmukh, MD, Department of Radiology, Thomas Jefferson University Hospital, Philadelphia, PA.)

with ultrasound-based elastography methods. An additional advantage to MRE is that it allows sampling of a much larger section of liver compared with biopsy, TE, or ARFI, an important point given that fat deposition in the liver is often nonuniform.[31] MRE is also less likely than ultrasound-based elastography methods to fail in obese patients or those with high degrees of hepatic inflammation. However, there are limitations to MRE, which include the possibility of failure in patients with iron deposition,[56] its relatively limited availability, its expense, and that some patients have contraindications to undergoing an MRI.

HEPATOCELLULAR CARCINOMA IN NONALCOHOLIC FATTY LIVER DISEASE

NAFLD is the most common liver disorder in the industrialized world, with a prevalence among adults of 30% in the general population and 90% in the morbidly obese population (body mass index $\geq$40 kg/m^2).[57] Furthermore, NAFLD is recognized as an increasingly common predisposing factor for the development of HCC.[58] Although the risk of developing HCC in an individual patient with NAFLD is less than that in an individual patient with chronic hepatitis C virus (HCV), the increasing prevalence of NAFLD may lead to this entity becoming the most frequent cause of HCC in the United States and other industrialized countries.[57]

Among patients with NAFLD, HCC occurs most commonly in those who have progressed to fibrosis or cirrhosis.[57] However, Piscaglia and colleagues[59] reported that up to 50% of patients with NAFLD newly diagnosed with HCC have no morphologic evidence of cirrhosis. Another study by Mittal and colleagues[60] noted that patients with NAFLD-related HCC were 5-fold more likely than patients with HCV-related HCC to have developed HCC in the absence of cirrhosis.

Beyond its frequency in noncirrhotic livers, NAFLD-related HCC typically presents differently than HCC related to other causes, occurring as a large solitary mass that is moderately to well differentiated.[57] NAFLD-related HCC is more likely to present at a later stage than HCV-related HCC.[58,59] The late presentation of NAFLD-related HCC relative to HCV-related HCC is thought to be secondary to delayed diagnosis of HCC in patients with NAFLD who, as a population, are under suboptimal HCC surveillance compared with the population of patients with hepatitis or alcohol-related liver disease.[58,59,61] The American Association for the Study of Liver Diseases' guidelines recommend that all patients with cirrhosis, regardless of cause, should undergo screening for HCC every 6 months.[62] HCC screening is most commonly performed using ultrasound. However, given the frequency with which HCC occurs in the noncirrhotic livers of patients with NAFLD, further research will be important to establish optimal screening protocols for all patients with NAFLD.

REFERENCES

1. Patel V, Sanyal AJ, Sterling R. Clinical presentation and patient evaluation in nonalcoholic fatty liver disease. Clin Liver Dis 2016;20(2):277–92.
2. Lee SS, Park SH. Radiologic evaluation of nonalcoholic fatty liver disease. World J Gastroenterol 2014;20(23):7392–402.
3. Marengo A, Jouness RI, Bugianesi E. Progression and natural history of nonalcoholic fatty liver disease in adults. Clin Liver Dis 2016;20(2):313–24.
4. Bellentani S. The epidemiology of non-alcoholic fatty liver disease. Liver Int 2017; 37(Suppl 1):81–4.
5. Ekstedt M, Franzen LE, Mathiesen UL, et al. Long-term follow-up of patients with NAFLD and elevated liver enzymes. Hepatology 2006;44(4):865–73.
6. Soderberg C, Stal P, Askling J, et al. Decreased survival of subjects with elevated liver function tests during a 28-year follow-up. Hepatology 2010;51(2):595–602.
7. Younossi ZM, Stepanova M, Rafiq N, et al. Pathologic criteria for nonalcoholic steatohepatitis: interprotocol agreement and ability to predict liver-related mortality. Hepatology 2011;53(6):1874–82.
8. Vuppalanchi R, Unalp A, Van Natta ML, et al. Effects of liver biopsy sample length and number of readings on sampling variability in nonalcoholic fatty liver disease. Clin Gastroenterol Hepatol 2009;7(4):481–6.
9. Ma X, Holalkere NS, Kambadakone RA, et al. Imaging-based quantification of hepatic fat: methods and clinical applications. Radiographics 2009;29(5):1253–77.
10. Hertzberg BS, Middleton WD. Ultrasound: the requisites. Philadelphia: Elsevier - Health Sciences Division; 2015.

11. Bril F, Ortiz-Lopez C, Lomonaco R, et al. Clinical value of liver ultrasound for the diagnosis of nonalcoholic fatty liver disease in overweight and obese patients. Liver Int 2015;35(9):2139–46.

12. de Moura Almeida A, Cotrim HP, Barbosa DB, et al. Fatty liver disease in severe obese patients: diagnostic value of abdominal ultrasound. World J Gastroenterol 2008;14(9):1415–8.

13. Hernaez R, Lazo M, Bonekamp S, et al. Diagnostic accuracy and reliability of ultrasonography for the detection of fatty liver: a meta-analysis. Hepatology 2011; 54(3):1082–90.

14. Lee SS, Park SH, Kim HJ, et al. Non-invasive assessment of hepatic steatosis: prospective comparison of the accuracy of imaging examinations. J Hepatol 2010;52(4):579–85.

15. Palmentieri B, de Sio I, La Mura V, et al. The role of bright liver echo pattern on ultrasound B-mode examination in the diagnosis of liver steatosis. Dig Liver Dis 2006;38(7):485–9.

16. van Werven JR, Marsman HA, Nederveen AJ, et al. Assessment of hepatic steatosis in patients undergoing liver resection: comparison of US, CT, T1-weighted dual-echo MR imaging, and point-resolved 1H MR spectroscopy. Radiology 2010;256(1):159–68.

17. Saadeh S, Younossi ZM, Remer EM, et al. The utility of radiological imaging in nonalcoholic fatty liver disease. Gastroenterology 2002;123(3):745–50.

18. Strauss S, Gavish E, Gottlieb P, et al. Interobserver and intraobserver variability in the sonographic assessment of fatty liver. AJR Am J Roentgenol 2007;189(6): W320–3.

19. Webb M, Yeshua H, Zelber-Sagi S, et al. Diagnostic value of a computerized hepatorenal index for sonographic quantification of liver steatosis. AJR Am J Roentgenol 2009;192(4):909–14.

20. Marshall RH, Eissa M, Bluth EI, et al. Hepatorenal index as an accurate, simple, and effective tool in screening for steatosis. AJR Am J Roentgenol 2012;199(5): 997–1002.

21. Hamer OW, Aguirre DA, Casola G, et al. Fatty liver: imaging patterns and pitfalls. Radiographics 2006;26(6):1637–53.

22. Lee SW, Park SH, Kim KW, et al. Unenhanced CT for assessment of macrovesicular hepatic steatosis in living liver donors: comparison of visual grading with liver attenuation index. Radiology 2007;244(2):479–85.

23. Limanond P, Raman SS, Lassman C, et al. Macrovesicular hepatic steatosis in living related liver donors: correlation between CT and histologic findings. Radiology 2004;230(1):276–80.

24. Park SH, Kim PN, Kim KW, et al. Macrovesicular hepatic steatosis in living liver donors: use of CT for quantitative and qualitative assessment. Radiology 2006; 239(1):105–12.

25. Boyce CJ, Pickhardt PJ, Kim DH, et al. Hepatic steatosis (fatty liver disease) in asymptomatic adults identified by unenhanced low-dose CT. AJR Am J Roentgenol 2010;194(3):623–8.

26. Lawrence DA, Oliva IB, Israel GM. Detection of hepatic steatosis on contrast-enhanced CT images: diagnostic accuracy of identification of areas of presumed focal fatty sparing. AJR Am J Roentgenol 2012;199(1):44–7.

27. Kodama Y, Ng CS, Wu TT, et al. Comparison of CT methods for determining the fat content of the liver. AJR Am J Roentgenol 2007;188(5):1307–12.

28. Pickhardt PJ, Park SH, Hahn L, et al. Specificity of unenhanced CT for non-invasive diagnosis of hepatic steatosis: implications for the investigation of the natural history of incidental steatosis. Eur Radiol 2012;22(5):1075–82.

29. Panicek DM, Giess CS, Schwartz LH. Qualitative assessment of liver for fatty infiltration on contrast-enhanced CT: is muscle a better standard of reference than spleen? J Comput Assist Tomogr 1997;21(5):699–705.

30. d'Assignies G, Ruel M, Khiat A, et al. Noninvasive quantitation of human liver steatosis using magnetic resonance and bioassay methods. Eur Radiol 2009; 19(8):2033–40.

31. Dulai PS, Sirlin CB, Loomba R. MRI and MRE for non-invasive quantitative assessment of hepatic steatosis and fibrosis in NAFLD and NASH: clinical trials to clinical practice. J Hepatol 2016;65(5):1006–16.

32. Tang A, Tan J, Sun M, et al. Nonalcoholic fatty liver disease: MR imaging of liver proton density fat fraction to assess hepatic steatosis. Radiology 2013;267(2): 422–31.

33. Kovanlikaya A, Guclu C, Desai C, et al. Fat quantification using three-point Dixon technique: in vitro validation. Acad Radiol 2005;12(5):636–9.

34. Lee SS, Lee Y, Kim N, et al. Hepatic fat quantification using chemical shift MR imaging and MR spectroscopy in the presence of hepatic iron deposition: validation in phantoms and in patients with chronic liver disease. J Magn Reson Imaging 2011;33(6):1390–8.

35. Yokoo T, Bydder M, Hamilton G, et al. Nonalcoholic fatty liver disease: diagnostic and fat-grading accuracy of low-flip-angle multiecho gradient-recalled-echo MR imaging at 1.5 T. Radiology 2009;251(1):67–76.

36. Yokoo T, Shiehmorteza M, Hamilton G, et al. Estimation of hepatic proton-density fat fraction by using MR imaging at 3.0 T. Radiology 2011;258(3):749–59.

37. Fischer MA, Raptis DA, Montani M, et al. Liver fat quantification by dual-echo MR imaging outperforms traditional histopathological analysis. Acad Radiol 2012; 19(10):1208–14.

38. Raptis DA, Fischer MA, Graf R, et al. MRI: the new reference standard in quantifying hepatic steatosis? Gut 2012;61(1):117–27.

39. Noureddin M, Lam J, Peterson MR, et al. Utility of magnetic resonance imaging versus histology for quantifying changes in liver fat in nonalcoholic fatty liver disease trials. Hepatology 2013;58(6):1930–40.

40. Le TA, Chen J, Changchien C, et al. Effect of colesevelam on liver fat quantified by magnetic resonance in nonalcoholic steatohepatitis: a randomized controlled trial. Hepatology 2012;56(3):922–32.

41. Stal P. Liver fibrosis in non-alcoholic fatty liver disease - diagnostic challenge with prognostic significance. World J Gastroenterol 2015;21(39):11077–87.

42. Jayakumar S, Harrison SA, Loomba R. Noninvasive markers of fibrosis and inflammation in nonalcoholic fatty liver disease. Curr Hepatol Rep 2016;15(2): 86–95.

43. Musso G, Gambino R, Cassader M, et al. Meta-analysis: natural history of non-alcoholic fatty liver disease (NAFLD) and diagnostic accuracy of non-invasive tests for liver disease severity. Ann Med 2011;43(8):617–49.

44. Barr RG, Ferraioli G, Palmeri ML, et al. Elastography assessment of liver fibrosis: society of radiologists in ultrasound consensus conference statement. Radiology 2015;276(3):845–61.

45. Liu H, Fu J, Hong R, et al. Acoustic radiation force impulse elastography for the non-invasive evaluation of hepatic fibrosis in non-alcoholic fatty liver disease patients: a systematic review & meta-analysis. PLoS One 2015;10(7):e0127782.

46. Yoneda M, Suzuki K, Kato S, et al. Nonalcoholic fatty liver disease: US-based acoustic radiation force impulse elastography. Radiology 2010;256(2):640–7.
47. Festi D, Schiumerini R, Marzi L, et al. Review article: the diagnosis of non-alcoholic fatty liver disease – availability and accuracy of non-invasive methods. Aliment Pharmacol Ther 2013;37(4):392–400.
48. Palmeri ML, Wang MH, Rouze NC, et al. Noninvasive evaluation of hepatic fibrosis using acoustic radiation force-based shear stiffness in patients with nonalcoholic fatty liver disease. J Hepatol 2011;55(3):666–72.
49. Friedrich-Rust M, Romen D, Vermehren J, et al. Acoustic radiation force impulse-imaging and transient elastography for non-invasive assessment of liver fibrosis and steatosis in NAFLD. Eur J Radiol 2012;81(3):e325–31.
50. Cui J, Heba E, Hernandez C, et al. Magnetic resonance elastography is superior to acoustic radiation force impulse for the diagnosis of fibrosis in patients with biopsy-proven nonalcoholic fatty liver disease: a prospective study. Hepatology 2016;63(2):453–61.
51. Tan CH, Venkatesh SK. Magnetic resonance elastography and other magnetic resonance imaging techniques in chronic liver disease: current status and future directions. Gut Liver 2016;10(5):672–86.
52. Singh S, Venkatesh SK, Loomba R, et al. Magnetic resonance elastography for staging liver fibrosis in non-alcoholic fatty liver disease: a diagnostic accuracy systematic review and individual participant data pooled analysis. Eur Radiol 2016;26(5):1431–40.
53. Runge JH, Bohte AE, Verheij J, et al. Comparison of interobserver agreement of magnetic resonance elastography with histopathological staging of liver fibrosis. Abdom Imaging 2014;39(2):283–90.
54. Imajo K, Kessoku T, Honda Y, et al. Magnetic resonance imaging more accurately classifies steatosis and fibrosis in patients with nonalcoholic fatty liver disease than transient elastography. Gastroenterology 2016;150(3):626–37.e7.
55. Park CC, Nguyen P, Hernandez C, et al. Magnetic resonance elastography vs transient elastography in detection of fibrosis and noninvasive measurement of steatosis in patients with biopsy-proven nonalcoholic fatty liver disease. Gastro-enterology 2017;152(3):598–607.e2.
56. Taouli B, Serfaty L. Magnetic resonance imaging/elastography is superior to tran-sient elastography for detection of liver fibrosis and fat in nonalcoholic fatty liver disease. Gastroenterology 2016;150(3):553–6.
57. Baffy G, Brunt EM, Caldwell SH. Hepatocellular carcinoma in non-alcoholic fatty liver disease: an emerging menace. J Hepatol 2012;56(6):1384–91.
58. Wong CR, Nguyen MH, Lim JK. Hepatocellular carcinoma in patients with non-alcoholic fatty liver disease. World J Gastroenterol 2016;22(37):8294–303.
59. Piscaglia F, Svegliati-Baroni G, Barchetti A, et al. Clinical patterns of hepatocellu-lar carcinoma in nonalcoholic fatty liver disease: a multicenter prospective study. Hepatology 2016;63(3):827–38.
60. Mittal S, El-Serag HB, Sada YH, et al. Hepatocellular carcinoma in the absence of cirrhosis in United States veterans is associated with nonalcoholic fatty liver dis-ease. Clin Gastroenterol Hepatol 2016;14(1):124–31.e1.
61. Mittal S, Sada YH, El-Serag HB, et al. Temporal trends of nonalcoholic fatty liver disease-related hepatocellular carcinoma in the veteran affairs population. Clin Gastroenterol Hepatol 2015;13(3):594–601.e1.
62. Margini C, Dufour JF. The story of HCC in NAFLD: from epidemiology, across pathogenesis, to prevention and treatment. Liver Int 2016;36(3):317–24.

The Use of Liver Biopsy in Nonalcoholic Fatty Liver Disease: When to Biopsy and in Whom

Nadege T. Gunn, MD[a], Mitchell L. Shiffman, MD[b,c],*

KEYWORDS

- Nonalcoholic fatty liver disease • Nonalcoholic steatohepatitis • Liver biopsy
- Elastography

KEY POINTS

- Liver biopsy remains the gold standard for the diagnosis of nonalcoholic fatty liver and is currently the only modality that can reliably differentiate benign fatty liver from nonalcoholic steatohepatitis.
- Liver biopsy remains a valuable tool for the assessment of liver disease progression or regression in patients with nonalcoholic steatohepatitis.
- Liver biopsy is the only tool that can correctly differentiate which process may be causing liver injury in patients with clinical features of the metabolic syndrome and serologic markers of another liver disorder.

INTRODUCTION

Nonalcoholic fatty liver disease (NAFLD) is the most common cause of liver disease worldwide.[1] NAFLD is most commonly observed in persons with obesity and the metabolic syndrome. In the United States, approximately one-third of persons are obese, approximately one-third of obese persons have NAFLD, and approximately one-third of persons with NAFLD have nonalcoholic steatohepatitis (NASH). This amount represents about 100, 33, and 11 million persons, respectively. NAFLD is

Disclosure Statement: Dr N.T. Gunn has received research grant support from Conatus, Cyma-Bay, Galectin, Gilead, and Immuron and has received speaker fees from Abbvie, Gilead, and Salix. Dr M.L. Shiffman receives research grant support from Abbvie, BMS, Conatus, CymaBay, Exalenz, Galectin, Genfit, Gilead, Intercept, Immuron, Merck, NGMBio, Novartis, and Shire; is an advisor to Abbvie, BMS, Gilead, Merck, Optum Rx, and Salix; and has received speaker fees from Abbvie, Bayer, BMS, Daiichi-Sankyo, Gilead, Intercept, and Merck.
[a] Pinnacle Clinical Research, 2001 Bee Caves Road, Suite 220, Rollingwood, TX 78746, USA;
[b] Liver Institute of Virginia, Bon Secours Health System, Newport News, VA, USA; [c] Liver Institute of Virginia, Bon Secours Health System, 5885 Bremo Road, Suite 509, Richmond, VA 23226, USA
* Corresponding author. 5885 Bremo Road, Suite 509, Richmond, VA 23226.
E-mail address: Mitchell_Shiffman@bshsi.org

Clin Liver Dis 22 (2018) 109–119
http://dx.doi.org/10.1016/j.cld.2017.08.006
1089-3261/18/© 2017 Elsevier Inc. All rights reserved.

liver.theclinics.com

suspected in persons with elevated liver transaminases when imaging (either ultrasound, computerized tomography [CT], or MRI) suggests fatty liver, serologic studies for all other causes of chronic liver disease are negative, patients have features of metabolic syndrome, and the clinical history suggests patients do not consume excessive amounts of alcohol.[2] However, the diagnosis of NAFLD, and especially that of NASH, can only be confirmed by histologic assessment of liver tissue. NAFLD is present when there is greater than 5% steatosis in the liver histologic specimen in the absence of excessive alcohol consumption.[3] NASH requires the presence of steatosis, inflammation, and ballooning of hepatocytes by steatosis.[4]

Noninvasive testing can be useful in predicting that patients suspected of having NAFLD have significant fibrosis and, therefore, NASH. These tests include scoring systems that are based on clinical findings and readily available biochemical tests.[5,6] Vibration controlled transient elastography (VCTE) with the controlled attenuation parameter (CAP) or shear wave elastography can assess liver stiffness and suggest this is due to NAFLD.[7–10] Imaging modalities, such as ultrasound and CT scan can suggest that patients have fatty liver; MRI can quantitate steatosis; and magnetic resonance (MR) elastography can assess liver stiffness, which in most situations reflects hepatic fibrosis.[4,11–14] However, neither ultrasound nor CT can determine if patients actually have NASH. In addition, the various scoring systems, elastography, and MRI techniques that attempt to diagnose NASH base this distinction on the assessment of fibrosis and presume that patients with suspected NAFLD and fibrosis have NASH. In reality, none of these tests can determine if liver injury and fibrosis is really due to NAFLD or to another coexistent liver disorder.

When to perform a liver biopsy in patients with suspected fatty liver remains controversial because no medication is available now to treat NAFLD when it is identified. Clinical guidelines suggest that only those patients who are suspected of having NASH based on clinical features, noninvasive testing, and imaging should undergo liver biopsy.[15,16] Clinicians are, therefore, often left debating the need for biopsy with their patients because, in the absence of enrolling in a clinical trial, the only treatment of NAFLD is dietary modification and weight reduction; clearly, patients do not need to undergo a liver biopsy in order to diet or lose weight.

This article discusses the role of liver biopsy in the management of patients with NAFLD and identifies which patients with NAFLD might benefit from liver biopsy and why. The role of noninvasive testing in patients suspected of having NAFLD and how these tests can be used to select patients who may benefit from biopsy are discussed. Finally, the pros, cons, and limitations of liver biopsy are also reviewed.

NATURAL HISTORY AND CLINICAL FEATURES OF NONALCOHOLIC FATTY LIVER DISEASE

NAFLD can be divided into 2 categories: benign steatosis, also referred to as isolated fatty liver or NAFL, and NASH. NAFL is present in about 66% to 80% of patients with NAFLD.[1,2,4] Long-term studies have demonstrated that patients with NAFL have less than a 1% chance of developing fibrosis progression to cirrhosis or liver-related mortality over 15 years.[17–21] Long-term survival is similar to that of the general population. In contrast, 20% to 33% of patients with NAFLD have NASH.[1,2,4] Patients with NASH have an 11% risk of developing progressive fibrosis, cirrhosis, hepatic decompensation, and liver cancer and a 7% risk of both liver-related and all-cause mortality over 15 years from the time of diagnosis.[17–21] The presence of fibrosis in patients with NAFLD is also associated with increased mortality regardless of whether or not patients have other histologic features of NASH. Given the increased risk of both morbidity and mortality associated with NASH and hepatic fibrosis, it seems prudent to determine on which end of the spectrum patients with NAFLD may reside. A liver biopsy may be required to determine if patients have NAFL or NASH.

Most patients with NAFLD have features of the metabolic syndrome, obesity, hypertension, dyslipidemia, and type 2 diabetes mellitus (T2DM). The more features of the metabolic syndrome patients have, the more likely they are to have NAFLD.[1,2,4] Patients with all 5 features of the metabolic syndrome have a 90% likelihood of having NAFLD.[22] However, neither the number of features of metabolic syndrome nor absolute body mass index (BMI) correlates with the severity of NAFLD. The strongest predictor of having NASH seems to be the combination of elevated liver transaminases and T2DM, which is associated with a 3.5-fold increased risk of having stage 3 to 4 fibrosis.[23,24] Thus, if the goal of liver biopsy is to identify patients with NASH, then patients with elevated liver transaminases and T2DM should be considered for liver biopsy.

In the past, we thought that NAFL and NASH acted as different diseases and patients either had NAFL or NASH.[1,2,4] We have recently realized that fatty liver is actually a continuum and that patients can histologically move between NAFL and NASH.[25] The only factor that seems to be associated with this is body weight. Patients with NAFL can develop NASH if they gain weight. Patients with NASH will regress to NAFL with weight loss. Other features of metabolic syndrome do not seem to have any significant impact on histologic changes in NAFLD but may also be impacted by changes in body weight. Performing a liver biopsy in patients who have had a marked change in body weight may, therefore, be important to ensure that NASH has regressed to NAFL or, more importantly, if NAFL has progressed to NASH.

Approximately 10% of persons with NASH have normal body weight.[1,26] Because diet and weight reduction is not a therapeutic option for patients with NASH and a normal BMI, performing a liver biopsy to determine whether these patients have NAFL or NASH also seems important.

RECOGNITION OF PATIENTS WITH NONALCOHOLIC FATTY LIVER DISEASE

An elevation in serum liver transaminases, either aspartate transaminase (AST) and/or alanine transaminase (ALT), is often the first hint that patients may have NAFLD. Serologic studies should be performed in such patients to exclude all other causes of chronic liver disease. NAFLD is suspected when all serologic studies are negative. However, many patients with NAFLD may have a moderate elevation in serum ferritin, some have a positive antinuclear (ANA) smooth muscle antibody (ASMA), and others may be heterozygotes for alpha-1-antitrypsin deficiency and have a somewhat low serum level of the enzyme.[27–29] In addition, approximately 20% of persons with autoimmune liver disease do not have positive serologic markers.[30] Performing a liver biopsy is the only way to confirm that these patients have NAFLD and that the elevation in liver transaminases is secondary to NAFLD. In 354 subjects with unexplained elevations in liver enzymes, 66% were found to have NAFLD on liver biopsy. However, 19% of these patients were found to have another treatable cause of chronic liver disease and 15% had either a normal liver biopsy or nonspecific findings.[31,32] Thus, simply assuming that patients have NAFLD instead of performing a liver biopsy for confirmation would misclassify up to 33% of patients with unexplained elevations in liver transaminases.

Assessing liver transaminases is not helpful in determining if patients with NAFLD have NAFL or NASH. Patients with NASH tend to have higher levels of liver transaminases than patients with NAFL. However, up to 60% of patients with NASH have persistently or intermittently normal liver transaminases; more than half of patients with NAFL have elevated liver transaminases.[33,34]

Another common way in which patients are found to have NAFLD is when ultrasonography is performed for evaluation of right upper quadrant abdominal pain or other abdominal symptoms. The most common ultrasound descriptions include *increased echogenicity consistent with fatty liver* or *changes consistent with hepatic steatosis*. However, the authors have also seen ultrasound reports stating *increased echogenicity suggestive of NAFLD* and *increased echogenicity consistent with NASH*. Unfortunately, increased echogenicity is a nonspecific finding that can be seen in any chronic liver disease. Fatty liver does give a very fine granular appearance to the liver, but this is not specific for NAFLD, does not allow for quantification of the degree of fat within the liver, and cannot differentiate alcoholic fatty liver from NAFL or NASH.[5] Radiologists should, therefore, refrain from making a histologic diagnosis based on nonspecific ultrasonographic findings. Such reports enable physicians to presume patients have NAFLD rather than performing a complete evaluation to identify the correct cause for the abnormal liver ultrasound. Previous studies have demonstrated that an isolated ultrasound report suggesting NAFLD in the absence of biochemical, serologic, and clinical data has a sensitivity of about 60% to 94% and a positive predictive value of 83% to 94%. When all other causes of chronic liver disease have been excluded by serologic testing, and alcohol has been excluded by history, the positive predictive value of NAFLD by ultrasound increases to about 80%. In a study whereby apparently healthy persons were found to have NAFLD by ultrasound, 18% had clinically insignificant steatosis (<5%) and another 3% had normal liver histology.[32]

Ultrasonography does not identify all persons with NAFLD. In a study in which 70 apparently healthy persons being evaluated as donors for living liver transplantation underwent liver biopsy, NAFLD was identified in 37% even though these patients had a normal liver ultrasound.[35] Seventy percent of these patients had less than 33% steatosis. However, 18% and 11% had grades 2 and 3 steatosis, respectively. Only 1 out of 22 patients with NAFLD and a normal liver ultrasound had NASH. In another study in which patients with normal liver transaminases underwent liver biopsy, 25% of patients with NASH had a normal liver ultrasound.[36]

NONINVASIVE MARKERS OF NONALCOHOLIC FATTY LIVER DISEASE

Once patients are suspected of having NAFLD, several noninvasive tests can be used to help confirm this is correct and to determine if this is NAFL or NASH. Cytokeratin (CK)-18 is a serum marker that is increased in patients with hepatocyte apoptosis and is thought to be relatively specific for NASH as opposed to being a general marker of apoptosis from other forms of chronic liver disease. Elevations in CK-18 greater than 210 u/L are suggestive of NASH.[32,37] Unfortunately, CK-18 is not a laboratory test that is readily available for routine clinical care. Various scoring systems have also been developed that assess the likelihood patients may have NASH. These systems are all based on various clinical findings and readily available biochemical tests and include the BARD score (includes BMI, AST/ALT ratio, presence or absence of diabetes), NAFLD fibrosis score (includes age, BMI, presence of absence of insulin resistance or diabetes, AST, ALT and serum albumin), and FIB-4 (includes age AST, ALT, and platelet count). Each of these tests provides a cutoff value greater than which patients with NAFLD have about an 80% chance of having significant fibrosis and, therefore, NASH.[5,6,38–40] The sensitivity of these tests to predict NASH with milder fibrosis is significantly lower.

VCTE (FibroScan, Echosens, Waltham, MA) can assess liver stiffness and is reported in kilopascals. In most cases, elevations in kilopascals are due to increased hepatic fibrosis.[5–7] The controlled attenuation parameter (CAP) assesses the degree of hepatic steatosis; in most cases, an elevation in CAP is due to increasing hepatic steatosis.[10] Patients with CAP values greater than 300 and liver stiffness greater than 7 kPa have a 90% chance of having NASH. Even without CAP, high values for VCTE or shear wave elastography in patients suspected of having NALFD suggests that patients have NASH. Patients with NALFD and obesity frequently have wide variation in the kilopascals values obtained with VCTE or shear wave elastography with a high interquartile range greater than 30% and a high standard error. The mean values obtained in these situations may be unreliable in predicting the degree of hepatic fibrosis.[41,42]

Advanced imaging modalities, such as MRI, can be used to quantitate the amount of hepatic steatosis by protein density fat fraction (PDFF); MR elastography (MRE) can assess hepatic fibrosis.[13,14,43] Values for both PDFF and MRE have been shown to closely correlate with the percent steatosis and the degree of fibrosis seen in a liver biopsy. Quantification of steatosis fibrosis by PDFF and MRE seem to be more accurate than with VCTE and CAP.[44] However, very few MRI scanners in the community are capable of performing PDFF and MRE. In addition, the cost of performing MRI for these purposes alone is unlikely to be funded by insurance carriers. As a result, these techniques will remain a research tool to monitor NAFLD in patients enrolled in clinical trials for the foreseeable future.

No pharmacologic therapy has been shown to be effective for patients with NAFLD and NASH. Selected patients can be enrolled in clinical trials to evaluate one of several promising therapies. Many of these therapies are discussed in Samer Gawrieh and Naga Chalasani's article, "Emerging Treatments for Nonalcoholic Fatty Liver Disease and Nonalcoholic Steatohepatitis," in this issue of *Clinics in Liver Disease*. Several of the noninvasive tests and imaging studies discussed earlier are being used to monitor the impact of these experimental medications in various clinical trials. In time, these studies will likely validate at least some of these tests and MRI techniques as being useful in the assessment of NAFLD and NASH. For now, a liver biopsy demonstrating NAFLD or NASH is required for enrollment in virtually all clinical trials and is the only technique that can reliably confirm that patients have NAFLD and whether this represents NAFL or NASH.[15,16]

WHAT IS LEARNED BY PERFORMING LIVER BIOPSY IN PATIENTS WITH SUSPECTED NONALCOHOLIC FATTY LIVER DISEASE

The goals of performing a liver biopsy in patients suspected of having NAFLD are to confirm this diagnosis, exclude other causes of chronic liver disease, determine if patients have NAFL or NASH, and to demonstrate if patients have cirrhosis. A diagnosis of NAFLD requires that there is at last 5% steatosis in the liver biopsy specimen.[1–3] The NAFLD Activity Score (NAS) is a useful system to assess liver injury in patients with NAFLD and response to therapy for patients enrolled in clinical trials.[45,46] According to this system, steatosis is graded as 1 to 3, with each grade representing 5% to 33%, 33% to 66%, and greater than 66% steatosis, respectively. Inflammation is graded 0 to 3 (none, mild, moderate, or severe) and ballooning is graded as 0 to 2 (none, mild, or severe). An NAS score of 4 with a score of at least 1 point in each of the 3 categories (steatosis, inflammation, and ballooning) is required for the diagnosis of NASH.[47] Fibrosis in patients with NAFLD is staged separately (0–4) and not included in the NAS score. In general, fibrosis staging in NAFLD is similar to that for other types of liver diseases: none, portal, portal with short septa extending into the hepatic parenchyma, bridging, and cirrhosis, respectively.[45,46] Patients with pericellular fibrosis are generally given a fibrosis stage of 2.

It is not absolutely necessary for pathologists to provide NAS and fibrosis scores in patients found to have NAFLD on liver biopsy. However, it is extremely useful for the clinician who has to manage patients with NAFLD to have a description of the NAFLD histology, which includes the percent steatosis, degree of inflammation, whether ballooning is present or not, and the stage of fibrosis. Pathology reports simply stating *fatty liver consistent with NAFLD* or *NASH with pericellular fibrosis* without this information does not help the clinician counsel patients regarding the severity of their disease, the risk they may progress to cirrhosis, or to know if patients might be eligible for enrollment into a clinical trial. It is, therefore, important to discuss these issues with your pathology colleagues if this information is not being provided.

It is not uncommon to find persons with serologic markers for other forms of chronic liver disease to also be obese and have features of the metabolic syndrome. Liver biopsy is essential to determine the actual cause for liver disease in these patients. For example, patients with several features of metabolic syndrome and a family history of immune disorders with or without a positive ANA or ASMA could have NAFLD, autoimmune liver disease, or both disorders. An elevation in ferritin is common in persons with NAFLD and does not typically represent hepatic iron overload.[27,28] However, marked elevations in ferritin and iron saturation in patients with metabolic syndrome and an abnormal liver ultrasound could be from iron overload, NAFLD, or both disorders. Patients with chronic hepatitis B virus (HBV) or hepatitis C virus (HCV) now only rarely undergo liver biopsy before initiating antiviral therapy. Patients with chronic HBV or HCV who continue to have a persistent elevation in liver transaminases despite effective antiviral therapy and viral suppression or eradication need to be evaluated for coexistent liver disorders, including NALFD.[48]

IN WHOM AND WHEN SHOULD A LIVER BIOPSY BE PERFORMED

It is not necessary to perform a liver biopsy in all patients suspected of having NAFLD.[15,16] A liver biopsy should only be performed if it will alter your treatment recommendations for patients, make patients aware they have a serious liver condition, or to confirm or exclude NAFLD in patients with conflicting clinical data. The data that you should use to decide on whether to perform a liver biopsy include liver transaminases, liver ultrasound, serologic studies for other causes of liver disease, and whether patients have features of metabolic syndrome or are overweight and, if so, whether there is a commitment to lose weight. For example, an obese patient with multiple clinical features of metabolic syndrome, an ultrasound suggesting fatty liver with negative serologic testing for all other causes of chronic liver disease, a low value for liver stiffness by one of the many fibrosis scoring systems or elastography, and who claims to be committed to modifying his or her diet and losing weight does not require a liver biopsy. Rather, this patient can be monitored at periodic intervals to see if he or she achieves weight reduction. If this patient is not successful, a biopsy can be performed at some point in the future to confirm NAFLD and determine if the patient has NAFL or NASH. In contrast, an obese patient with T2DM, elevated liver transaminases, an ultrasound suggesting fatty liver, and a family history of immune disorders but negative serologic studies for autoimmune liver disease probably needs a liver biopsy to determine if this is NAFLD or an autoimmune liver disorder.

Box 1 lists factors whereby a biopsy would be useful in patients suspected of having NAFLD and others whereby a biopsy could be deferred with monitoring. In general, you should consider performing a liver biopsy when you suspect patients have

---

Box 1
Clinical scenarios in patients suspected of having nonalcoholic fatty liver disease where a liver biopsy is useful or can be deferred

Liver biopsy now: likely to find NASH or be useful in patient management:
    All features of metabolic syndrome and obesity
    T2DM and elevated liver transaminases
    Normal BMI with elevated liver transaminases
    Elastography greater than 6 kPa
    Elevated value with a fibrosis scoring system
    Reliable elastography value cannot be obtained because of obesity
    Patients are not motivated to lose weight

Liver biopsy deferred: likely to find NAFL or not be useful in patient management:
    Two or fewer features of metabolic syndrome
    Normal liver transaminases and absence of T2DM
    Elastography less than 6 kPa
    Low value with a fibrosis scoring system
    Patients are motivated to lose weight

NASH. Although there is currently no defined treatment of NASH, a biopsy demonstrating NASH may be the motivating factor patients require to change their diet and lifestyle and lose weight. Patients who are motivated to diet and lose weight may wish to defer liver biopsy. These patients should be monitored to see if weight loss does occur and, if not, liver biopsy can be performed at a later date. The goal for weight reduction would be to lose about 10% of body weight.[49] A liver biopsy should also be considered in patients when you suspect NASH based on clinical features but the elastography cannot obtain a reproducible value. A biopsy demonstrating NASH enables motivated patients to enroll in a clinical trial to assess an experimental medical therapy for NASH. If advanced fibrosis or cirrhosis is identified, then screening for hepatocellular carcinoma can be implemented.

A liver biopsy is not needed in patients you strongly suspect have NAFL. Elastography can be very useful in deciding which patients are likely to have NAFL and can avoid liver biopsy.[50,51] Patients with an elastography value less than 6 kPa have none or minimal fibrosis and are, therefore, likely to have NAFL and can simply be monitored as illustrated in **Fig. 1**. If these patients do not lose weight, the authors

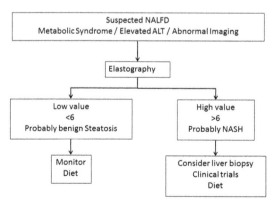

Fig. 1. Algorithm for evaluation of patients with suspected NAFLD to determine who is likely to have NASH and undergo liver biopsy for confirmation.

would recommend repeat elastography every 1 to 2 years to ensure they have not developed NASH and fibrosis.

When performing a liver biopsy, it is important to obtain an adequate tissue specimen. Unfortunately, most liver biopsies are now performed by radiologists who frequently use thin-gauge needles that may make it difficult to assess the degree of fibrosis if the specimen is of insufficient length or fragmented.[52] Liver biopsy does have a small but real risk of complications, including pneumothorax and pain. Significant bleeding occurs in less than 0.3% of persons with a normal platelet count and clotting factors.[53] Variations in how liver biopsy specimens are interpreted by pathologists also occurs. NAS scores may vary by 1 to 2 points even with expert liver pathologists, and fibrosis scores may vary by 1 point in up to 30% to 40% of patients.[54,55]

SUMMARY

NAFLD is common in the United States and throughout the world and leads to cirrhosis in a significant percentage of patients. Most patients with NAFLD are identified because they are found to have a liver ultrasound or other imaging study suggesting fatty liver with or without an elevation in liver transaminases. A presumptive diagnosis of NAFLD is correct once other causes of chronic liver disease have been excluded with appropriate serologic testing. NAFLD can exist as NAFL, which does not seem to cause liver injury, or as NASH, which can cause progressive fibrosis and progress to cirrhosis. Changes in body weight can lead patients to shift between NAFL and NASH. Noninvasive tests that assess fibrosis can suggest that patients have NAFL or NASH. Elastography, using either VCTE or shear wave ultrasound, seems to be the best way to make this distinction in clinical practice. Patients with NAFL should have none of minimal fibrosis. Liver biopsy is currently the only reliable method to confirm NAFLD and to determine if this is NAFL or NASH. However, because no medical therapy is currently available, it is not always necessary to perform a liver biopsy for diagnosis of NAFLD. The authors think that patients with clinical features and noninvasive testing suggesting NASH should undergo liver biopsy to confirm this diagnosis. This biopsy will provide confirmation to patients that they have a serious liver disease and that lifestyle changes are important.

REFERENCES

1. Yilmaz Y, Younossi ZM. Obesity-associated nonalcoholic fatty liver disease. Clin Liver Dis 2014;18:19–31.
2. Lazo M, Clark JM. The epidemiology of nonalcoholic fatty liver disease: a global perspective. Semin Liver Dis 2008;28:339–50.
3. Kleiner DE, Makhlouf HR. Histology of nonalcoholic fatty liver disease and nonalcoholic steatohepatitis in adults and children. Clin Liver Dis 2016;20:293–312.
4. Paredes AH, Torres DM, Harrison SA. Nonalcoholic fatty liver disease. Clin Liver Dis 2012;16:397–419.
5. Grandison GA, Angulo P. Can NASH be diagnosed, graded and staged non-invasively? Clin Liver Dis 2012;16:567–85.
6. Musso G, Gambino R, Cassader M, et al. Meta-analysis: natural history of nonalcoholic fatty liver disease (NAFLD) and diagnostic accuracy of non-invasive tests for liver disease severity. Ann Med 2011;43:617–49.
7. Myers RP, Pomier-Layrargues G, Kirsch R, et al. Feasibility and diagnostic performance of the FibroScan XL probe for liver stiffness measurement in overweight and obese patients. Hepatology 2012;55:199–208.

8. Palmeri ML, Wang MH, Rouze NC, et al. Noninvasive evaluation of hepatic fibrosis using acoustic radiation force-based shear stiffness in patients with nonalcoholic fatty liver disease. J Hepatol 2011;55:666–72.

9. Cassinotto C, Boursier J, de Ledinghen V, et al. Liver stiffness in nonalcoholic fatty liver disease: a comparison of supersonic shear imaging, Fibro Scan, and ARFI with liver biopsy. Hepatology 2016;63:1817–27.

10. de Lédinghen V, Wong GL, Vergniol J, et al. Controlled attenuation parameter for the diagnosis of steatosis in non-alcoholic fatty liver disease. J Gastroenterol Hepatol 2016;31:848–55.

11. Mottin CC, Moretto M, Padoin AV, et al. The role of ultrasound in the diagnosis of hepatic steatosis in morbidly obese patients. Obes Surg 2004;14:635–7.

12. Kodama Y, Ng CS, Wu TT, et al. Comparison of CT methods for determining the fat content of the liver. Am J Roentgenol 2007;188:1307–12.

13. Fishbein M, Castro F, Cheruku S, et al. Hepatic MRI for fat quantitation: its relationship to fat morphology, diagnosis, and ultrasound. J Clin Gastroenterol 2005;39:619–25.

14. Paige JS, Bernstein GS, Heba E, et al. A pilot comparative study of quantitative ultrasound, conventional ultrasound, and MRI for predicting histology-determined steatosis grade in adult nonalcoholic fatty liver disease. AJR Am J Roentgenol 2017;208:W168–77.

15. Chalasani N, Younossi Z, Lavine JE, et al. The diagnosis and management of non-alcoholic fatty liver disease: practice guideline by the American Gastroenterological Association, American Association for the Study of Liver Diseases, and American College of Gastroenterology. Gastroenterology 2012;142:1592–609.

16. Ratziu V, Bellentani S, Cortez-Pinto H, et al. A position statement on NAFLD/NASH based on the EASL 2009 special conference. J Hepatol 2010;53:372–84.

17. Younossi ZM, Stepanova M, Rafiq N, et al. Pathologic criteria for nonalcoholic steatohepatitis: interprotocol agreement and ability to predict liver-related mortality. Hepatology 2011;53:1874–82.

18. Singh S, Allen AM, Wang Z, et al. Fibrosis progression in nonalcoholic fatty liver vs nonalcoholic steatohepatitis: a systematic review and meta-analysis of paired biopsy studies. Clin Gastroenterol Hepatol 2015;13:643–54.

19. Angulo P, Kleiner DE, Dam-Larsen S, et al. Liver fibrosis but no other histologic features, is associated with long term outcomes of patients with non alcoholic fatty liver disease. Gastroenterology 2015;149:389–97.e10.

20. Ekstedt M, Franzen LE, Mathiesen UL, et al. Long-term follow up of patients with NAFLD and elevated liver enzymes. Hepatology 2006;44:865–73.

21. Ekstedt M, Hagstrom H, Nasr P, et al. Fibrosis stage is strongest predictor of disease specific mortality in NAFLD after up to 33 years of follow up. Hepatology 2015;61:1547–54.

22. Smits MM, Ioannou GN, Boyko EJ, et al. Non-alcoholic fatty liver disease as an independent manifestation of the metabolic syndrome: results of a US national survey in three ethnic groups. J Gastroenterol Hepatol 2013;28:664–70.

23. Marchesini G, Bugianesi E, Forlani G, et al. Nonalcoholic fatty liver, steatohepatitis, and the metabolic syndrome. Hepatology 2003;37:917–23.

24. Kanwar P, Kowdley KV. The metabolic syndrome and its influence on nonalcoholic steatohepatitis. Clin Liver Dis 2016;20:225–43.

25. Kleiner DE, Brunt EM, Belt PH, et al. Diagnostic pattern and disease activity are related to disease progression and regression in non-alcoholic fatty liver disease. Hepatology 2016;64(Suppl 1):19A.

26. Yilmaz Y. NAFLD in the absence of metabolic syndrome: different epidemiology, pathogenetic mechanisms, risk factors for disease progression? Semin Liver Dis 2012;32:14–21.

27. Manousou P, Kalambokis G, Grillo F, et al. Serum ferritin is a discriminant marker for both fibrosis and inflammation in histologically proven non-alcoholic fatty liver disease patients. Liver Int 2011;31:730–9.

28. Jehn M, Clark JM, Guallar E. Serum ferritin and risk of the metabolic syndrome in U.S. adults. Diabetes Care 2004;27:2422–8.

29. Cotler SJ, Kanji K, Keshavarzian A, et al. Prevalence and significance of autoantibodies in patients with non-alcoholic steatohepatitis. J Clin Gastroenterol 2004; 38:801–4.

30. Czaja AJ. Behavior and significance of autoantibodies in type 1 autoimmune hepatitis. J Hepatol 1999;30:394–401.

31. Skelly MM, James PD, Ryder SD. Findings on liver biopsy to investigate abnormal liver function tests in the absence of diagnostic serology. J Hepatol 2001;35: 195–9.

32. Williams CD, Stengel J, Asike MI, et al. Prevalence of nonalcoholic fatty liver disease and nonalcoholic steatohepatitis among a largely middle-aged population utilizing ultrasound and liver biopsy: a prospective study. Gastroenterology 2011;140:124–31.

33. Fracanzani AL, Valenti L, Bugianesi E, et al. Risks of severe liver disease in nonalcoholic fatty liver disease with normal aminotransferase levels: role for insulin resistance and diabetes. Hepatology 2008;48:792–8.

34. Verma S, Jensen D, Hart J, et al. Predicative value of ALT levels for non-alcoholic steatohepatitis (NASH). Liver Int 2013;33:1398–405.

35. Tran TT, Changsri C, Shackleton CR, et al. Living donor liver transplantation: histological abnormalities found on liver biopsies of apparently healthy potential donors. J Gastroenterol Hepatol 2006;21:381–3.

36. Mofrad P, Contos MJ, Haque M, et al. Clinical and histologic spectrum of nonalcoholic fatty liver disease associated with normal ALT values. Hepatology 2003; 37:1286–92.

37. Lebensztejn DM, Wierzbicka A, Socha P, et al. Cytokeratin-18 and hyaluronic acid levels predict liver fibrosis in children with non-alcoholic fatty liver disease. Acta Biochim Pol 2011;58:563–6.

38. Angulo P, Bugianesi E, Bjornsson ES, et al. Simple noninvasive systems predict long-term outcomes of patients with nonalcoholic fatty liver disease. Gastroenterology 2013;145:782–9.

39. Raszeja-Wyszomirska J, Szymanik B, Ławniczak M, et al. Validation of the BARD scoring system in Polish patients with nonalcoholic fatty liver disease (NAFLD). BMC Gastroenterol 2010;10:67–73.

40. Angulo P, Hui JM, Marchesini G, et al. The NAFLD fibrosis score. A noninvasive system that identifies liver fibrosis in patients with NAFLD. Hepatology 2007;45: 846–54.

41. Myers RP, Pomier-Layrargues G, Kirsch R, et al. Discordance in fibrosis staging between liver biopsy and transient elastography using the FibroScan XL probe. J Hepatol 2012;56:564–70.

42. Mahadeva S, Mahfudz AS, Vijayanathan A, et al. Performance of transient elastography (TE) and factors associated with discordance in non-alcoholic fatty liver disease. J Dig Dis 2013;14:604–10.

43. Dulai PS, Sirlin CB, Loomba R. MRI and MRE for non-invasive quantitative assessment of hepatic steatosis and fibrosis in NAFLD and NASH: clinical trials to clinical practice. J Hepatol 2016;65:1006–16.

44. Park CC, Nguyen P, Hernandez C, et al. Magnetic resonance elastography vs transient elastography in detection of fibrosis and noninvasive measurement of steatosis in patients with biopsy-proven nonalcoholic fatty liver disease. Gastroenterology 2017;152:598–607.

45. Brunt EM, Janney CG, Di Bisceglie AM, et al. Nonalcoholic steatohepatitis: a proposal for grading and staging the histological lesions. Am J Gastroenterol 1999; 94:2467–74.

46. Kleiner DE, Brunt EM, Van Natta M, et al. Design and validation of a histological scoring system for nonalcoholic fatty liver disease. Hepatology 2005;41:1313–21.

47. Brunt EM, Kleiner DE, Wilson LA, et al. Nonalcoholic fatty liver disease (NAFLD) activity score and the histopathologic diagnosis in NAFLD: distinct clinicopathologic meanings. Hepatology 2011;53:810–20.

48. Shiffman ML, Benhamou Y. Cure of HCV related disease. Liver Int 2015; 35(suppl 1):71–7.

49. Hannah WN Jr, Harrison SA. Effect of weight loss, diet, exercise, and bariatric surgery on nonalcoholic fatty liver disease. Clin Liver Dis 2016;20:339–50.

50. Boursier J, Vergniol J, Guillet A, et al. Diagnostic accuracy and prognostic significance of blood fibrosis tests and liver stiffness measurement by FibroScan in non-alcoholic fatty liver disease. J Hepatol 2016;65:570–8.

51. Tapper EB, Sengupta N, Hunink MG, et al. Cost-effective evaluation of nonalcoholic fatty liver disease with NAFLD fibrosis score and vibration controlled transient elastography. Am J Gastroenterol 2015;110:1298–304.

52. Colloredo G, Guido M, Sonzogni A, et al. Impact of liver biopsy size on the histological evaluation of chronic viral hepatitis: the smaller the sample, the milder the disease. J Hepatol 2003;39:239–44.

53. Piccinino F, Sagnelli E, Pasquale G, et al. Complications following percutaneous liver biopsy. A multicentre retrospective study on 68,276 biopsies. J Hepatol 1986;2:165–73.

54. Ratziu V, Charlotte F, Heurtier A, et al. Sampling variability of liver biopsy in nonalcoholic fatty liver disease. Gastroenterology 2005;128:1898–906.

55. Janiec DJ, Jacobson ER, Freeth A, et al. Histologic variation of grade and stage of non-alcoholic fatty liver disease in liver biopsies. Obes Surg 2005;15:497–501.

The Intestinal Microbiome in Nonalcoholic Fatty Liver Disease

Puneet Puri, MBBS, MD, Arun J. Sanyal, MBBS, MD*

KEYWORDS

- Nonalcoholic fatty liver disease • Nonalcoholic steatohepatitis • Cirrhosis
- Microbiome • 16S pyrosequencing • Microbiota • Intestinal permeability
- Innate immune system

KEY POINTS

- Nonalcoholic fatty liver disease is a clinicopathologic spectrum with aggressive phenotype nonalcoholic steatohepatitis (NASH) and rapidly rising cause of cirrhosis, liver cancer and liver transplant.
- NAFLD and NASH are commonly associated with obesity and other components of the metabolic syndrome, which are linked to the changes in the intestinal microbiome.
- Although few studies have demonstrated compositional changes intestinal microbiome in both pediatric and adult NAFLD, no consistent signature can be defined.
- Bacteroidetes and Firmicutes are major phyla altered in NAFLD in different studies, and Proteobacteria are among others that are increased in NAFLD.
- Predictive functional changes related to compositional intestinal microbial shifts reflect changes associated with carbohydrate, lipid and amino acid metabolism.

INTRODUCTION

There is growing realization that the human body is a "super" ecosystem where the host that is the body lives in harmony with a large number of microbes. Not only does the body live in harmony but also there is a symbiotic relationship between the

Grant Support: National Institute of Diabetes and Digestive and Kidney Diseases (NIDDK, RO1 DK 105961) and National Institute on Alcohol Abuse and Alcoholism (NIAAA, K23 AA 021179).
Disclosure: Dr A.J. Sanyal is President of Sanyal Bio and has stock options in Genfit, Exhalenz, Tiziana, Akarna, Hemoshear, and Indalo. He serves on the following advisory boards with remuneration: Lilly, Pfizer, Allergan, Novartis, Ardelyx, Sanofi, and General Electric. He has served on the following advisory boards without remuneration: Merck, Bristol Myers Squibb, Intercept, Syntlogic, Fractyl, Galectin, Gilead, Nitto Denko, Zydus, Janssen, Nordic BioSiences, and Immuron. He is a consultant to Salix, Cumberland Pharmaceuticals, Nordic Biosciences, Octeta, and Novo Nordisk. Dr P. Puri has nothing to disclose.
Department of Internal Medicine, Virginia Commonwealth University School of Medicine, MCV Box 980341, Richmond, VA 23298-0341, USA
* Corresponding author.
E-mail address: arun.sanyal@vcuhealth.org

liver.theclinics.com

microbes and the body, which is essential for good health. Recently developed tools have allowed the identification of bacteria not previously feasible due to the inability to grow a large number of bacteria in traditional culture media. This has led to new information on changes in the microbiome in various disease states and a growing number of diseases from developmental disorders and behavioral diseases to type 2 diabetes mellitus and autoimmune disorders have been shown to be associated with an altered microflora in the intestine.[1]

Nonalcoholic fatty liver disease (NAFLD) is the most common cause of chronic liver disease in North America and is growing as a cause of chronic liver disease in many other parts of the world as well. It has 2 principal clinical-pathologic phenotypes: (1) nonalcoholic fatty liver, which is characterized by hepatic steatosis with or without minimal lobular inflammation, and (2) nonalcoholic steatohepatitis (NASH), which is characterized by steatosis, lobular inflammation, and hepatocellular ballooning with varying degrees of fibrosis.[2] The development of both phenotypes is tightly linked to excess body weight and insulin resistance. It thus shares several common clinical and physiologic features with type 2 diabetes mellitus and as with diabetes it too has been associated with specific changes in the intestinal microbiome. This review discusses the emerging tools for the analysis of the microbiome, their limitations, and the existing literature with respect to the intestinal microbiome and their role in NAFLD.

METHODS USED FOR INTERROGATING THE INTESTINAL MICROBIOME

Louis Pasteur and Robert Koch pioneered the original concepts about the microbiome along with Eli Metchnikoff. In the early days of microbiology, the identification of bacteria required their isolation by culture, which was established as the gold standard. This technique was limited, however, by the fact that less than 1% of bacteria can be cultured in traditional aerobic and anaerobic culture conditions.

The ability to clone and sequence polymerase chain reaction (PCR) amplicons of the 16S ribosomal RNA (rRNA) gene from a complex community of bacteria allows generating an abundant profile of different bacterial species in the community. This has been used to further generate community fingerprinting of the microbial diversity using denaturing gradient gel electrophoresis or length heterogeneity fingerprinting to derive the bacterial abundance in terms of operational taxonomic units (OTUs) in a sample. Although this allows profiling of the entire community in 1 run on a sequencer, it does not, however, identify individual species in the OTUs.

Next-generation sequencing technology, for example, the Roche 454 technology, essentially clones 16S rRNA PCR amplicons onto beads producing up to 500,000 reads in a single run. Another innovation was the use of sample bar-coding where multiple samples can be mixed and given unique bar codes and then run on a next-generation sequencer followed by sorting of the sequences in to bins. The current ion torrent technology (Thermo Fisher, MA, USA) and polytomy (Illumina, CA, USA) can produce an even higher number of reads,[3,4] and the ability to generate reads of the microbial sequences is no longer the rate-limiting step in the study of the microbiome, and the main challenges remain in the application of bioinformatics to make sense of the large amount of data generated and ascribe mechanistic roles in various disease states.

Bioinformatics in the Study of the Microbiome

One approach is the identification of raw 16S rRNA sequences and comparing them to bacterial databases to build relative abundance tables. Computational limitations restrict this approach to algorithms that can compare millions of sequences against the bacterial databases. In this context, the Bayesian analysis tool provided by the Ribosomal Database Project[5] can be used to annotate the raw reads and build relative abundance tables.[6] The limitation of this tool is that it only identifies taxa down to the genus level although this is usually sufficient taxonomic resolution to analyze most projects.

Another approach involves comparison of taxa diversity between samples from various clinical states (controls vs disease). The Quantitative Insights in to Microbial Ecology[6,7] and mothur[8] are 2 commonly used tools for this purpose. Both tools clusters the raw reads, identify representative sequences for each cluster to define the OTUs and construct the relative abundance tables to construct a phylogenetic tree from the OTUs, and compare the trees using nonparametric and multivariable analytical methods.[6] Inferences about the function of the changes in the microbiome are made by linking the abundance tables to whole-genome annotations of fully sequenced taxa for example, by the Phylogenetic Investigation of Communities by Reconstruction of Unobserved States.[9] In this method, the relative abundance tables of functional pathways is created from the Kyoto Encyclopedia of Genes and Genomes (KEGG) database.[10] The Linear Discriminant Analysis Effect Size is another such tool, which performs a Kruskal-Wallis nonparametric t test followed by linear discriminant analysis to identify the taxa that have changed significantly from controls to disease state.[11] Metastats is yet another tool where a Fisher exact test is used to determine the differences in the proportion of the taxa from one clinical state to another.[12]

Metagenomics is another approach where shotgun sequencing of all of the DNA in a sample is performed and the taxa abundance tables constructed after identification of the reads against genome databases.[13] The accuracy of the this method has been questioned due to the ligation bias inherent in this process, and 16S rRNA amplification using fusion adapter is currently preferred as bar codes and adaptors are introduced in the PCR process, thereby avoiding the biases in the ligation based-methods.[14]

A fourth approach to assessing the functional complexity of the microbiome in the context of disease pathogenesis is to use correlation network and correlation difference network analyses.[15] Here, correlations between various microbiota and microbiota versus metabolites or changes in immune function, are determined by creating feature tables and calculation of Spearman correlation coefficients between all the features. This is visualized by tools such as Cytoscape[16] to generate hypotheses about which microbial changes are linked to the physiologic parameter of interest. Further changes in these correlation matrices between disease and control state can be further leveraged by subtraction analysis (correlation-difference analyses) of these matrices to determine which changes (loss of correlations in the control state or gain of correlations in the disease state) are most closely linked to alterations in the disease-related pathophysiologic parameter of interest.

The most recent tools used include machine-learning tools. Several open source, tools, such as Orange, are available and others are in development. These take advantage of advances in computational sciences to perform inferential analyses. This remains a technology that is still evolving.

LIMITATIONS OF CURRENT APPROACHES TO ASSESSING THE ROLE OF THE MICROBIOME AND THEIR RELEVANCE TO NONALCOHOLIC STEATOHEPATITIS

Historically, the linkage between an organism and disease state was established from the Koch postulates of identification of the bacteria in the diseased state, improvement of disease with eradication of the bacteria, and reproduction of the disease with reintroduction of the bacteria. This is not entirely feasible any more for ethical reasons. Moreover, when there are large numbers of bacteria present, the role of a given bacteria is hard to account for, especially because there is substantial redundancy of function across bacteria. Also, given the myriad bacterial sequences and potential correlates, there is a high probability of false discovery, especially when traditional P values are used. This requires additional statistical approaches to minimize false discovery. Finally, current approaches generate hypotheses and are unable to test the mechanistic role of specific bacteria by the usual loss of function and gain-of-function approaches.

In the context of NAFLD, it is important for interested clinicians who are not necessarily involved in microbiome research to be cognizant of the approaches taken, the complexity of the approaches to appreciate the potential pitfalls in the process, and the boundaries around the conclusions drawn from various articles. As causal inferential analytical tools are developed and validated, these will allow a clearer picture of the role of the microbiome in NAFLD to emerge.

PATHOPHYSIOLOGY OF NONALCOHOLIC FATTY LIVER DISEASE AND THE POTENTIAL EFFECTS OF INTESTINAL MICROBIOTA ON THESE PROCESSES

There is now a substantial body of literature on the mechanisms involved in the pathogenesis of NAFLD and its progression through steatohepatitis to cirrhosis and hepatocellular cancer (**Fig.1**). A useful construct links this to the onset of obesity and insulin resistance, which then triggers a cascade of events in the liver, which results in the development of progressive steatohepatitis.

The development of insulin resistance requires an increase in adipose tissue mass along with activation of the innate immune system within adipose tissue and other affected organs. The innate immune system can be activated by altered gut microbiome and changes in intestinal permeability, which lead to endotoxemia. It can also be activated from the cell stress induced by the increased lipid load. When adipose tissue becomes inflamed and insulin resistant, there is a decrease in insulin-mediated suppression of lipolysis, resulting in increased release of free fatty acids (FFAs), which are delivered to the liver, where they can be toxic

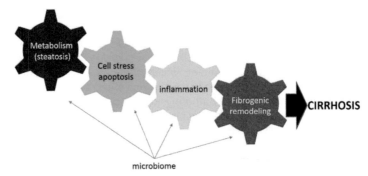

Fig. 1. The current paradigm of disease pathogenesis in NAFLD. Metabolic stress due to lipid and carbohydrate overload causes oxidative stress, endoplasmic reticulum stress, and other forms of cell stress. These lead to cell death or adaptive responses, which together trigger inflammatory responses. These are amplified by the innate immune system. Eventually inflammation drives fibrosis and progression to cirrhosis. The intestinal microbiome can affect each of these pathways and modulate the development of NASH.

(lipotoxicity). FFAs also impair insulin signaling in striated muscle and reduce the ability to clear glucose from circulation. The pancreas responds to these changes by ramping up insulin production and release and hyperinsulinemia is a hallmark feature of the insulin resistant state until pancreatic β-cell exhaustion sets in and insulin levels drop to the point where they can no longer maintain glycemic control and diabetes sets in.

A combination of increased FFAs load and hyperinsulinemia lead to an increased lipid load in the liver, where the lipogenic machinery is still sensitive to insulin and responds by increasing triglyceride and cholesterol synthesis.[17] Also there is initial increase in mitochondrial lipid oxidation, which generates reactive oxygen species. Over time, mitochondrial DNA is subject to oxidative injury and due to poor repair mechanisms in the mitochondria, there is mitochondrial DNA loss further decreasing electron transport chain activity and enhancing oxidative stress.[18] Oxidative stress and other cellular stress, for example, endoplasmic reticulum stress, activate stress signaling, which leads to either adaptation or apoptosis. This process also triggers additional inflammatory signals, which recruit macrophages to the liver. Progressive inflammation triggers fibrogenic remodeling of the liver ultimately culminating in cirrhosis.

Thus, a 4-step process, where metabolic perturbation leads to cell stress, which triggers cell death and regeneration versus adaptation, both of which can trigger inflammation, which in turn triggers fibrosis, has emerged as a general paradigm for the pathogenesis of NASH and currently serves as the basis for drug development approaches. The microbiome can affect extraintestinal organs by direct translocation, gut-derived neurohormonal signaling, altering the profile of metabolites and nutritional substrates absorbed from the intestine and activation of immune responses (**Fig. 2**).

Via these functional outputs, the microbiome can affect each of the individual steps in NASH pathogenesis, and the data for such relationships are reviewed.

The Intestinal Microbiome and Obesity/Steatosis

Increased fat and carbohydrate load in the diet lead to changes in the microbiome, such as an increase in Proteobacteria.[19] The functional consequences of these

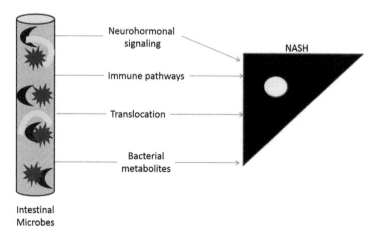

Fig. 2. The potential mechanisms by which the gut microbiome can influence development of obesity and NAFLD.

changes include increased extraction of nutrition from even traditionally less nutrition-ally dense sources.[20] For example, many complex carbohydrates, which are normally not metabolized, can be broken down by altered bacteria to release fatty acids and sugars that can be absorbed and contribute to the dietary caloric load. Thus, for the same diet, affected individuals extract more calories and have a greater caloric load compared with lean healthy individuals.

Another important mechanism by which the microbiome can potentially modulate hepatic steatosis is by affecting both farsenoid X receptor (FXR) and G protein-coupled receptor (TGR5) mediating signaling from the intestine. Primary bile acids are converted in to secondary bile acids by bacterial dihydroxylation reactions in the intestine. This is mediated by intestinal bacterial, in particular *Clostridium* spe-cies, such as *C scindens*.[21] FXR activation in the intestine releases FGF19, which has multiple metabolic effects that improve insulin sensitivity. TGR5 signaling in the intestine releases GLP-1 (glucagon-like peptide), which also promotes insulin signaling.[22] Recently, TGR5 has also been shown to modulate the pancreatic response to hyperglycemia.[23] Studies on the potential role of the bile acid biome are currently under way to elucidate the specific mechanisms by which these bacteria modify the metabolic milieu in obesity, type 2 diabetes mellitus, and in NAFLD.

The Intestinal Microbiome and Hepatic Inflammation

Toll-like receptors and the microbiome

Toll-like receptors (TLRs) are critical elements of the innate immune system and TLR4 is the most studied TLR. Lipopolysaccharide (LPS), a bacterial wall constituent from gram-negative bacteria, is a natural ligand for TLR4s, which are ubiquitously present. The TLR4-LPS association also involves LPS-binding protein, CD14, and myeloid dif-ferentiation protein 2 to recognize LPS. The cell signaling consequent to activation of TLR4 is now well established and involves both myeloid differentiation primary response 88 (MyD88)-dependent and MyD88-independent signaling, which converge on inflammatory activation via nuclear factor κB, mitogen-activated protein kinases, and JNK and ERK pathways. Cell death induced by these pathways also further trig-gers recruitment of neutrophils and other inflammatory cells to the liver. The intestinal microbiome affects the intestinal permeability and increases the endotoxin load in the portal circulation in obesity and may be critical drivers of initial adipose tissue and he-patic inflammation. This level of endotoxemia does not produce a sepsis syndrome but creates a systemic proinflammatory profibrogenic milieu where insulin signaling is impaired leading to increased net lipolysis in adipose tissue, and the delivery of FFAs from adipose tissue to the liver. Once excess hepatic stores of lipids generate cell stress,[24,25] these can be further amplified by the intrahepatic and systemic proin-flammatory milieu. This is manifest as the acute phase reaction where the liver gener-ates additional inflammatory signals, such as interleukin (IL)-6 and high-sensitivity C-reactive proetin.[26] TLR4 activation by FFAs and flagellin are other potential mech-anisms by which the innate immune system can modulate the hepatic inflammatory response.

There is growing awareness of the potential role of other TLRs, especially intracel-lular TLRs in NASH. Cytosine phosphate guanine–containing DNA have been shown to activate the inflammasome in the liver.[27]

Nucleotide-binding oligomerization domain–like receptors

These intracellular receptors bind pathogen-derived nuclear material via pathogen-associated pattern recognition or danger signal–associated pathways. They activate a cytosolic multiprotein complex called the inflammasome. The inflammasome serves as a platform for activating caspase-1 that, in turn, results in the maturation of proinflammatory cytokines, predominantly IL-1b.[28] Activation of the inflammasome is a 2-step process in which the priming step (injury, infection, or sterile inflammation) results in up-regulation of inflammasome expression and the second step triggers functional inflammasome activation by an inflammasome activator.[29] LPS is a potent inducer of the inflammasome and leads to a profound inflammatory response in the liver.[30]

The Intestinal Microbiome and Fibrosis

Hepatic stellate cells and portal myofibroblasts are key cellular drivers of hepatic fibrosis, a principal component of the tissue remodeling that leads to cirrhosis in NASH. Two major mechanisms linking the microbiome to hepatic fibrosis have emerged.

First, TLR signaling in hepatocytes and hepatic stellate cells have been shown to increase the expression of a variety of chemokines, such as monocyte chemotactic protein (MCP)-1, macrophage inflammatory protein-1α, and RANTES.[31] They also enhance expression of adhesion molecules (intercellular adhesion molecule 1, vascular cell adhesion molecule 1, and E-selectin).[31] Stellate cell–derived MCP-1 acts in an autocrine manner to activate these cells.[32] MCP-1 is a particularly important cytokine because it is the ligand for the chemokines CCR2–CCR5 and amplifies the inflammatory response and also links the inflammation to the fibrogenesis. Inhibition of this step has been leveraged in clinical trials to specifically block fibrosis in NASH.[33]

A second mechanism involves transforming growth factor (TGF)-β signaling. TGF-β is the prototypic classic profibrogenic cytokine and is closely linked to hepatic fibrogenesis across many chronic liver diseases, including NASH.[34] TGF-β receptor activation is normally held in check by expression of a decoy receptor bone morphogenetic protein (BMP) and activin membrane-bound receptor (BAMBI) in quiescent stellate cells. BAMBI interacts with Smad7 to interfere with transduction of TGF receptor I and II–mediated signals to Smad3.[35] TLR4-mediated activation of hepatic stellate cells is followed by down-regulation of BAMBI in a nuclear factor κB–dependent manner, thus releasing the cells from the fibrogenic brake.[31]

CHANGES IN THE MICROBIOME IN OBESITY

Excess body weight is the most common risk factor for the development of NAFLD. A causal link between the intestinal microflora and the consequences of obesity are supported by humanized mice where fecal transplant has been shown to increase obesity. Obesity is associated with (1) a lower ratio of Bacteroidetes to Firmicutes phyla[36,37] and (2) decreased bacterial diversity.[38] These data have been disputed by other studies.[39,40] A recent analyses from Human Microbiome Project (HMP) and MetaHIT (Metagenomics of the Human Intestinal Tract) data[41] demonstrate that (1) the ratio of Bacteroidetes:Firmicutes is not associated with obesity or body mass index (BMI) (**Fig. 3**A); (2) there is no relationship between BMI and the phylum-level composition of the microbiome (see **Fig. 3**B); (3) there is no association between intestinal microbiome diversity and BMI; and (4) obesity effects on relative abundance of Bacteroidetes and Firmicutes are not consistent across studies (**Fig. 3**C). Moreover, the interstudy variability far exceeds the differences in composition between lean and obese individuals within any study. These results underscore the evolving nature of the science in the field and caution must be exercised in overinterpreting the data as noted above in the section of methodology.

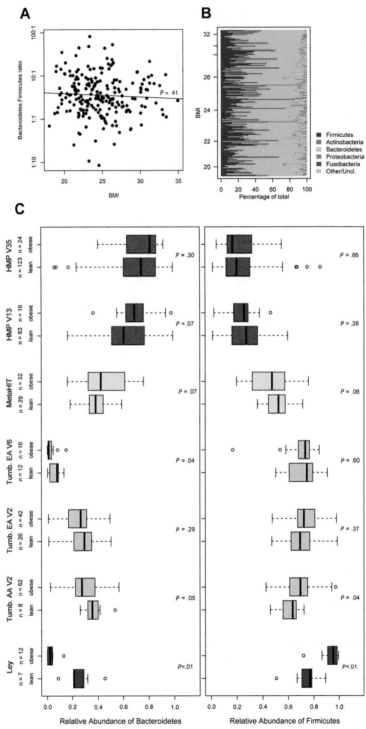

Fig. 3. (*A*) There is no association between BMI and the Bacteroidetes:Firmicutes ratio in HMP stool microbiomes. (*B*) There is no relationship between BMI and the phylum-level

CHANGE IN THE INTESTINAL MICROBIOME IN NONALCOHOLIC FATTY LIVER DISEASE

Several studies on changes in the intestinal microbiome have been published to date; all have been in adults with a couple exceptions.[42–48] These studies vary in the definitions used, availability of standardized histologic assessments, methods used, and bioinformatics approach and are all of inadequate sample size to make generalizable conclusions about the changes in the microbiome and the role of specific changes in the pathophysiologic cascade of NASH.

In 1 human study, a choline-deficient diet was related to a shift in microbial communities and development of hepatic steatosis.[42] In this trial, higher baseline levels of Proteobacteria protected against steatosis whereas bacteria in the class Erysipelotrichia (phylum Firmicutes) correlated with a higher risk. On the other hand, a pediatric study found that obese children with biopsy-proved NASH had decreased Firmicutes and increased Bacteroidetes phyla along with abundant Escherichia (Proteobacteria).[43] Endogenous alcohol levels were increased and endotoxin levels were not increased in this study. The finding of increased alcohol levels have not been reproduced by others. Other studies in adults noted increased *C coccoides* and decreased fecal Bacteroidetes, independent of BMI and daily fat intake.[45] Another study of adult patients with clinically defined NAFLD without histology compared with nonobese healthy subjects[46] demonstrated increased Lachnospiraceae and Lactobacillaceae and lower proportion of Ruminococcaceae family, and these changes were associated with elevated levels of fecal volatile compounds. Given the absence of obese controls and histology, the effect of BMI and distinct profile for NASH could not be ascertained. Moreover, none of these studies rigorously evaluated diet or prior dietary manipulations before engaging in the microbiome analysis.

A recent study demonstrated an increased abundance of Bacteroides and Ruminococcus and decreased proportion of Prevotella.[47] Bacteroides was independently associated with NASH and Ruminococcus with significant fibrosis. Furthermore, a significant relationship with dysbiosis to carbohydrate, lipid, and amino acid metabolism was observed on KEGG pathway analysis. Thus, gut microbiota analysis adds information to classic predictors of NAFLD severity and potential metabolic targets for prebiotics/probiotics therapies.

From a mechanistic point of view, the changes in the microbiome have been linked to the pathogenesis of NASH by (1) increased energy extraction both in the gut and by modulation of the fasting endotoxin-induced adipose factor, which impairs lipoprotein lipase function and increased FFA availability for hepatic uptake, (2) altered gut barrier function with consequent endotoxemia and activation of TLR4 mediated pathways and inflammasomes with downstream proinflammatory and

---

composition of the microbiome. Each row shows the relative abundance of major gut bacterial phyla in an individual. Individuals are ordered according to their BMI. (C) The between-study variability in the relative abundance of Bacteroidetes and Firmicutes is greater than the within-study differences between lean and obese individuals. The "Turnb." data are from Turnbaugh from African Americans (AA) and European Americans (EA), from variable regions (V) 2 and 6. The MetaHIT data are from the Danish subjects who do not have inflammatory bowel disease. The HMP data are from V13 and V35. The primary results from this article were generated using data from HMP V35. All *P* values by *t* test. Uncl, unclassified. (*From* Finucane MM, Sharpton TJ, Laurent TJ, et al. A taxonomic signature of obesity in the microbiome? getting to the guts of the matter. PLoS One 2014;9:e84689; with permission.)

profibrogenic signaling, (3) modulation of choline metabolism, (4) altered bile acid metabolism and modulating levels of secondary bile acids that affect FXR and TGR5 signaling, which have important effects on metabolic homeostasis, and (5) endogenous alcohol production. While plausible, the endogenous alcohol production, however, has not been reproduced and may be a function of excess carbohydrate (pasta and breads) intake in the single study that reported it.

In summary, there is a growing body of evidence implicating the microbiome in the development of NASH. Altogether, these human studies demonstrate measurable differences in the microbiome in NAFLD and NASH, but, due to the great variability in study design, methods, and clinical endpoints, several aspects of what is known may change and there remain many open questions. Further work is needed to explore the mechanisms, pathologic significance, and diagnostic and therapeutic potential of intestinal microbiome in the context of human NAFLD.

REFERENCES

1. Lynch SV, Pedersen O. The human intestinal microbiome in health and disease. N Engl J Med 2016;375:2369–79.
2. Kleiner DE, Brunt EM, Van Natta M, et al. Design and validation of a histological scoring system for nonalcoholic fatty liver disease. Hepatology 2005;41:1313–21.
3. Eid J, Fehr A, Gray J, et al. Real-time DNA sequencing from single polymerase molecules. Science 2009;323:133–8.
4. Berglund EC, Kiialainen A, Syvanen AC. Next-generation sequencing technologies and applications for human genetic history and forensics. Investig Genet 2011;2:23.
5. Wang Q, Garrity GM, Tiedje JM, et al. Naïve bayesian classifier for rapid assignment of rRNA sequences into the new bacterial taxonomy. Appl Environ Microbiol 2007;73:5261–7.
6. Naqvi A, Rangwala H, Spear G, et al. Analysis of multitag pyrosequence data from human cervical lavage samples. Chem Biodivers 2010;7:1076–85.
7. Caporaso JG, Kuczynski J, Stombaugh J, et al. QIIME allows analysis of high-throughput community sequencing data. Nat Methods 2010;7:335–6.
8. Schloss PD, Westcott SL, Ryabin T, et al. Introducing mothur: open-source, platform-independent, community-supported software for describing and comparing microbial communities. Appl Environ Microbiol 2009;75:7537–41.
9. Langille MGI, Zaneveld J, Caporaso JG, et al. Predictive functional profiling of microbial communities using 16S rRNA marker gene sequences. Nat Biotech 2013; 31:814–21.
10. Kanehisa M, Goto S. KEGG: kyoto encyclopedia of genes and genomes. Nucleic Acids Res 2000;28:27–30.
11. Segata N, Izard J, Walron L, et al. Metagenomic biomarker discovery and explanation. Genome Biol 2011;12:R60.
12. White JR, Nagarajan N, Pop M. Statistical methods for detecting differentially abundant features in clinical metagenomic samples. PLoS Comput Biol 2009;5:e1000352.
13. Sunagawa S, Mende DR, Zeller G, et al. Metagenomic species profiling using universal phylogenetic marker genes. Nat Methods 2013;10:1196–9.
14. Jones MB, Highlander SK, Anderson EL, et al. Library preparation methodology can influence genomic and functional predictions in human microbiome research. Proc Natl Acad Sci USA 2015;112:14024–9.
15. Naqvi A, Rangwale H, Keshavarzian A, et al. Network-based modeling of the human gut microbiome. Chem Biodiversity 2010;7:1040–50.

16. Shannon P, Markiel A, Ozier O, et al. Cytoscape: a software environment for integrated models of biomolecular interaction networks. Genome Res 2003;13: 2498–504.
17. Sanyal AJ. Mechanisms of disease: pathogenesis of nonalcoholic fatty liver disease. Nat Clin Pract Gastroenterol Hepatol 2005;2:46–53.
18. Sanyal AJ, Campbell-Sargent C, Mirshahi F, et al. Nonalcoholic steatohepatitis: association of insulin resistance and mitochondrial abnormalities. Gastroenterology 2001;120:1183–92.
19. Turnbaugh PJ, Backhed F, Fulton L, et al. Diet-induced obesity is linked to marked but reversible alterations in the mouse distal gut microbiome. Cell Host Microbe 2008;3:213–23.
20. Turnbaugh PJ, Ley RE, Mahowald MA, et al. An obesity-associated gut microbiome with increased capacity for energy harvest. Nature 2006;444:1027–31.
21. Ridlon JM, Ikegawa S, Alves JM, et al. Clostridium scindens: a human gut microbe with a high potential to convert glucocorticoids into androgens. J Lipid Res 2013;54:2437–49.
22. Thomas C, Gioiello A, Noriega L, et al. TGR5-mediated bile acid sensing controls glucose homeostasis. Cell Metab 2009;10:167–77.
23. Kumar DP, Asgharpour A, Mirshahi F, et al. Activation of transmembrane bile acid receptor TGR5 modulates pancreatic islet alpha cells to promote glucose homeostasis. J Biol Chem 2016;291:6626–40.
24. Glass CK, Olefsky JM. Inflammation and lipid signaling in the etiology of insulin resistance. Cell Metab 2012;15:635–45.
25. Fu S, Watkins SM, Hotamisligil GS. The role of endoplasmic reticulum in hepatic lipid homeostasis and stress signaling. Cell Metab 2012;15:623–34.
26. Boga S, Alkim H, Koksal AR, et al. Increased plasma levels of asymmetric dimethylarginine in nonalcoholic fatty liver disease: relation with insulin resistance, inflammation, and liver histology. J Investig Med 2015;63:871–7.
27. Csak T, Pillai A, Ganz M, et al. Both bone marrow-derived and non-bone marrow-derived cells contribute to AIM2 and NLRP3 inflammasome activation in a MyD88-dependent manner in dietary steatohepatitis. Liver Int 2014;34:1402–13.
28. Dinarello CA. Immunological and inflammatory functions of the interleukin-1 family. Annu Rev Immunol 2009;27:519–50.
29. Ratsimandresy RA, Dorfleutner A, Stehlik C. An update on PYRIN domain-containing pattern recognition receptors: from immunity to pathology. Front Immunol 2013;4:440.
30. Ganz M, Csak T, Nath B, et al. Lipopolysaccharide induces and activates the Nalp3 inflammasome in the liver. World J Gastroenterol 2011;17:4772–8.
31. Seki E, De Minicis S, Osterreicher CH, et al. TLR4 enhances TGF-beta signaling and hepatic fibrosis. Nat Med 2007;13:1324–32.
32. Marra F, Romanelli RG, Giannini C, et al. Monocyte chemotactic protein-1 as a chemoattractant for human hepatic stellate cells. Hepatology 1999;29:140–8.
33. Friedman S, Sanyal A, Goodman Z, et al. Efficacy and safety study of cenicriviroc for the treatment of non-alcoholic steatohepatitis in adult subjects with liver fibrosis: CENTAUR Phase 2b study design. Contemp Clin Trials 2016;47:356–65.
34. Fabregat I, Moreno-Caceres J, Sanchez A, et al. TGF-beta signalling and liver disease. FEBS J 2016;283:2219–32.
35. Yan X, Lin Z, Chen F, et al. Human BAMBI cooperates with Smad7 to inhibit transforming growth factor-beta signaling. J Biol Chem 2009;284:30097–104.
36. Ley RE, Turnbaugh PJ, Klein S, et al. Microbial ecology: human gut microbes associated with obesity. Nature 2006;444:1022–3.

37. Turnbaugh PJ, Hamady M, Yatsunenko T, et al. A core gut microbiome in obese and lean twins. Nature 2009;457:480–4.
38. Le Chatelier E, Nielsen T, Qin J, et al. Richness of human gut microbiome correlates with metabolic markers. Nature 2013;500:541–6.
39. Arumugam M, Raes J, Pelletier E, et al. Enterotypes of the human gut microbiome. Nature 2011;473:174–80.
40. Human Microbiome Project Consortium. Structure, function and diversity of the healthy human microbiome. Nature 2012;486:207–14.
41. Finucane MM, Sharpton TJ, Laurent TJ, et al. A taxonomic signature of obesity in the microbiome? getting to the guts of the matter. PLoS One 2014;9:e84689.
42. Spencer MD, Hamp TJ, Reid RW, et al. Association between composition of the human gastrointestinal microbiome and development of fatty liver with choline deficiency. Gastroenterology 2011;140:976–86.
43. Zhu L, Baker SS, Gill C, et al. Characterization of gut microbiomes in nonalcoholic steatohepatitis (NASH) patients: a connection between endogenous alcohol and NASH. Hepatology 2013;57:601–9.
44. Yuan J, Baker SS, Liu W, et al. Endotoxemia unrequired in the pathogenesis of pediatric nonalcoholic steatohepatitis. J Gastroenterol Hepatol 2014;29:1292–8.
45. Mouzaki M, Comelli EM, Arendt BM, et al. Intestinal microbiota in patients with nonalcoholic fatty liver disease. Hepatology 2013;58:120–7.
46. Raman M, Ahmed I, Gillevet PM, et al. Fecal microbiome and volatile organic compound metabolome in obese humans with nonalcoholic fatty liver disease. Clin Gastroenterol Hepatol 2013;11:868–75.e1–3.
47. Boursier J, Mueller O, Barret M, et al. The severity of nonalcoholic fatty liver disease is associated with gut dysbiosis and shift in the metabolic function of the gut microbiota. Hepatology 2016;63:764–75.
48. Loomba R, Seguritan V, Li W, et al. Gut microbiome-based metagenomic signature for non-invasive detection of advanced fibrosis in human nonalcoholic fatty liver disease. Cell Metab 2017;25:1054–62.e5.

Nonalcoholic Fatty Liver Disease and Metabolic Syndrome

Donghee Kim, MD, PhD, Alexis Touros, BA, W. Ray Kim, MD*

KEYWORDS

- Nonalcoholic fatty liver disease • Low-density lipoprotein • Metabolic syndrome
- Hyperglycemia • Abdominal obesity • Hypertension • Nonalcoholic steatohepatitis

KEY POINTS

- Nonalcoholic fatty liver disease (NAFLD) and metabolic syndrome (MS) are highly prevalent, affecting approximately a third of the US population.
- Common pathogenetic mechanisms for NAFLD and the MS are associated with the development of cardiovascular disease, type 2 diabetes, and severe forms of liver disease.
- NAFLD is associated with MS and the abdominal obesity, hyperglycemia, hypertension, and dyslipidemia as each component of MS.
- NAFLD associated with the *PNPLA3* G allele variant is not associated by MS and insulin resistance.

INTRODUCTION

Nonalcoholic fatty liver disease (NAFLD) is known as the most common chronic liver disease in the United States.[1] With the advent of effective antiviral therapy for hepatitis C and the ongoing epidemic of obesity, the significance of NAFLD as the dominant cause of chronic liver disease is expected to increase over the next 20 years.[2] The increasing prevalence of NAFLD, specifically nonalcoholic steatohepatitis (NASH) with fibrosis, is concerning, because patients appear to experience higher mortality from liver-related and non-liver-related causes compared with the general population.[3] This has occurred within the greater context of prevalent metabolic syndrome (MS), both in the United States and worldwide.

MS is a cluster of metabolic derangements that predicts risk of type 2 diabetes and cardiovascular disease. There is robust evidence in support of common pathogenetic

Conflicts of Interests: The authors have nothing to disclose.
Division of Gastroenterology and Hepatology, Stanford University School of Medicine, 300 Pasteur Drive, Stanford, CA 94304, USA
* Corresponding author. Division of Gastroenterology and Hepatology, Stanford University School of Medicine, 300 Pasteur Drive, Stanford, CA 94304.
E-mail address: wrkim@stanford.edu

Clin Liver Dis 22 (2018) 133–140
http://dx.doi.org/10.1016/j.cld.2017.08.010
1089-3261/18/© 2017 Elsevier Inc. All rights reserved.

liver.theclinics.com

mechanisms for NAFLD and the MS, which are associated with the development of type 2 diabetes, cardiovascular disease, and severe forms of liver disease including cirrhosis and hepatocellular carcinoma (HCC). However, not all patients with NAFLD exhibit the typical features of MS; approximately 30% of NAFLD patients are estimated to lack metabolic abnormalities. For example, NAFLD patients who carry at least 1 palatin-like phospholipase domain-containing 3 (PNPLA3) gene variant allele display a favorable metabolic profile, characterized by normal triglycerides and insulin sensitivity.

PREVALENCE AND DIAGNOSIS OF NONALCOHOLIC FATTY LIVER DISEASE

NAFLD is estimated to affect as many as a third of the general population and up to 70% of diabetic and obese subjects in the United States.[1] As a result of the obesity epidemic in many parts of the world and lack of effective therapy, the global burden of NAFLD is projected to increase over the next decade, raising concerns that an increasing proportion of the population will develop cirrhosis and end-stage liver disease with age.

NAFLD is defined as the presence of fatty infiltration in the liver, determined either by imaging or by histology after the exclusion of other causes of hepatic fat accumulation (eg, significant alcohol consumption, medications known to cause fatty liver, and other causes of liver disease). Hepatic ultrasonography, computed tomography, and MRI are accepted modalities for detecting hepatic fatty infiltration. For the evaluation of advanced fibrosis, 2 modalities, namely transient elastography[4,5] and magnetic resonance elastography,[6,7] are often useful in differentiating NAFLD with or without advanced fibrosis.

PREVALENCE AND DIAGNOSIS OF METABOLIC SYNDROME

MS is highly prevalent in the United States and becoming increasingly common worldwide. In the National Health and Nutrition Examination Survey (NHANES), the overall prevalence of the MS increased from 32.9% in 2003 to 2004 to 34.7% in 2011 to 2012, with significantly higher prevalence in women compared with men, and in Hispanics compared with non-Hispanic whites and blacks.[8]

MS consists of a cluster of inter-related factors, including central obesity, dysglycemia, dyslipidemia, and raised blood pressure. It increases the risk for type 2 diabetes and cardiovascular disease. Over the past few decades, various societies have proposed diagnostic criteria, albeit with considerable heterogeneity. In 2009, representatives from the International Diabetes Federation; American Heart Association; National Heart, Lung, and Blood Institute; World Heart Federation; International Atherosclerosis Society; and the International Association for the Study of Obesity developed consensus criteria (**Table 1**).[9] Salient differences compared with prior definitions include: 3 abnormalities out of 5 diagnostic criteria would qualify a person for the MS; sex and ethnicity-specific thresholds for waist circumference were recommended for defining abdominal obesity; and abdominal obesity would not be a prerequisite for diagnosis, but it is 1 of 5 criteria.[9]

METABOLIC SYNDROME AND NONALCOHOLIC FATTY LIVER DISEASE

It is well known that NAFLD often occurs in the context of MS. The prevalence of MS in patients with NAFLD increases with higher body mass index (BMI), from 18% in non-obese NAFLD to 67% in obese NAFLD in a series of 304 patients.[10] In the same series, the presence of MS was associated with a higher risk of NASH and severe fibrosis; 88% of patients with NASH met the criteria for MS, compared with 53% of patients

Table 1	
Diagnosing criteria for metabolic syndrome	
Criteria	**Categorical Cut Points**
Elevated waist circumference	Ethnicity-specific definitions
Elevated fasting glucose	$\geq$100 mg/dL and/or drug treatment of elevated glucose
Elevated triglycerides	$\geq$150 mg/dL and/or drug treatment for elevated triglycerides
Reduced HDL cholesterol	<40 mg/dL in men; <50 mg/dL in women
Elevated blood pressure	Systolic $\geq$130 and/or diastolic $\geq$85 mm Hg

Definition of MS: meeting at least 3 of the 5 criteria. Ethnicity specific definitions of elevated waist circumference: (1) Caucasian: 102 cm or greater in men and 88 cm or greater in women (2) Asian: 90 cm or greater in men and 80 cm or greater in women (3) Middle East, Mediterranean, African: 94 cm or greater in men and 80 cm or greater in women (4) Ethnic Central and South American: 90 cm or greater in men and 80 cm or greater in women.

Data from Alberti KG, Eckel RH, Grundy SM, et al. Harmonizing the metabolic syndrome: a joint interim statement of the International Diabetes Federation Task Force on Epidemiology and Prevention; National Heart, Lung, and Blood Institute; American Heart Association; World Heart Federation; International Atherosclerosis Society; and International Association for the Study of Obesity. Circulation 2009;120:1640–5.

with NAFLD.[10] In the NASH Clinical Research Network data, MS conferred an increase in risk of histology-confirmed NASH by 40%.[11] In the NHANES data, MS, but not obesity, was independently associated with increased risk of overall mortality among patients with NAFLD.[12]

Conversely, NAFLD is also strongly associated with development of MS. A recent meta-analysis including a pooled population of 81,411 patients showed that NAFLD, as diagnosed by either liver enzymes or ultrasonography, significantly increased the risk of incident MS during a 5-year follow-up period, with a relative risk of 1.80 for alanine aminotransferase (ALT) (last vs first quartile or quintile), 1.98 for gamma-glutamyltransferase (GGT), and 3.22 for ultrasonography.[13] Kwon and colleagues[14] reported a stronger association of MS for nonobese NAFLD than for obese NAFLD; patients with nonobese NAFLD had higher adjusted prevalence ratios for certain components of MS (high triglycerides for both genders and high blood pressure, impaired fasting glucose, and low high density lipoprotein [HDL]-cholesterol for women) than those with obese NAFLD.

NONALCOHOLIC FATTY LIVER DISEASE AND COMPONENTS OF METABOLIC SYNDROME
Abdominal Obesity

As a determinant of NAFLD, the distribution of adiposity may be more important than the total adipose mass.[15–20] NAFLD is correlated more with abdominal obesity, a component of the MS, than BMI.[21] A higher fat mass, greater central obesity, and increased visceral fat are associated with MS.[22,23] Visceral adipose tissue (VAT) area is increased in patients with NAFLD (with and without significant fibrosis) and is independently associated with increased risks of NASH and NAFLD with significant fibrosis.[24] In another recent cohort study of 2017 subjects with a median follow-up time of 4.4 years, the VAT area was associated with incident NAFLD in a dose-dependent manner, with an adjusted hazard ratio (HR, per 1-standard deviation [SD] increase) for incident NAFLD of 1.36 (95% confidence interval [CI] 1.16–1.59).[25] Higher subcutaneous adipose tissue area was associated with NAFLD regression (HR per 1 SD increase 1.36, 95% CI 1.08–1.72), independent of visceral adiposity.[25]

This finding provides evidence that a certain type of body adiposity may be a risk factor for NAFLD, whereas other types may be protective against NAFLD.[25] Visceral adiposity accounts for only 7% to 15% of the total body fat; however, it plays a more important role than subcutaneous fat in the development of insulin resistance, which may be because the liver receives portal venous blood containing free fatty acids and cytokines secreted by VAT.[26]

Dyslipidemia (Hypertriglyceridemia and Low High-Density Lipoprotein Cholesterol)

The rate of secretion of fatty acid and triglycerides-rich very low-density lipoprotein (VLDL) into the plasma is higher in subjects with NAFLD and/or MS compared with those without.[27] In these patients, there is a marked increase in the contribution of nonsystemic fatty acids, presumably derived from lipolysis of intrahepatic and visceral fat and de novo lipogenesis, to triglycerides-rich VLDL secretion.[27] In general, insulin reduces the production of VLDL by suppressing adipose tissue lipolysis and hepatic production of VLDL.[28,29] However, in patients with NAFLD or MS, insulin fails to inhibit both lipolysis and production of triglycerides-rich VLDL from the liver, leading to an increase in serum triglycerides and lowering of HDL cholesterol.[29] In a recent large cohort study, 23% of patients with NAFLD had isolated hypertriglyceridemia, 10% isolated low HDL cholesterol, and 18% dyslipidemia of MS (both low HDL cholesterol and high triglycerides), providing evidence for higher prevalence of dyslipidemia in patients with NAFLD.[30]

Hyperglycemia

The ability of insulin to suppress glucose production is impaired in patients with NAFLD and/or MS.[31] This results in hyperglycemia and increased insulin secretion.[29] A recent meta-analysis with a pooled population of 117,020 patients demonstrated a significantly increased risk of incident type 2 diabetes in patients with NAFLD, with a pooled relative risk of 1.97 (95% CI 1.80–2.15) for alanine aminotransferase (ALT, last vs first quartile or quintile) and 1.86 (95% CI 1.76–1.95) for ultrasonography, respectively.[13] However, the relationship between type 2 diabetes and NAFLD is complex and may be bi-directional. Once type 2 diabetes develops, it may promote progression of NAFLD to NASH, advanced fibrosis, cirrhosis, and hepatocellular carcinoma.[32]

Hypertension

Although hypertension is a controversial component of the MS, several mechanisms linking MS to hypertension are proposed, including increased stimulation of the sympathetic nervous system, enhanced renal sodium reabsorption by hyperinsulinemia, and impaired vasodilation due to insulin stimulation.[29,33] Several longitudinal studies have shown that NAFLD at baseline or incident NAFLD is associated with an increased risk of incident hypertension.[34,35]

NONALCOHOLIC FATTY LIVER DISEASE NOT ASSOCIATED WITH METABOLIC SYNDROME

Although NAFLD and MS are closely associated, the 2 conditions do not always coexist in the same individual. This discrepancy may be attributed to the arbitrary definitions of MS and various diagnostic tools of NAFLD. However, recent evidence suggests that pathogenetic processes beyond MS and insulin resistance may also lead to NAFLD. A classic example is genetic variants in the PNPLA3 gene.

In 2008, a genome-wide association study as part of the Dallas Heart Study found that an allele (rs738409) of *PNPLA3*, caused by a missense mutation (I148 M), was strongly associated with increased hepatic fat levels and hepatic inflammation.[36] The allele was most common in Hispanics, the group most susceptible to NAFLD, and the hepatic fat content was more than twofold higher in *PNPLA3* rs738409[G] homozygotes than in noncarriers.[36] A recent meta-analysis showed that rs738409 exerts a strong influence, not only on hepatic fat accumulation, but also on the susceptibility to more aggressive liver disease.[37] These associations were maintained independent of the degree of obesity or the presence of diabetes.[38–40]

NAFLD associated with the *PNPLA3* G allele does not feature the typical metabolic abnormalities of NAFLD, including insulin resistance, hyperglycemia, hypertriglyceridemia, low HDL cholesterol concentration, or inflammation in adipose tissue.[38–41] This was first shown in a German study, in which *PNPLA3* was strongly associated with NAFLD but not with insulin resistance independent of visceral adiposity.[42] Similarly, a recent Finnish study compared patients with *PNPLA3* variant NAFLD versus obese NAFLD against *PNPLA3* wild-type controls. *PNPLA3* variant NAFLD and controls had similar BMI and insulin levels, which were significantly different from obese NAFLD patients.[41] Adipose tissue gene expression was also similar in the *PNPLA3* NAFLD and control groups. Liver fat, however, was increased in patients with *PNPLA3* NAFLD and obese NAFLD.[41] *PNPLA3* NAFLD is characterized by an increase in hepatic fat without insulin resistance or adipose tissue inflammation, whereas obese NAFLD have all 3 of these features.[41]

PNPLA3 NAFLD is characterized by deficiencies of distinct circulating triacylglycerols, suggesting that the G allele variant impairs lipolysis rather than stimulates synthesis of intrahepatocellular triacylglycerols.[43] In contrast, obese NAFLD is associated with increase in triacylglycerol concentrations, in the context of insulin resistance and/or obesity.[43] Bariatric surgery patients carrying the *PNPLA3* G allele variant have been found to have paradoxically lower triglyceride concentrations and a higher susceptibility to type 2 diabetes compared with noncarriers.[44] Among subjects without MS, the presence of the *PNPLA3* G allele is associated with a risk of NAFLD.[45] Given the evidence from current literature, subjects with variant *PNPLA3* are at increased risk for the development and progression of NAFLD, but spared from insulin resistance, adipose tissue inflammation, and MS.[41,45]

SUMMARY

NAFLD and MS are highly prevalent, affecting approximately a third of the US population. The relationship between NAFLD and MS is complex and may be bi-directionally associated. NAFLD is strongly associated with MS, the components of which include abdominal obesity, hyperglycemia, hypertension, and dyslipidemia. NAFLD associated with certain genetic factors such as the *PNPLA3* G allele variant is not accompanied by insulin resistance and MS. Lifestyle modification, including diet and physical activity targeting visceral adiposity, remains the standard of care for patients with NAFLD and MS.

REFERENCES

1. Younossi ZM, Stepanova M, Afendy M, et al. Changes in the prevalence of the most common causes of chronic liver diseases in the United States from 1988 to 2008. Clin Gastroenterol Hepatol 2011;9:524–30.e1 [quiz: e60].
2. Wong RJ, Cheung R, Ahmed A. Nonalcoholic steatohepatitis is the most rapidly growing indication for liver transplantation in patients with hepatocellular carcinoma in the U.S. Hepatology 2014;59:2188–95.

3. Kim D, Kim WR, Kim HJ, et al. Association between noninvasive fibrosis markers and mortality among adults with nonalcoholic fatty liver disease in the United States. Hepatology 2013;57:1357–65.

4. Nobili V, Vizzutti F, Arena U, et al. Accuracy and reproducibility of transient elastography for the diagnosis of fibrosis in pediatric nonalcoholic steatohepatitis. Hepatology 2008;48:442–8.

5. Wong VW, Vergniol J, Wong GL, et al. Diagnosis of fibrosis and cirrhosis using liver stiffness measurement in nonalcoholic fatty liver disease. Hepatology 2010;51:454–62.

6. Chen J, Talwalkar JA, Yin M, et al. Early detection of nonalcoholic steatohepatitis in patients with nonalcoholic fatty liver disease by using MR elastography. Radiology 2011;259:749–56.

7. Kim D, Kim WR, Talwalkar JA, et al. Advanced fibrosis in nonalcoholic fatty liver disease: noninvasive assessment with MR elastography. Radiology 2013;268: 411–9.

8. Aguilar M, Bhuket T, Torres S, et al. Prevalence of the metabolic syndrome in the United States, 2003-2012. JAMA 2015;313:1973–4.

9. Alberti KG, Eckel RH, Grundy SM, et al. Harmonizing the metabolic syndrome: a joint interim statement of the International Diabetes Federation Task Force on Epidemiology and Prevention; National Heart, Lung, and Blood Institute; American Heart Association; World Heart Federation; International Atherosclerosis Society; and International Association for the Study of Obesity. Circulation 2009;120:1640–5.

10. Marchesini G, Bugianesi E, Forlani G, et al. Nonalcoholic fatty liver, steatohepatitis, and the metabolic syndrome. Hepatology 2003;37:917–23.

11. Brunt EM, Kleiner DE, Wilson LA, et al. Nonalcoholic fatty liver disease (NAFLD) activity score and the histopathologic diagnosis in NAFLD: distinct clinicopathologic meanings. Hepatology 2011;53:810–20.

12. Stepanova M, Rafiq N, Younossi ZM. Components of metabolic syndrome are independent predictors of mortality in patients with chronic liver disease: a population-based study. Gut 2010;59:1410–5.

13. Ballestri S, Zona S, Targher G, et al. Nonalcoholic fatty liver disease is associated with an almost twofold increased risk of incident type 2 diabetes and metabolic syndrome. Evidence from a systematic review and meta-analysis. J Gastroenterol Hepatol 2016;31:936–44.

14. Kwon YM, Oh SW, Hwang SS, et al. Association of nonalcoholic fatty liver disease with components of metabolic syndrome according to body mass index in Korean adults. Am J Gastroenterol 2012;107:1852–8.

15. Farrell GC, Chitturi S, Lau GK, et al. Guidelines for the assessment and management of non-alcoholic fatty liver disease in the Asia-Pacific region: executive summary. J Gastroenterol Hepatol 2007;22:775–7.

16. Finelli C, Tarantino G. Is visceral fat reduction necessary to favour metabolic changes in the liver? J Gastrointestin Liver Dis 2012;21:205–8.

17. Park BJ, Kim YJ, Kim DH, et al. Visceral adipose tissue area is an independent risk factor for hepatic steatosis. J Gastroenterol Hepatol 2008;23:900–7.

18. Hamaguchi M, Kojima T, Itoh Y, et al. The severity of ultrasonographic findings in nonalcoholic fatty liver disease reflects the metabolic syndrome and visceral fat accumulation. Am J Gastroenterol 2007;102:2708–15.

19. Kim D, Park BJ, Kim W, et al. Visceral fat as a strong and independent risk factor of nonalcoholic fatty liver disease. Gastroenterology 2008;134:A782–3.

20. Eguchi Y, Eguchi T, Mizuta T, et al. Visceral fat accumulation and insulin resistance are important factors in nonalcoholic fatty liver disease. J Gastroenterol 2006;41:462–9.

21. van der Poorten D, Milner KL, Hui J, et al. Visceral fat: a key mediator of steatohepatitis in metabolic liver disease. Hepatology 2008;48:449–57.

22. Conus F, Allison DB, Rabasa-Lhoret R, et al. Metabolic and behavioral characteristics of metabolically obese but normal-weight women. J Clin Endocrinol Metab 2004;89:5013–20.

23. Katsuki A, Sumida Y, Urakawa H, et al. Increased visceral fat and serum levels of triglyceride are associated with insulin resistance in Japanese metabolically obese, normal weight subjects with normal glucose tolerance. Diabetes Care 2003;26:2341–4.

24. Yu SJ, Kim W, Kim D, et al. Visceral obesity predicts significant fibrosis in patients with nonalcoholic fatty liver disease. Medicine (Baltimore) 2015;94:e2159.

25. Kim D, Chung GE, Kwak MS, et al. Body fat distribution and risk of incident and regressed nonalcoholic fatty liver disease. Clin Gastroenterol Hepatol 2016;14:132–8.e4.

26. McLaughlin T, Lamendola C, Liu A, et al. Preferential fat deposition in subcutaneous versus visceral depots is associated with insulin sensitivity. J Clin Endocrinol Metab 2011;96:E1756–60.

27. Fabbrini E, Mohammed BS, Magkos F, et al. Alterations in adipose tissue and hepatic lipid kinetics in obese men and women with nonalcoholic fatty liver disease. Gastroenterology 2008;134:424–31.

28. Adiels M, Olofsson SO, Taskinen MR, et al. Overproduction of very low-density lipoproteins is the hallmark of the dyslipidemia in the metabolic syndrome. Arterioscler Thromb Vasc Biol 2008;28:1225–36.

29. Yki-Jarvinen H. Non-alcoholic fatty liver disease as a cause and a consequence of metabolic syndrome. Lancet Diabetes Endocrinol 2014;2:901–10.

30. Du T, Sun X, Yuan G, et al. Lipid phenotypes in patients with nonalcoholic fatty liver disease. Metabolism 2016;65:1391–8.

31. Gastaldelli A, Cusi K, Pettiti M, et al. Relationship between hepatic/visceral fat and hepatic insulin resistance in nondiabetic and type 2 diabetic subjects. Gastroenterology 2007;133:496–506.

32. Anstee QM, Targher G, Day CP. Progression of NAFLD to diabetes mellitus, cardiovascular disease or cirrhosis. Nat Rev Gastroenterol Hepatol 2013;10:330–44.

33. Kotronen A, Yki-Jarvinen H. Fatty liver: a novel component of the metabolic syndrome. Arterioscler Thromb Vasc Biol 2008;28:27–38.

34. Ryoo JH, Suh YJ, Shin HC, et al. Clinical association between non-alcoholic fatty liver disease and the development of hypertension. J Gastroenterol Hepatol 2014;29:1926–31.

35. Sung KC, Wild SH, Byrne CD. Development of new fatty liver, or resolution of existing fatty liver, over five years of follow-up, and risk of incident hypertension. J Hepatol 2014;60:1040–5.

36. Romeo S, Kozlitina J, Xing C, et al. Genetic variation in PNPLA3 confers susceptibility to nonalcoholic fatty liver disease. Nat Genet 2008;40:1461–5.

37. Sookoian S, Pirola CJ. Meta-analysis of the influence of I148M variant of patatin-like phospholipase domain containing 3 gene (PNPLA3) on the susceptibility and histological severity of nonalcoholic fatty liver disease. Hepatology 2011;53:1883–94.

38. Rotman Y, Koh C, Zmuda JM, et al. The association of genetic variability in patatin-like phospholipase domain-containing protein 3 (PNPLA3) with histological severity of nonalcoholic fatty liver disease. Hepatology 2010;52:894–903.
39. Speliotes EK, Butler JL, Palmer CD, et al. PNPLA3 variants specifically confer increased risk for histologic nonalcoholic fatty liver disease but not metabolic disease. Hepatology 2010;52:904–12.
40. Valenti L, Al-Serri A, Daly AK, et al. Homozygosity for the patatin-like phospholipase-3/adiponutrin I148M polymorphism influences liver fibrosis in patients with nonalcoholic fatty liver disease. Hepatology 2010;51:1209–17.
41. Lallukka S, Sevastianova K, Perttila J, et al. Adipose tissue is inflamed in NAFLD due to obesity but not in NAFLD due to genetic variation in PNPLA3. Diabetologia 2013;56:886–92.
42. Kantartzis K, Peter A, Machicao F, et al. Dissociation between fatty liver and insulin resistance in humans carrying a variant of the patatin-like phospholipase 3 gene. Diabetes 2009;58:2616–23.
43. Hyysalo J, Gopalacharyulu P, Bian H, et al. Circulating triacylglycerol signatures in nonalcoholic fatty liver disease associated with the I148M variant in PNPLA3 and with obesity. Diabetes 2014;63:312–22.
44. Palmer CN, Maglio C, Pirazzi C, et al. Paradoxical lower serum triglyceride levels and higher type 2 diabetes mellitus susceptibility in obese individuals with the PNPLA3 148M variant. PLoS One 2012;7:e39362.
45. Shen J, Wong GL, Chan HL, et al. PNPLA3 gene polymorphism accounts for fatty liver in community subjects without metabolic syndrome. Aliment Pharmacol Ther 2014;39:532–9.

The Role of Nonalcoholic Fatty Liver Disease on Cardiovascular Manifestations and Outcomes

Alexander J. Kovalic, MD[a], Sanjaya K. Satapathy, MBBS, MD, DM[b,c],*

KEYWORDS

- Nonalcoholic fatty liver disease • NAFLD • Cardiovascular disease • Atherosclerosis
- Cardiac dysfunction • Conduction abnormalities • Atrial fibrillation
- Thromboembolic risk • Cardiovascular mortality

KEY POINTS

- There have been numerous studies confirming the association between nonalcoholic fatty liver disease (NAFLD) and atherosclerosis, cardiac dysfunction, conduction abnormalities, atrial fibrillation, and thromboembolic risk.
- NAFLD is associated with increased CV events and mortality.
- The key pathogenetic link between NAFLD and cardiovascular events appears to be related insulin resistance.

INTRODUCTION

Nonalcoholic fatty liver disease (NAFLD) is rapidly becoming one of the most common forms of liver disease worldwide.[1] Given the concomitant increase in obesity and the metabolic syndrome, the number of patients with this disease will only increase in the

Author Contribution: A.J. Kovalic was responsible for the initial draft of the article, critical revision of the article, approval of the article S.K. Satapathy was responsible for the concept/design, drafting the article, critical revision of the article, approval of the article.
The authors have nothing to disclose.
a Department of Internal Medicine, Wake Forest Baptist Medical Center, Medical Center Boulevard, Winston-Salem, NC 27103, USA; b Transplant Hepatology, Methodist University Hospital Transplant Institute, University of Tennessee Health Science Center, 1211 Union Avenue, Memphis, TN 38104, USA; c Division of Surgery, Methodist University Hospital Transplant Institute, University of Tennessee Health Science Center, 1211 Union Avenue, Memphis, TN 38104, USA
* Corresponding author. Methodist University Hospital Transplant Institute, University of Tennessee Health Sciences Center, 1211 Union Avenue, Suite #340, Memphis, TN 38104, USA.
E-mail address: ssatat@uthsc.edu

years to come. It has been postulated that a leading cause of mortality among patients with NAFLD is due to cardiovascular (CV) disease, rather than complications directly from liver disease. As more effective and targeted treatment strategies emerge, not only will the size of the NAFLD patient population increase, but also their longevity. Therefore, the incidence of CV sequelae of this disease process will undoubtedly be increasing.

LITERATURE REVIEW

A comprehensive PubMed search was performed, which queried English articles among human patients through February 1, 2017. This literature search included patients with NAFLD, as defined by either "NAFLD," "NAFLD (MeSH Terms)," or "nonalcoholic fatty liver disease," and cross-referenced with other concomitant pathologies that will be listed here in detail. First, atherosclerosis was queried by searching for the terms "atherosclerosis," "coronary artery disease (CAD)," "carotid artery disease," "carotid artery stenosis," "aortic aneurysm," "abdominal aortic aneurysm (AAA)," "endothelial dysfunction," "intima media thickness," "peripheral vascular disease (PVD)," and "peripheral artery disease (PAD)." Upon searching the primary literature, cardiac dysfunction was defined as "cardiac dysfunction," "heart failure," "diastolic dysfunction," "diastolic heart failure," "heart failure with preserved ejection fraction (HFpEF)," and "left ventricular hypertrophy (LVH)." To assess thromboembolic risk, articles were queried for patients with NAFLD with "thromboembolism," "venothromboembolism (VTE)," "deep venous thrombosis (DVT)," or "pulmonary embolism (PE)." Most important, subjects with NAFLD were evaluated on their effect of CV events and mortality, as defined by "myocardial infarction (MI)," "acute coronary syndrome (ACS)," "cerebrovascular accident (CVA)," "transient ischemic attack (TIA)," or "stroke." The endpoint of mortality was assessed using the terms "mortality," "death," "cardiac arrest," or "cardiopulmonary arrest."

ATHEROSCLEROSIS

There are a litany of studies linking NAFLD to atherosclerosis. It is imperative to tease out the influence of NAFLD as an independent risk factor. **Table 1** outlines the current studies with the largest impact on the connection between these two entities.

Earlier systematic reviews provided a comprehensive outlook on studies, noting this association of NAFLD with atherosclerosis. The two reviews listed herein used a large sample size across a multitude of studies and ethnicities. In the review by Sookoian and colleagues,[2] NAFLD was correlated with carotid atherosclerosis. NAFLD was primarily established via ultrasound imaging, with 3 of the 7 studies implementing liver biopsy. In establishing the diagnosis of NAFLD, the liver biopsy remains the gold standard, not only for the detection of hepatic steatosis, but also to assess the presence of NASH. Although ultrasound imaging is a good, noninvasive tool to detect hepatic steatosis, its sensitivity is poor when the degree of hepatic steatosis is less than 30%.[3] Despite liver biopsy remaining the gold standard for the diagnosis of NAFLD, it too is limited by its invasiveness and potential sampling error. Nevertheless, 1 study in this review stratified their results based on liver histology and found that carotid atherosclerosis is more pronounced in cases of more severe NAFLD, such as NASH. The second systematic review by Oni and colleagues[4] validated this affiliation, not only between NAFLD and carotid atherosclerosis, but also coronary artery calcifications, endothelial dysfunction, and arterial stiffness. This systematic review implemented a large sample size including 27 different studies, but did not comment on the degree of atherosclerosis in relation to the

Table 1
Evidence demonstrating association between NAFLD and atherosclerosis

Reference	Key Findings	Study Design/ Nationality	Number of Subjects	Notable Cohort Characteristics	Diagnostic Modality	% NASH Based on Liver Biopsy	Limitations
Bhatia et al,[7] 2016	Primary endpoint found PUFA decreased CIMT progression; reduced hepatic steatosis and lower CK-18 levels were independently associated with reduced CIMT progression	RCT/United Kingdom	92 total 45 in treatment group, 47 in placebo group	Mean age 54.2 in placebo group vs 48.6 in PUFA cohort Placebo group 66% males vs 49% in PUFA cohort	MRS	n/a	CIMT progression a secondary outcome as a substudy of the WELCOME trial, and no sample size or power calculations were calculated in this study
Puchner et al,[10] 2015	NAFLD more frequently correlated with high-risk coronary plaques, independent of CAD severity and traditional CV risk factors	Retrospective case-control analysis of one arm of RCT/ United States	182 NAFLD cases, 263 controls	34.1% females in NAFLD group vs 55.5% in non-NAFLD group	CT scan	N/A	Study performed in patients with acute chest pain in ED, most likely with higher prevalence of CV risk factors and atherosclerosis than the general population. Alcohol history was obtained through chart review and not validated questionnaire, which may have underreported alcohol consumption in this patient population

(continued on next page)

Table 1
(continued)

Reference	Key Findings	Study Design/ Nationality	Number of Subjects	Notable Cohort Characteristics	Diagnostic Modality	% NASH Based on Liver Biopsy	Limitations
Madan et al,[6] 2015	NAFLD-associated with increased CIMT in both children and adults	Metaanalysis/ United States	20 adult studies 8652 NAFLD, 10,622 controls	5 hospital-based studies, all others are population-based or from outpatient clinics	Liver biopsy in 4 studies and US imaging in 16 studies	Only 1 of the 4 studies that used liver biopsy reports NASH cases separately; 43 out of 50 NAFLD cases had biopsy-proven NASH, which was associated with significantly increased CIMT compared with both controls and simple hepatic steatosis	Heterogeneity of studies with respect to carotid plaques, based on variation of definitions of CIMT via US imaging
Ampuero et al,[5] 2015	NAFLD associated with increased CIMT and CAD, as defined by coronary artery stenosis >50%	Metaanalysis/ Spain	14 studies (10 to assess CIMT, 4 to assess coronary artery stenosis >50%)	Atherosclerosis group: 2932 total CAD group: 999 NAFLD, 948 controls	Atherosclerosis group: Liver biopsy in 2 studies, US imaging in 8 studies CAD group: US imaging in all 4 studies	N/A	Studies selected somewhat limited owing to endpoints of CIMT and carotid plaques

Oni et al,[4] 2013	NAFLD associated with increased CIMT, coronary artery calcifications, endothelial dysfunction, and arterial stiffness	Systematic review/ United States	27 studies analyzing CIMT, coronary artery calcifications, endothelial dysfunction, and arterial stiffness	Numerous studies reported across a multitude of ethnic cohorts	Liver biopsy 6/16 studies assessing CIMT, 0/7 measuring coronary artery calcification, 4/7 studies comparing endothelial dysfunction, 1/6 studies observing arterial stiffness	Not universally analyzed, only calculated in limited studies	Primary endpoint was measurement of atherosclerotic risk factors. Patients with NAFLD were not stratified, but merely an association with these factors.
Sookoian et al,[2] 2008	NAFLD associated with increased CIMT and carotid atherosclerosis	Systematic review/ Argentina	7 studies 1427 NAFLD, 2070 controls	Italian, Turkish, Spanish, and German cohorts 5 hospital and 2 population based	Liver biopsy in 3/7 studies, US imaging in remaining studies	N/A	Only 1 study differentiated CIMT based on liver histology, in which NASH associated with increased carotid atherosclerosis than simple hepatic steatosis and control patients

Abbreviations: CAD, coronary artery disease; CIMT, carotid intima-media thickness; CK-18, cytokeratin 18; CT, computed tomography; CV, cardiovascular; ED, emergency department; MRS, magnetic resonance spectroscopy; N/A, not applicable; NAFLD, nonalcoholic fatty liver disease; NASH, nonalcoholic steatohepatitis; PUFA, polyunsaturated fatty acid; RCT, randomized, controlled trial; US, ultrasound.

severity of liver histology in those studies that implemented liver biopsy. In summation, these large systematic reviews provide the necessary foundation substantiating the affinity of NAFLD and atherosclerosis.

Two major metaanalyses have been performed to date regarding the relationship between atherosclerosis and NAFLD. In the first metaanalysis by Ampuero and colleagues,[5] NAFLD was identified as a risk factor for atherosclerosis as defined by measurements of carotid intima-media thickness (CIMT) and coronary artery stenosis of greater than 50%. A large sample size was used in this study; however, most of the studies used ultrasound imaging to establish NAFLD with no mention of the prevalence of NASH. Another metaanalysis analyzed more than 8000 patients with NAFLD across 20 adult studies.[6] This review also found a significant link between the presence of NAFLD and increased CIMT. Although the majority of the studies used ultrasound imaging, there were 4 studies that analyzed patients who underwent liver biopsy. One of these studies found a significant association between patients with biopsy-proven NASH and increased CIMT compared with both simple hepatic steatosis and controls. Significant heterogeneity exists among the wide range of studies analyzed in this metaanalysis. Much of this discrepancy lies within the variation of defining carotid plaques as measured by CIMT. This lack of uniformity among studies has the potential to convolute results; however, the large sample size and reproducible nature of these findings provides compelling evidence for the association between NAFLD and increased CIMT.

Since the release of these metaanalyses and systematic reviews, two retrospective case-control studies targeting subgroups of major randomized, controlled trials have been published observing NAFLD and atherosclerotic risk. One randomized, controlled trial analyzed the effect of polyunsaturated fatty acids on CIMT.[7] It was observed that 15 to 18 months of polyunsaturated fatty acid therapy caused a decrease in CIMT. In a predefined substudy among this cohort, antihypertensive use, lower cytokeratin 18 levels, and reduced hepatic steatosis, as detected by ^{1}H magnetic resonance spectroscopy (^{1}H-MRS), were found to be in conjunction with reduced CIMT progression across this cohort. Cytokeratin 18 has proven to be a novel biomarker in the assessment of NAFLD, and also demonstrated to accurately correlate with liver histology.[8,9] Overall, this study suggests that the presence or severity of NAFLD is correlated with the progression of atherosclerosis.

Another study observed this relationship among patients of one arm of the randomized, controlled trial of ROMICAT II trial (Multicenter Study to Rule Out Myocardial Infarction by Cardiac Computed Tomography). Between 182 patients with NAFLD and 263 matched controls presenting with ACS, patients with NAFLD were found to have increased frequency of high-risk coronary plaques independent of other CV risk factors.[10] Although this study provides strong evidence of this association, several limitations exist. First, there was a discrepancy between the NAFLD group, which was composed of 34.1% females, and 55.5% in the non-NAFLD group. Second, this study established NAFLD via CT scan, which, much like ultrasound imaging, has a poor sensitivity when the degree of hepatic steatosis is low.[11] It is not inconceivable that a number of patients with a low amount of hepatic steatosis went undetected and were then placed in the non-NAFLD group. However, it is difficult to assess for NAFLD in the presence of ACS, or patients presenting with acute chest pain. It is not practical, nor is there time, to undergo liver biopsy. Last, alcohol history was obtained through chart review. No active interview or validated questionnaire was performed in this setting. This methodology perhaps could underreport alcohol consumption, which could confound results with the presence of alcoholic liver disease. Although limitations are apparent in this study, they do not overturn the clear evidence supporting the cooperation between the presence of NAFLD and atherosclerosis.

Nonalcoholic Steatohepatitis and Atherosclerosis

Two recent studies have set out to specifically assess the effects of NASH on atherosclerosis. One cross-sectional study out of Japan observed a higher low-density lipoprotein (LDL) migration index among patients with NASH as compared with the rest of patients with NAFLD.[12] The LDL migration index is an indicator for small dense LDL, and, therefore, higher levels suggest increased atherosclerotic risk. This analysis was performed among a small sample size. Furthermore, no liver biopsy was performed in controls, who simply underwent US examination to rule out the presence of hepatic steatosis. As mentioned, US examination is unable to definitely rule out hepatic steatosis, and some of these control subjects could potentially have had mild steatosis undetected on noninvasive imaging.

In a retrospective case-control study, an American cohort was shown to have increased atherosclerogenic profile among patients with NALFD.[13] This profile included insulin, triglycerides, apolipoprotein B, very low-density lipoprotein size, LDL, and small dense LDL. However, patients with NASH displayed a nonsignificant increase in these measurements. Not only was this study performed in almost exclusively in Caucasian subjects, but it also implemented liver biopsy only after hepatic steatosis was detected on noninvasive imaging, either with US examination or ^{1}H-MRS. Therefore, the control subjects did not undergo liver biopsy, which presents a similar limitation to the previous study.

CARDIAC DYSFUNCTION

The effects on cardiac structure and function have long been analyzed among patients with NAFLD. Studies analyzing systolic or diastolic dysfunction in this patient population are detailed in **Table 2**.

In the first study observing this effect, Goland and colleagues[14] revealed an association between NAFLD and diastolic dysfunction and left ventricular (LV) mass, which can be a sign of increased heart strain or LV hypertrophy. This study included nondiabetic, normotensive subjects who were not morbidly obese. Patients with an abnormal exercise stress test were also excluded. Eleven patients underwent liver biopsy, 6 of whom were found to have NASH on histology. However, outcomes were not differentiated among the histologic subtypes. This was somewhat of a selective cohort in that subjects had US findings of hepatic steatosis and sent to a hepatology clinic for further evaluation. Yet, it was an important, prospective examination of cardiac dysfunction in patients with NAFLD that would serve as a benchmark for future studies.

Multiple further studies across a vast array of ethnicities and study populations have been analyzed for their effect on cardiac function in patients with NAFLD. In a prospective case-control study, Fotbolcu and colleagues[15] demonstrated a relationship with systolic and diastolic dysfunction in addition to increased LV mass among nondiabetic patients with NAFLD. However, even among nondiabetic patients there was significantly increased homeostatic model assessment of insulin resistance (HOMA-IR) among subjects with NAFLD (3.1) versus controls (1.28). HOMA-IR is a diagnostic quantification of insulin resistance, and values greater than 2.0 to 2.5 have been shown independently to enhance the diagnostic value of distinguishing insulin resistance in subjects with NAFLD versus controls.[16] Similarly, Granér and colleagues[17] illustrated that nondiabetic subjects with NAFLD

Table 2
The link between NAFLD and cardiac dysfunction

Reference	Key Findings	Study Design/ Nationality	Number of Subjects	Notable Cohort Characteristics	Diagnostic Modality	% NASH Based on Liver Biopsy	Limitations
Psychari et al,[56] 2016	NAFLD was not associated with increased thickness of epicardial adipose tissue	Cross-sectional/ Greece	57 NAFLD, 48 controls	BMI significantly higher in NAFLD group (31.9) vs control group (26.5)	US imaging	N/A	No uniform modality to quantify epicardial adipose tissue. This study used echocardiography; however, more sensitive tests are available, such as cardiac MRI.
VanWagner et al,[57] 2015	NAFLD associated with impaired diastolic relaxation, increased LV filling pressure, and increased heart strain than controls based on echocardiography	Cross-sectional/ United States	271 NAFLD, 2442 control	58.8% females 48% African Americans Prevalence of T2DM 42.4% in NAFLD group vs 11.0% in controls	CT scan	N/A	Disparity in prevalence of T2DM between groups

Granér et al,[17] 2014	NAFLD results in higher amounts of epicardial adipose tissue and associated diastolic dysfunction	Cross-sectional/ Finland	75 subjects, stratified into 3 groups based on hepatic triglyceride content	100% nondiabetic males HOMA-IR in the low, moderate, and high hepatic triglyceride content groups were 0.6, 1.0, and 3.0, respectively	1H-MRS	N/A	Diabetes excluded based on 2-h glucose tolerance test, no measurement of HgA1c Ischemic cardiomyopathy was essentially excluded in this study based on adenosine MR perfusion cardiac stress test More aberrations at baseline with respect to age, BMI, smoking, and dyslipidemia among groups with higher amount of hepatic steatosis
Kim et al,[58] 2014	Subjects with NAFLD and/or metabolic syndrome exhibited higher incidence of subclinical diastolic dysfunction based on echocardiography	Cross-sectional/ Korea	1886 total subjects, then stratified by presence of NAFLD and/ or metabolic syndrome	Groups with metabolic syndrome had significantly higher prevalence of insulin resistance and diabetes	CT scan	N/A	Did not rule out CAD or ischemic cardiomyopathy HOMA-IR used to establish insulin resistance, no HgA1c

(continued on next page)

Table 2
(continued)

Reference	Key Findings	Study Design/ Nationality	Number of Subjects	Notable Cohort Characteristics	Diagnostic Modality	% NASH Based on Liver Biopsy	Limitations
Karabay et al,[20] 2014	Systolic dysfunction observed in NAFLD group compared with controls; however, no difference found between NAFLD severity No significant difference in cardiac function was observed in a subgroup analysis between controls and 11 patients with NAFLD who were normotensive, nondiabetic, nonobese, and without insulin resistance	Cross-sectional/ Italy and Turkey	55 NAFLD, 21 controls	Based on baseline histology, BMI, insulin resistance, and dyslipidemia were significantly pronounced as NAFLD severity increased	Liver biopsy	40%	Potential role of insulin resistance seen with increased incidence of comorbidities with increasing severity of liver histology HOMA-IR to establish insulin resistance, no HgA1c noted
Hallsworth et al,[19] 2013	NAFLD associated with systolic and diastolic dysfunction based on cardiac MRI; however, no difference in LV mass and myocardial metabolism based on 31P-MRS	Cross-sectional/ United Kingdom	19 NAFLD, 19 controls	Nondiabetic, overweight subjects Fasting blood glucose levels similar in both groups and within normal reference range	1H-MRS	N/A	Noncomprehensive measurement of insulin resistance; however, this study observed nonobese patients with no history of diabetes

Fotbolcu et al,[15] 2010	Prospective case-control/ Turkey	35 NAFLD, 30 control	NAFLD associated with systolic and diastolic dysfunction in addition to increased LV mass	Nondiabetic, normotensive subjects HOMA-IR significantly increased in NAFLD group (3.59) vs controls (1.28)	US	N/A	Patients with T2DM were excluded; however, disparity in insulin resistance was present
Fallo et al,[59] 2009	Cross-sectional/ Italy	48 NAFLD, 38 controls	NAFLD associated with diastolic dysfunction based on echocardiography; however, no significant difference in LV mass	Untreated patients with newly diagnosed hypertension HOMA-IR significantly increased in NAFLD group (3.1) vs controls (1.6)	US	N/A	Disparity in prevalence of T2DM between groups
Goland et al,[14] 2006	Prospective case-control/ Israel	38 NAFLD, 25 controls	NAFLD associated with diastolic dysfunction based on echocardiography and increased LV mass	Nondiabetic, normotensive subjects who were not morbidly obese Significantly increased fasting glucose in subjects with NAFLD (100.3) vs controls (83.0)	US, with 11 subjects undergoing further liver biopsy	NASH confirmed in 6 out of 11 patients who underwent liver biopsy, however did not differentiate outcomes	Study only included a select patient population who had elevated liver enzymes or US findings of fatty liver and referred to hepatology clinic Excluded patients with morbid obesity (BMI > 40) or an abnormal exercise stress test

Abbreviations: BMI, body mass index; CAD, coronary artery disease; CT, computed tomography; HgA1c, hemoglobin A1c; HOMA-IR, homeostatic model assessment of insulin resistance; LV, left ventricular; MRS, magnetic resonance spectroscopy; N/A, not applicable; NAFLD, nonalcoholic fatty liver disease; NASH, nonalcoholic steatohepatitis; T2DM, type 2 diabetes mellitus; US, ultrasound.

have higher amounts of epicardial adipose tissue as well as diastolic dysfunction. Although these patients were nondiabetic, HOMA-IR increased proportionately with the degree of hepatic steatosis between groups. Furthermore, hepatic steatosis in this study was diagnosed via ^{1}H-MRS, whose sensitivity approaches that of liver biopsy and is more effectively able to detect steatosis even when less pronounced, unlike the usefulness of US imaging or CT scanning.[18] Although ^{1}H-MRS provides increased diagnostic yield in the assessment of NAFLD, its global operation for everyday practice is restricted by its expense and limited availability. Even though the relationship between NAFLD and cardiac dysfunction is well-documented, most of these studies implement a cross-sectional design. Therefore, no causality or temporal relationships can be gleaned from these studies, and further analysis using prospective trials are necessary to confirm this relationship.

Given the presence of this phenomenon seen in nondiabetics, a predictable association also exists among diabetic patients with NAFLD and cardiac dysfunction, primarily regarding LV mass, impaired diastolic relaxation, and perhaps systolic dysfunction. However, impaired insulin resistance is observed more frequently in patients with NAFLD as compared with control subjects, which could certainly factor into cardiac function. Two exceptions seem to exist here. First, in the study by Hallsworth and colleagues,[19] nondiabetic, overweight subjects with NAFLD with no significant difference in fasting blood glucose levels compared with controls were found to have impaired systolic and diastolic dysfunction. However, this was a very small study, and fasting blood glucose levels do not serve as an accurate barometer of insulin resistance. Second, a subgroup analysis was performed in the study by Karabay and colleagues[20] between controls and 11 normotensive, nondiabetic, nonobese subjects with NAFLD without insulin resistance. In this subgroup analysis, there was no difference in cardiac function. Although an analysis of 11 NAFLD represents a small and selective patient group, this finding is worth pursuing in larger future studies. Overall, cardiac dysfunction is widely observed in patients with NAFLD; however, this finding may be attributed to the increased prevalence of type 2 diabetes mellitus (T2DM), or at least insulin resistance, in this at-risk patient population.

Finally, NAFLD also has been demonstrated to impact morbidity directly in patients with cardiac dysfunction. Among patients initially admitted for exacerbation of acute heart failure, NAFLD was found to be an independent risk factor for readmission rates in a prospective 1-year follow-up study.[21] This study was performed among an older cohort, average around 80 years of age, and patients who were readmitted had a significantly higher incidence of both NAFLD and atrial fibrillation.

Nonalcoholic Steatohepatitis and Cardiac Dysfunction

There have been a paucity of studies exclusively observing patients with NASH via liver biopsy and their corresponding association with cardiac dysfunction. One prospective Turkish study found an association with NASH and subclinical systolic and diastolic LV dysfunction as compared with controls.[22] However, a rather small sample size was conducted and there were significant differences in insulin resistance at baseline, as measured by HOMA-IR, between the NASH group (5.29) and the control group (2.1). Another cross-sectional study analyzed liver biopsies from an obese, predominantly male cohort from southern Italy.[23] They concluded that the severity of NAFLD correlated with epicardial adipose tissue thickness, which was an indicator for diastolic dysfunction.

AUTONOMIC DYSFUNCTION, CONDUCTION ABNORMALITIES, AND ARRHYTHMIAS

Independent of systolic and diastolic dysfunction, patients with NAFLD also have a predilection for cardiac autonomic dysfunction and conduction abnormalities. The underlying insulin resistance commonly seen in NAFLD predisposes these patients to increased free fatty acid and adipose tissue deposition among remote tissues, such as the liver or even the heart.[24] This increase in epicardial adipose tissue deposition, also mentioned previously in the Graner and Petta studies, could potentially serve as the mechanism for this phenomenon. Cardiac autonomic dysfunction has been documented among patients with NAFLD.[25–27] Recently, Balcioğlu and colleagues[28] demonstrated that increased epicardial adipose tissue thickness is associated with sympathovagal imbalance, and is, therefore, a strong predictor of cardiac arrhythmias. Other studies have also revealed a correlation with QTc prolongation in this patient population.[29,30]

The increased propensity for cardiac autonomic abnormalities and arrhythmias set the stage for the development of atrial fibrillation. There have been 3 major studies observing the prevalence of atrial fibrillation in patients with NAFLD that have been described in **Table 3**.

A cross-sectional study of hospitalized, diabetic patients with atrial fibrillation demonstrated an association with NAFLD.[31] However, this study carries the burden of selection bias within a highly restricted group, including inpatient diabetics. There was a significant difference in the mean age and prevalence of NAFLD in patients with atrial fibrillation as compared with those without atrial fibrillation.

Another prospective study followed diabetics without atrial fibrillation at baseline for 10 years.[32] At the end of this study, it was found that patients with NAFLD had increased development of atrial fibrillation as compared with controls. However, even in the presence of a strong, prospective study design, there is a large disparity between the comorbidities among patients. Patients who developed atrial fibrillation had advanced age, longer duration of diabetes, higher blood pressure, increased heart failure, and increased carotid artery stenosis after the 10-year follow-up as compared with patients who did not develop atrial fibrillation. Nevertheless, a sound prospective study design following patients over a 10-year span represents the strongest evidence to date regarding this topic.

In another prospective study of nondiabetic, normotensive patients, findings confirming increased atrial fibrillation were upheld among patients with NAFLD.[33] This finding was primarily defined by an increase in impaired atrial conduction and left atrial volume. In this study, there was a relatively small sample size as well as significant differences in insulin resistance, as defined by HOMA-IR, between the NAFLD and control groups. Despite these limitations, there certainly seems to be an association between atrial fibrillation and NAFLD based on current data.

THROMBOEMBOLIC RISK

Independent of their increased propensity for atrial fibrillation, patients with NAFLD are also at increased risk of thromboembolic events. The major trials discussing this association are listed in **Table 4**.

In the first major study on this topic, it was demonstrated that patients with NAFLD had increased activity of factors VIII, IX, XI, and XII.[34] These findings were independent of age, gender, body mass index (BMI), and presence of diabetes. In a follow-up study, NAFLD was found to be associated with idiopathic, unprovoked VTE.[35] In this prospective Italian study, all patients were referred for suspicion of VTE. Obvious insults such as recent surgery or trauma, pregnancy, contraceptive use, history of

Table 3
Association of NAFLD with AF

Reference	Key Findings	Study Design/ Nationality	Number of Subjects	Notable Cohort Characteristics	Diagnostic Modality	% NASH Based on Liver Biopsy	Limitations
Ozveren et al,[33] 2016	Impaired atrial conduction more prevalent in patients with NAFLD compared with controls Increased left atrial volume suggests an increased risk of AF among patients with NAFLD, even independent from cardiac disease, diabetes, or hypertension	Prospective case-control/Turkey	59 NAFLD, 22 controls	Nondiabetic, nonhypertensive patients with no prior history of cardiac disease HOMA-IR elevated in NAFLD group (3.9) vs controls (1.5)	US imaging	N/A	Relatively small sample size and difficulty to identify patients with isolated NAFLD without coexisting diabetes, hypertension, or cardiac disease
Targher et al,[32] 2013	Increased prevalence of AF in hospitalized patients with NAFLD with T2DM	Cross-sectional/Italy	702 total patients	Significantly increased mean age of patients in the AF group (75) vs controls (65) NAFLD prevalent in 88.2% of patient with AF and 71.1% without	US imaging	N/A	Selection bias of hospitalized patients with T2DM

| Targgher et al,[32] 2013 | After 10 years of follow-up of T2DM patients without AF at baseline, there is an increased development of AF in patients with NAFLD | Prospective cohort/ Italy | 400 total patients, 42 developed AF and 358 did not | Patients with AF after 10 years of follow-up had increased age, longer duration of diabetes, higher SBP, increased history of HF, increased concomitant carotid artery stenosis, and NAFLD as compared with patients who did not develop AF | US imaging | N/A | Selection bias of patients with T2DM Large disparity of comorbidities between 2 groups |

Abbreviations: AF, atrial fibrillation; HF, heart failure; HOMA-IR, homeostatic model assessment of insulin resistance; LV, left ventricular; N/A, not applicable; NAFLD, nonalcoholic fatty liver disease; NASH, nonalcoholic steatohepatitis; SBP, systolic blood pressure; T2DM, type 2 diabetes mellitus; US, ultrasound.

Table 4
NAFLD and increased risk of thromboembolism

Reference	Key Findings	Study Design/Nationality	Number of Subjects	Notable Cohort Characteristics	Diagnostic Modality	% NASH Based on Liver Biopsy	Limitations
Tripodi et al,[37] 2014	Increased activity of factor VIII and decreased activity of protein C promote a procoagulant state in patients with NAFLD, with least severe forms in isolated hepatic steatosis and progressing to most severe in the presence of cirrhosis	Cross-sectional/Italy	113 NAFLD (32 hepatic steatosis, 51 NASH, 30 cirrhosis), 54 alcoholic/viral liver disease, 179 controls	76% male subjects with NAFLD Controls were selected from patients with normal liver enzymes, BMI <30, and no evidence of diabetes	Liver biopsy	45%	Poorly matched controls
Yu et al,[36] 2014	Early atherosclerotic changes increased proportionally to whole blood viscosity, which is elevated in NAFLD even after adjusting for CV risk factors	Cross-sectional/China	2032 subjects with NAFLD	50.9% males Average BMI 24	US imaging	N/A	Patients with hypertension, diabetes, lipid-lowering agents, or any other etiology for liver disease were excluded

Study	Conclusion	Design/Country	Sample	Notes	Imaging		Limitations
Di Minno et al,[35] 2010	NAFLD associated with idiopathic VTE	Prospective case control/Italy	138 cases idiopathic VTE, 276 controls	58.7% of VTE cases reported smoking, but only 39% in controls Patients with active malignancy; pregnancy; recent surgery, trauma, of immobilization, oral contraceptive use; history of repeated birth loss; or history of VTE were excluded	US imaging	N/A	Disparity in smoking history between groups Control group may not represent healthy population, because they were initially referred for suspicion of VTE, but then ruled out Cancer was a part of the exclusion criteria, but occult cancer still a possibility
Kotronen et al,[34] 2011	Increased activity of factors VIII, IX, XI, and XII are seen in NAFLD and show to be independent of age, gender, and BMI	Retrospective case control/ Finland	54 NAFLD, 44 controls	None of the subjects had T2DM	1H-MRS	N/A	Small sample size

Abbreviations: BMI, body mass index; MRS, magnetic resonance spectroscopy; N/A, not applicable; NAFLD, nonalcoholic fatty liver disease; NASH, nonalcoholic steatohepatitis; SBP, systolic blood pressure; T2DM, type 2 diabetes mellitus; US, ultrasound; VTE, venous thromboembolism.

VTE, and active malignancy were excluded in addition to genetic culprits for VTE. However, there was a large disparity in smoking between patients who had VTE (58.7%) as compared with controls (39%). Also, even the control patients were initially referred for suspicion of VTE and may not represent a normal, healthy control population. Cancer was one component of the exclusion criteria; however, occult cancer was not ruled out. Despite these limitations, this prospective study put forward a strong level of evidence in support of an association for thrombo-embolic events in NAFLD patients.

One cross-sectional study out of China established that early atherosclerotic changes were increased in proportion to whole blood viscosity, which was found to be increased in patients with NAFLD.[36] This held true even when adjusting for CV risk factors, such as obesity. The mean BMI in this study was 24 kg/m². Again, this was merely an association and no firm relationship can be established from this cross-sectional design.

Another recent study found a prothrombotic state in NAFLD patients with an increase in factor VIII and decrease in protein C activity.[37] This study analyzed varying degrees of NAFLD severity as established via liver biopsy, and revealed that the degree of coagulopathy increased with histologic severity of NAFLD. However, this study used a poor selection of controls, who were defined by normal liver enzymes, a BMI of less than 30 kg/m², and no underlying diabetes. No liver biopsy was performed in the controls, which potentially could misrepresent accurate results in this study. Meanwhile, the patients with NAFLD were compared not only with controls, but also with patients with alcoholic and viral liver disease. It was established that patients with NAFLD had increased incidence of VTE as compared with control subjects and those with other forms of liver disease. This finding is novel, substantiating the prothrombotic state among patients with NAFLD.

CARDIOVASCULAR EVENTS AND MORTALITY

All of these factors among subjects with NAFLD, such as atherosclerosis, cardiac dysfunction, cardiac conduction abnormalities, arrhythmias, and thromboembolism, place these patients at significantly increased risk of mortality from CV events. Endpoints such as MI, ACS, CVA, or stroke were analyzed with the outcome of mortality, death, cardiac arrest, or cardiopulmonary arrest. The effects of NAFLD on resultant CV events are listed in **Table 5**.

There have been 2 systematic reviews to date on this topic. In the most recent review by Luo and colleagues,[38] NAFLD was found to be associated with both increased CV and all-cause mortality. This analysis was performed across 13 prospective and primarily American studies; however, multiple other studies were included worldwide and included more than 241,000 patients. Liver biopsy was performed in 4 studies in addition to ultrasound examination in 4 others. One major limitation of this review is that the majority of the patients in this analysis come from 5 studies that established the diagnosis of NAFLD based on liver enzymes. Liver enzymes, including aspartate aminotransferase and alanine aminotransferase, have been proven to be a poor diagnostic tool for NAFLD.[39] Although it is true that increased liver enzymes can be seen in NAFLD, the specificity for this disease is very poor. Furthermore, it has been proven that patients with NAFLD may have normal levels of liver enzymes, which, in effect, indicates the poor usefulness for this measure as a diagnostic modality.[40,41] Overall, the remaining studies in which patients underwent liver biopsy or ultrasound examination still provide ample evidence for increased CV and all-cause mortality among patients with NAFLD.

Table 5
Increased incidence of CV events among patients with NAFLD

Reference	Key Findings	Study Design/ Nationality	Number of Subjects	Notable Cohort Characteristics	Diagnostic Modality	% NASH Based on Liver Biopsy	Limitations
Zeb et al,[45] 2016	Patients with NAFLD have increased incidence of nonfatal coronary heart disease (as defined by MI, resuscitated cardiac arrest, or angina with or without revascularization) and all-cause mortality over median 7.6 y follow-up	Prospective cohort/ United States	728 NAFLD, 3391 controls	Not reported	CT scan	N/A	Poor characterization of baseline characteristics Excluded patients with self-reported cirrhosis
Perera et al,[44] 2016	Patients with NAFLD presenting with ACS had higher GRACE score as well as increased inpatient and 6-mo postdischarge mortality	Retrospective case-control/ Sri Lanka	120	62.5% males	US imaging	N/A	Small sample size

(continued on next page)

Table 5
(continued)

Reference	Key Findings	Study Design/ Nationality	Number of Subjects	Notable Cohort Characteristics	Diagnostic Modality	% NASH Based on Liver Biopsy	Limitations
Fracanzani et al,[43] 2016	Patients with NAFLD at increased risk for CV events than controls with presence of carotid plaques and hepatic steatosis the strongest predictors of CV events; grade of steatosis, ALT, and GGT significantly higher in those Patients with NAFLD who developed CV events	10-y prospective case-control/ Italy	125 NAFLD, 250 controls	87% males in NAFLD cohort	Abdominal and carotid artery US imaging, liver biopsy in 54 patients with NAFLD	N/A	25% of all patients lost to follow-up 37% of controls developed steatosis
Emre et al,[51] 2015	Among nondiabetic patients undergoing PCI for STEMI, patients with NAFLD had increased incidence of multivessel CAD Higher NAFLD severity correlated with absent myocardial perfusion, lack of resolution of ST segment elevation, higher peak CK-MB levels, lower postprocedural LVEF, in-hospital major adverse cardiac events, and death	Prospective cohort/ Turkey	186 nondiabetic patients undergoing PCI for STEMI, 149 of whom were found to have NAFLD	76% males Cohort stratified based on semiquantitative severity score based on US imaging, from 0 to 8 51% severity score <3 were smokers compared with 61% in >3 group (possibly skewing less severe patients with NAFLD with worse CAD)	US imaging	N/A	Specific patients presenting with acute chest pain Patients stratified by severity based on US examination, which is not standard of care CK-MB used as cardiac biomarker

Study	Design/Location	N	Findings	Demographics	Imaging		Limitations
Wong et al,[60] 2016	5-y prospective cohort/Hong Kong	612	In patients requiring heart catheterization, patients with NAFLD were more likely to have >50% coronary artery stenosis and requiring PCI, but NAFLD was not associated with increased mortality or CV complications vs controls	70% males Average BMI 25.7 in NAFLD, 23.2 in control group	US imaging	N/A	Lack of liver biopsy performed among study group, but not practical in setting of ACS
Mellinger et al,[48] 2015	Cross-sectional study of Framingham Heart Study offspring and third generation cohorts/United States	3014	No association between hepatic steatosis and CV events However, there was a significant association between hepatic steatosis and subclinical CVD, which includes coronary artery calcium and abdominal artery calcium, especially in males	50.5% females	CT scan	N/A	Cross-sectional study, inability to conclude causality Low prevalence of clinical CVD outcomes Mean age of CVD group was 62.3 while in the no CVD group, mean age was 50.4 T2DM prevalent in 20.9% of CVD group while 5.1% in no CVD group
Luo et al,[38] 2015	Systematic review/China	13 prospective studies 241,404 total subjects	NAFLD associated with CV mortality and all-cause mortality	Primarily American studies; however, included 1 study from each of the following: Sweden, Austria, Canada, Finland, the Netherlands	Liver biopsy in 4 studies US imaging in 4 studies Liver enzymes in 5 studies	3 studies comment on influence of NASH on mortality (see **Table 6**)	5 of 13 studies assumed NAFLD based off of liver enzymes

(continued on next page)

Table 5
(continued)

Reference	Key Findings	Study Design/ Nationality	Number of Subjects	Notable Cohort Characteristics	Diagnostic Modality	% NASH Based on Liver Biopsy	Limitations
Pickhardt et al,[47] 2014	NAFLD cases demonstrated no progression to symptomatic liver disease (eg, NASH or cirrhosis), but was associated with increased subsequent CV events after 5- to 10-y follow-up	Retrospective case control/ United States	282 NAFLD, 768 controls	Diabetes prevalent in 35.5% of NAFLD group vs 12.5% in control	CT scan	N/A	After controlling for diabetes mellitus and BMI, hepatic steatosis was not found to be an independent risk factor for CV events
Pisto et al,[46] 2014	Increase in hepatic steatosis increases the risk of CV events after 19 y of follow-up	Retrospective case control/ Finland	268 NAFLD, 720 controls	Groups 0, 1, and 2 have 2.4%, 12.1%, and 36.8% diabetic subjects, respectively	US imaging	N/A	Subjective severity of hepatic steatosis based on liver echogenicity on US imaging CV events heavily influenced by diabetes

Study	Results	Design/Country	Population	Characteristics	Imaging		Comments
Dunn et al,[49] 2013	Hepatic steatosis was not shown to be a strong predictor of liver-related or CV outcomes at 5 y of follow-up in diabetic patients	Retrospective cohort/United States	2343 total diabetic patients, 233 with NAFLD and 2110 without	54% females Predominantly Caucasian cohort Mean age at baseline significantly higher in <30% steatosis group (66.6) vs >30% steatosis group (58.1) Mean BMI at baseline significantly higher in >30% steatosis group (36.7) vs <30% steatosis group (30.8)	CT scan, but 41 patients underwent liver biopsy	N/A	NAFLD defined as >30% hepatic steatosis, which is not standard definition Other forms of hepatic steatosis and liver disease were not actively excluded, but not included in this study if they carried the corresponding ICD-9 code (ie, alcohol abuse, alcoholic liver disease, hepatitis B or C) Some nonfatal outcomes (eg, angina, arrhythmia, encephalopathy) can occur more than once, and will become more prevalent in a population with longer survival
Vilar et al,[42] 2013	NAFLD associated with increased rates of CV events and mortality	Review/Brazil	10 studies 2585 total subjects	Primarily Asian subjects, including Japan, Korea, China, Taiwan, Turkey, Israel	CT scan or US imaging	N/A	Primarily cross-sectional studies, some with a low level of evidence Mainly Asian subjects, quite polarized from typical American population

(continued on next page)

Table 5
(continued)

Reference	Key Findings	Study Design/ Nationality	Number of Subjects	Notable Cohort Characteristics	Diagnostic Modality	% NASH Based on Liver Biopsy	Limitations
Boddi et al,[50] 2013	Elevated prevalence of NAFLD in nondiabetic patients with STEMI, and furthermore, severe NAFLD associated with more cases of multivessel CAD	Retrospective case control/ Italy	83 NAFLD, 12 controls	78.9% males	US imaging	N/A	Stratified based on semiquantitative severity score based on US imaging, from 0 to 8. Other diagnostic modalities not as appropriate in setting of STEMI with patients in cardiac intensive care unit
Targher et al,[61] 2007	NAFLD associated with increased CV events in diabetic patients	Retrospective case control/ Italy	384 NAFLD, 1719 controls	63% males	US imaging	N/A	Diabetic cohort, mainly with male subjects
Hamaguchi et al,[62] 2007	NAFLD associated with increased CV events	Prospective case control/ Japan	231 NAFLD, 990 controls	80% males among subjects with NAFLD	US imaging	N/A	Predominantly male cohort
Targher et al,[63] 2005	T2DM in NAFLD significantly increases CV events after 5 y of follow-up	Prospective case control/ Italy	248 NAFLD, 496 controls	62% males	US imaging	N/A	Focused on diabetic patients

Abbreviations: ACS, acute coronary syndrome; ALT, alanine aminotransferase; BMI, body mass index; CAD, coronary artery disease; CK-MB, creatine kinase myocardial band; CT, computed tomography; CV, cardiovascular; GGT, gamma glutamyl transferase; GRACE, Global Registry of Acute Coronary Events; ICD-9, *International Classification of Diseases*, 9th edition; LVEF, left ventricular ejection fraction; MI, myocardial infarction; N/A, not applicable; NAFLD, nonalcoholic fatty liver disease; NASH, nonalcoholic steatohepatitis; PCI, percutaneous coronary intervention; STEMI, ST-elevation myocardial infarction; T2DM, type 2 diabetes mellitus; US, ultrasound.

The second review by Vilar and colleagues[42] also reported increased rates of CV events and mortality among patients with NAFLD across 10 different studies. These studies were primarily cross-sectional in nature and mainly composed of Asian subjects, which can be quite polarized from typical American subjects with respect to comorbidities and BMI. These studies used CT scan or US imaging, which again, are poor modalities for detecting hepatic steatosis when less pronounced, in addition to the inability to assess for NAFLD severity and the presence of NASH.

Since the data from these reviews were published, there have been several studies continuing to detail this relationship between NAFLD and CV events and mortality. One Italian study performed with 10-year follow-up via a prospective case-control design demonstrated that patients with NAFLD were at increased risk for CV events, such as ACS and CVA, as compared with controls.[43] The presence of carotid plaques and hepatic steatosis were the strongest predictors for such events. A predominantly male cohort was used, which does not depict a representative patient population. Also, 37% of the control subjects went on to develop hepatic steatosis as defined by the endpoints of their follow-up. Another study out of Sri Lanka observed patients presenting with ACS, and found that NAFLD was associated with higher risk coronary plaques, increased inpatient mortality, and a higher prevalence of mortality at 6 months after discharge.[44] This relatively small, retrospective study used US examination for the diagnosis of NAFLD. Also, typical Sri Lankan patients serve as a stark contrast to Americans with regard to comorbidities and BMI. Nevertheless, this study coincides with a great wealth of data supporting the association between NAFLD and increased CV events. Most recently, in an analysis of the MESA study (Mutli-Ethnic Study of Atherosclerosis), 728 American subjects with NAFLD were observed prospectively and found to have an increased incidence of nonfatal MI, cardiac arrest, angina with or without revascularization, and all-cause mortality after median 7.6-year follow-up as compared with controls.[45] Although this study excluded patients with self-reported cirrhosis and had a poor characterization of cohort characteristics at baseline, this was a sound study design in terms of its large number of representative, American subjects.

Although the data supporting NAFLD and CV events are ample, this association seems to be closely entangled with the presence of the metabolic syndrome, namely T2DM. This relationship is better characterized by studies specifically stratifying patients with diabetes and insulin resistance. Among a Finnish cohort observing 268 patients with NAFLD and 720 controls, there was an increase in CV events proportional to the amount of hepatic steatosis as quantified by ultrasound imaging.[46] However, this study used a subjective severity scale for hepatic steatosis based on the liver echogenicity on ultrasound examination. Based on this scale, there was great discord among the prevalence of diabetes, which were 2.4%, 12.1%, and 36.8% among respective groups of with increasing steatosis. A subsequent retrospective American study identified patients with NAFLD with an increased frequency of CV events after the 5- and 10-year follow-up examinations.[47] However, after further analysis, it was established that hepatic steatosis was not an independent risk factor after adjusting for diabetes and BMI among this patient cohort. In a recent cross-sectional study involving third-generation offspring from the Framingham Heart Study, no association existed between CV events and NAFLD, as diagnosed via CT scan.[48] However, several limitations of this study are evident. Not only were there significantly more diabetic patients within the CV group, but the ages of these patients were also much older than the controls who did not develop CV events. Also, there were a low prevalence of CV events overall, as defined by nonfatal MI, heart failure, CVA, transient ischemic attack, or peripheral artery disease among this selective patient population. Despite these drawbacks, there remained an association between hepatic steatosis and sub-clinical CV disease, which included coronary artery calcium and abdominal artery calcium, especially among male subjects.

One retrospective, American study was performed that revealed hepatic steatosis did not correlate with liver-related or CV-related outcomes among diabetic patients after 5 years of follow-up.[49] This study consisted of 2343 patients, predominantly Caucasian female subjects. Of these patients, 233 were diagnosed with NAFLD based on CT scans, defined by hepatic steatosis of greater than 30% on noninvasive imaging, which is not a standard definition that is widely used. Polarity between NAFLD cases and their respective controls were evident. The average BMI was significantly higher in the NAFLD group at 36.7 kg/m^2 as compared with 30.8 kg/m^2 in the controls. Also, the control subjects were significantly older than their NAFLD counterparts with mean ages of 66.6 and 58.1 years, respectively. This distinction is profound because this study set out to observe numerous nonfatal outcomes, such as angina and arrhythmia. These endpoints are not singular in nature and undoubtedly may occur more than once for a single patient. The dichotomy between the 2 study groups potentially places the control population at increased risk for these repeated nonfatal outcomes, given their significantly advanced age. Overall, this is a poor study design that should be noted when analyzing the primary literature regarding this topic.

Although identifying patients with NAFLD without T2DM remains challenging, it is important to distinguish the two, given the increase in vascular pathology seen in diabetic patients. There has been relatively limited analysis exclusively within nondiabetic patient populations to assess the relationship between NAFLD and CV events. In a retrospective Italian study, NAFLD was found to be an independent risk factor for patients presenting with ST-elevation MI.[50] However, this study used ultrasound imaging to assess for hepatic steatosis and stratified patients into degrees of severity based on a semiquantitative score. Another prospective study from Turkey exclusively analyzed nondiabetic patients undergoing percutaneous coronary intervention for ST-elevation MI.[51] Increased hepatic steatosis was associated with poor resolution of cardiac function, major adverse cardiac events, and mortality. However, this study had a 51% prevalence of smoking in the decreased hepatic steatosis group versus 61% in the increased steatosis group. This study also used ultrasound examination for the detection of hepatic steatosis and attempted to stratify patients based on their severity of steatosis on ultrasound imaging. These studies may present some bias in only observing patients presenting with ST-elevation MI and, therefore, may not accurately depict a representative patient population. Also, both studies used a rather large error in methodology, because ultrasound examination has a decreased sensitivity for less pronounced hepatic steatosis and is unable to quantify the severity of NAFLD. Although difficult to assess for hepatic steatosis using other tools for patients presenting with acute chest pain, the stratification of these patients based on ultrasound examination seems to be flawed.

Nonalcoholic Steatohepatitis and Cardiovascular Events and Mortality

Multiple studies have been performed to disentangle the relationship between CV events and varying NAFLD severity (**Table 6**). These studies were performed primarily in patients with NAFLD who underwent liver biopsy, with some portion of the cohort carrying the diagnosis of NASH. In the earliest study regarding this topic, a retrospective American study concluded that increasing severity of NAFLD histology was correlated with increased liver-related mortality, but not all-cause mortality.[52] These 132 NAFLD cases were almost exclusively analyzed in a Caucasian cohort. Also, the prevalence of T2DM was decreased in patients with isolated hepatic steatosis versus

Table 6
Presence of NASH exacerbates CV risk

Reference	Key Findings	Study Design/ Nationality	Number of Subjects	Notable Cohort Characteristics	Diagnostic Modality	% NASH Based on Liver Biopsy	Limitations
Atherosclerosis							
Siddiqui et al,[13] 2015	NAFLD associated with increased insulin, TG, ApoB, VLDL size, LDL, small dense LDL; patients with NASH had nonsignificant increase in these parameters	Retrospective case-control/ United States	81 controls, 81 obese subjects without NAFLD, 81 NAFLD cases	94.6% Caucasian subjects	Liver biopsy after steatosis detected on US imaging or MRS	43% based on NASH-CRN criteria	Lack of histology or noninvasive imaging in control group
Imajo et al,[12] 2014	LDL migration index, an indicator of sdLDL, is higher in patients with NASH compared with NAFLD, suggesting an increased atherosclerotic risk	Cross-sectional/ Japan	30 controls, 53 NAFLD, and 103 NASH subjects with a validation cohort of 25 and 44 of NAFLD and patients with NASH, respectively	59% male subjects	Liver biopsy for NAFLD cases; however, only US imaging to rule out NAFLD for controls	66% of NAFLD cases	No liver biopsy in controls
Cardiac dysfunction							
Petta et al,[23] 2015	NAFLD severity proportional to epicardial fat thickness, which is associated with diastolic dysfunction	Cross-sectional/ Italy	147 NAFLD cases	64% male subjects	Liver biopsy	51.70%	Select population of obese, southern Italian subjects

(continued on next page)

Table 6
(continued)

Reference	Key Findings	Study Design/ Nationality	Number of Subjects	Notable Cohort Characteristics	Diagnostic Modality	% NASH Based on Liver Biopsy	Limitations
Baktir et al,[64] 2015	NASH associated with subclinical systolic and diastolic LV dysfunction	Prospective cohort/Turkey	28 NASH, 28 controls	Mean HOMA-IR 5.29 in NASH group vs 2.1 in controls	Liver biopsy	100%	Small sample size
CV events and mortality							
Domanski et al,[55] 2012	Compared with patients with only NAFLD, NASH is not associated with increased CV risk	Retrospective case-control/ United States	158 NAFLD only, 219 NASH	Diabetes prevalent in 22.8% patients with NAFLD only and 47.5% NASH subjects	Liver biopsy	58%	Retrospective analysis using "presence or history" of primary endpoint of CV events, which include CHF, MI, unstable angina, revascularization, or stroke
Rafiq et al,[54] 2009	NASH increases liver-related mortality compared with patients with NAFLD alone; patients with NAFLD and T2DM are at increased risk for liver-related mortality	Prospective cohort/United States	101 NAFLD only, 72 NASH	39.9% male, 80.8% Caucasian subjects	Liver biopsy	41.60%	No difference in overall mortality between NASH and all patients with NAFLD

Ekstedt et al,[53] 2006	NASH associated with increased CV- and liver-related mortality, but not simple hepatic steatosis, as compared with control population	Prospective cohort/ Sweden	129 NAFLD cases	67% male subjects	Liver biopsy	55%	Swedish, predominantly male cohort
Matteoni et al,[52] 1999	Severity of NAFLD histology is found to be significantly correlated to increased liver-related mortality; however, there were no significant differences in all-cause mortality across NAFLD histologic subtypes	Retrospective cohort/United States	132 NAFLD cases	87% Caucasian subjects	Liver biopsy	55%	Selective cohort of Caucasian, primarily male subjects

Abbreviations: ApoB, apolipoprotein B; CHF, congestive heart failure; CV, cardiovascular; HOMA-IR, homeostatic model assessment of insulin resistance; LDL, low-density lipoprotein; LV, left ventricular; MI, myocardial infarction; MRS, magnetic resonance spectroscopy; NAFLD, nonalcoholic fatty liver disease; NASH, nonalcoholic steatohepatitis; NASH-CRN, NASH Clinical Research Network; sdLDL, small dense low-density lipoprotein; TG, triglycerides; T2DM, type 2 diabetes mellitus; US, ultrasound; VLDL, very low-density lipoprotein.

patients with steatohepatitis. A later prospective cohort study out of Sweden found that NASH was associated with both increased liver-related and all cause-mortality as compared with controls.[53] The investigators also concluded that this association did not hold true for other forms of NAFLD. This study was performed in a specific population in that all subjects were patients initially referred for persistently elevated liver enzymes for at least 6 months. Although this was performed among nonobese subjects, the majority of these patients developed T2DM after a mean follow-up time of 13.7 years. Another prospective American study stated that NASH increases liver-related mortality, but not overall mortality when compared with all patients with NAFLD.[54] Independent risk factors for liver-related mortality included T2DM, increased age, lower albumin, and increased alkaline phosphatase levels. In a recent study, NASH was not found to be associated with an increase in CV events after adjusting for BMI and T2DM.[55] However, there was a low prevalence of CV events overall in this analysis. Also, this study was a retrospective chart review that defined CVD as "the presence or history of" congestive heart failure, MI, unstable angina, revascularization, or stroke. Although this definition may result in easier methods for data gathering in the electronic medical record, these parameters are not adequate for inclusion criteria for such an endpoint. Overall, NASH definitely has been demonstrated to increase liver-related mortality; however, its effect on CV events and CV-related mortality as compared with less severe forms of NAFLD remain controversial and unproven.

SUMMARY

There have been numerous studies confirming the association between NAFLD and several CV conditions, including atherosclerosis, cardiac dysfunction, conduction abnormalities, atrial fibrillation, and thromboembolic risk. These underlying comorbidities increase CV risk among patients with NALFD, which ultimately leads to an increased incidence of CV events and mortality.

Although studies have been performed validating this association in nondiabetic patients, the confounding factor of T2DM is profound. There is currently a vast amount of data supporting the association between NAFLD and CV disease risk. However, it seems that this link depends on the coexistence of T2DM or, at least, insulin resistance. Among the majority of studies that do not differentiate subjects based on their inclusion criteria, there seems to be an overwhelming disparity between patients with reported T2DM between patients with NAFLD and controls. These investigations expose a general trend of a greater proportion of diabetics comprising these NAFLD cohorts. Even among the trials exclusively analyzing nondiabetic patients, there are discrepancies of insulin resistance between NAFLD and control groups. These data suggest that, even in patients without documented T2DM, there is some degree of smoldering insulin resistance that could be contributing to this increased CV risk.

Nevertheless, it is difficult to isolate a large number of subjects with NAFLD without concomitant T2DM. One possible explanation for this effect is the lack of early detection of NAFLD in clinical practice. Often, NAFLD becomes an incidental finding, only uncovered on noninvasive imaging performed for some other workup or etiology. Because the isolation of nondiabetic patients with NAFLD is a formidable undertaking, the early detection of both T2DM and NAFLD should be emphasized. The aim is not only to proactively treat these conditions to prevent the progression of hepatic steatosis and NAFLD, but also to protect these patients against the CV sequelae for which this population is at high risk.

In conclusion, there is ample evidence validating the association between NAFLD and increased CV comorbidities, cardiac events, and mortality. However, current data present a challenge in attributing this effect solely to NAFLD, given the common presence of insulin resistance and T2DM. Small cohorts among nondiabetic patients with NAFLD have yielded mixed results. Although evidence in support of NAFLD and CV risk is mounting, the endpoint of increased CV risk remains tightly linked to the concomitant presence of insulin resistance and T2DM. Prospective studies accentuating early detection of NAFLD are imperative to institute early intervention and prevent future cardiovascular events.

REFERENCES

1. Sayiner M, Koenig A, Henry L, et al. Epidemiology of nonalcoholic fatty liver disease and nonalcoholic steatohepatitis in the United States and the rest of the world. Clin Liver Dis 2016;20(2):205–14.
2. Sookoian S, Pirola CJ. Non-alcoholic fatty liver disease is strongly associated with carotid atherosclerosis: a systematic review. J Hepatol 2008;49(4):600–7.
3. Dasarathy S, Dasarathy J, Khiyami A, et al. Validity of real time ultrasound in the diagnosis of hepatic steatosis: a prospective study. J Hepatol 2009;51(6):1061–7.
4. Oni ET, Agatston AS, Blaha MJ, et al. A systematic review: burden and severity of subclinical cardiovascular disease among those with nonalcoholic fatty liver; should we care? Atherosclerosis 2013;230(2):258–67.
5. Ampuero J, Gallego-Durán R, Romero-Gómez M. Association of NAFLD with subclinical atherosclerosis and coronary-artery disease: meta-analysis. Rev Espanola Enfermedades Dig 2015;107(1):10–6.
6. Madan SA, John F, Pyrsopoulos N, et al. Nonalcoholic fatty liver disease and carotid artery atherosclerosis in children and adults: a meta-analysis. Eur J Gastroenterol Hepatol 2015;27(11):1237–48.
7. Bhatia L, Scorletti E, Curzen N, et al. Improvement in non-alcoholic fatty liver disease severity is associated with a reduction in carotid intima-media thickness progression. Atherosclerosis 2016;246:13–20.
8. Kawanaka M, Nishino K, Nakamura J, et al. Correlation between serum cytokeratin-18 and the progression or regression of non-alcoholic fatty liver disease. Ann Hepatol 2015;14(6):837–44.
9. Jayakumar S, Harrison SA, Loomba R. Noninvasive markers of fibrosis and inflammation in nonalcoholic fatty liver disease. Curr Hepatol Rep 2016;15(2): 86–95.
10. Puchner SB, Lu MT, Mayrhofer T, et al. High-risk coronary plaque at coronary CT angiography is associated with nonalcoholic fatty liver disease, independent of coronary plaque and stenosis burden: results from the ROMICAT II trial. Radiology 2015;274(3):693–701.
11. Cho CS, Curran S, Schwartz LH, et al. Preoperative radiographic assessment of hepatic steatosis with histologic correlation. J Am Coll Surg 2008;206(3):480–8.
12. Imajo K, Hyogo H, Yoneda M, et al. LDL-migration index (LDL-MI), an indicator of small dense low-density lipoprotein (sdLDL), is higher in non-alcoholic steatohepatitis than in non-alcoholic fatty liver: a multicenter cross-sectional study. PLoS One 2014;9(12):e115403.
13. Siddiqui MS, Fuchs M, Idowu MO, et al. Severity of nonalcoholic fatty liver disease and progression to cirrhosis are associated with atherogenic lipoprotein profile. Clin Gastroenterol Hepatol 2015;13(5):1000–8.e3.

14. Goland S, Shimoni S, Zornitzki T, et al. Cardiac abnormalities as a new manifestation of nonalcoholic fatty liver disease: echocardiographic and tissue Doppler imaging assessment. J Clin Gastroenterol 2006;40(10):949–55.
15. Fotbolcu H, Yakar T, Duman D, et al. Impairment of the left ventricular systolic and diastolic function in patients with non-alcoholic fatty liver disease. Cardiol J 2010; 17(5):457–63.
16. Salgado AL, Carvalho LD, Oliveira AC, et al. Insulin resistance index (HOMA-IR) in the differentiation of patients with non-alcoholic fatty liver disease and healthy individuals. Arq Gastroenterol 2010;47(2):165–9.
17. Granér M, Nyman K, Siren R, et al. Ectopic fat depots and left ventricular function in nondiabetic men with nonalcoholic fatty liver disease. Circ Cardiovasc Imaging 2015;8(1). pii:e001979.
18. Springer F, Machann J, Claussen CD, et al. Liver fat content determined by magnetic resonance imaging and spectroscopy. World J Gastroenterol 2010;16(13): 1560–6.
19. Hallsworth K, Hollingsworth KG, Thoma C, et al. Cardiac structure and function are altered in adults with non-alcoholic fatty liver disease. J Hepatol 2013; 58(4):757–62.
20. Karabay CY, Kocabay G, Kalayci A, et al. Impaired left ventricular mechanics in nonalcoholic fatty liver disease: a speckle-tracking echocardiography study. Eur J Gastroenterol Hepatol 2014;26(3):325–31.
21. Valbusa F, Bonapace S, Grillo C, et al. Nonalcoholic fatty liver disease is associated with higher 1-year all-cause rehospitalization rates in patients Admitted for acute heart failure. Medicine (Baltimore) 2016;95(7):e2760.
22. Baktır AO, Şarlı B, Altekin RE, et al. Non alcoholic steatohepatitis is associated with subclinical impairment in left ventricular function measured by speckle tracking echocardiography. Anatol J Cardiol 2015;15(2):137–42.
23. Petta S, Argano C, Colomba D, et al. Epicardial fat, cardiac geometry and cardiac function in patients with non-alcoholic fatty liver disease: association with the severity of liver disease. J Hepatol 2015;62(4):928–33.
24. Holm C. Molecular mechanisms regulating hormone-sensitive lipase and lipolysis. Biochem Soc Trans 2003;31(6):1120–4.
25. Liu YC, Hung CS, Wu YW, et al. Influence of non-alcoholic fatty liver disease on autonomic changes evaluated by the time domain, frequency domain, and symbolic dynamics of heart rate variability. PLoS One 2013;8(4):e61803.
26. Pimenta NM, Santa-Clara H, Cortez-Pinto H, et al. Body composition and body fat distribution are related to cardiac autonomic control in non-alcoholic fatty liver disease patients. Eur J Clin Nutr 2014;68(2):241–6.
27. Sun W, Zhang D, Sun J, et al. Association between non-alcoholic fatty liver disease and autonomic dysfunction in a Chinese population. QJM 2015;108(8): 617–24.
28. Balcioğlu AS, Çiçek D, Akinci S, et al. Arrhythmogenic evidence for epicardial adipose tissue: heart rate variability and turbulence are influenced by epicardial fat thickness. Pacing Clin Electrophysiol 2015;38(1):99–106.
29. Targher G, Valbusa F, Bonapace S, et al. Association of nonalcoholic fatty liver disease with QTC interval in patients with type 2 diabetes. Nutr Metab Cardiovasc Dis 2014;24(6):663–9.
30. Hung CS, Tseng PH, Tu CH, et al. Nonalcoholic fatty liver disease is associated with QT prolongation in the general population. J Am Heart Assoc 2015;4(7). pii:e001820.

31. Targher G, Mantovani A, Pichiri I, et al. Non-alcoholic fatty liver disease is associated with an increased prevalence of atrial fibrillation in hospitalized patients with type 2 diabetes. Clin Sci (Lond) 2013;125(6):301–9.
32. Targher G, Valbusa F, Bonapace S, et al. Non-alcoholic fatty liver disease is associated with an increased incidence of atrial fibrillation in patients with type 2 diabetes. PLoS One 2013;8(2):e57183.
33. Ozveren O, Izgi C, Eroglu E, et al. Doppler tissue evaluation of atrial conduction properties in patients with non-alcoholic fatty-liver disease. Ultrason Imaging 2016;38(3):225–35.
34. Kotronen A, Joutsi-Korhonen L, Sevastianova K, et al. Increased coagulation factor VIII, IX, XI and XII activities in non-alcoholic fatty liver disease. Liver Int 2011; 31(2):176–83.
35. Di Minno MND, Tufano A, Rusolillo A, et al. High prevalence of nonalcoholic fatty liver in patients with idiopathic venous thromboembolism. World J Gastroenterol 2010;16(48):6119–22.
36. Yu KJ, Zhang MJ, Li Y, et al. Increased whole blood viscosity associated with arterial stiffness in patients with non-alcoholic fatty liver disease. J Gastroenterol Hepatol 2014;29(3):540–4.
37. Tripodi A, Fracanzani AL, Primignani M, et al. Procoagulant imbalance in patients with non-alcoholic fatty liver disease. J Hepatol 2014;61(1):148–54.
38. Luo J, Xu L, Li J, et al. Nonalcoholic fatty liver disease as a potential risk factor of cardiovascular disease. Eur J Gastroenterol Hepatol 2015;27(3):193–9.
39. Sonsuz A, Basaranoglu M, Ozbay G. Relationship between aminotransferase levels and histopathological findings in patients with nonalcoholic steatohepatitis. Am J Gastroenterol 2000;95(5):1370–1.
40. Mofrad P, Contos MJ, Haque M, et al. Clinical and histologic spectrum of nonalcoholic fatty liver disease associated with normal ALT values. Hepatology 2003; 37(6):1286–92.
41. Amarapurkar DN, Patel ND. Clinical spectrum and natural history of non-alcoholic steatohepatitis with normal alanine aminotransferase values. Trop Gastroenterol 2004;25(3):130–4.
42. Vilar CP, Cotrim HP, Florentino GS, et al. Association between nonalcoholic fatty liver disease and coronary artery disease. Rev Assoc Med Bras (1992) 2013; 59(3):290–7.
43. Fracanzani AL, Tiraboschi S, Pisano G, et al. Progression of carotid vascular damage and cardiovascular events in non-alcoholic fatty liver disease patients compared to the general population during 10 years of follow-up. Atherosclerosis 2016;246:208–13.
44. Perera N, Indrakumar J, Abeysinghe WV, et al. Non alcoholic fatty liver disease increases the mortality from acute coronary syndrome: an observational study from Sri Lanka. BMC Cardiovasc Disord 2016;16:37.
45. Zeb I, Li D, Budoff MJ, et al. Nonalcoholic fatty liver disease and incident cardiac events: the multi-ethnic study of atherosclerosis. J Am Coll Cardiol 2016;67(16): 1965–6.
46. Pisto P, Santaniemi M, Bloigu R, et al. Fatty liver predicts the risk for cardiovascular events in middle-aged population: a population-based cohort study. BMJ Open 2014;4(3):e004973.
47. Pickhardt PJ, Hahn L, Muñoz del Rio A, et al. Natural history of hepatic steatosis: observed outcomes for subsequent liver and cardiovascular complications. AJR Am J Roentgenol 2014;202(4):752–8.

48. Mellinger JL, Pencina KM, Massaro JM, et al. Hepatic steatosis and cardiovascular disease outcomes: an analysis of the Framingham heart study. J Hepatol 2015;63(2):470–6.

49. Dunn MA, Behari J, Rogal SS, et al. Hepatic steatosis in diabetic patients does not predict adverse liver-related or cardiovascular outcomes. Liver Int Off J Int Assoc Study Liver 2013;33(10):1575–82.

50. Boddi M, Tarquini R, Chiostri M, et al. Nonalcoholic fatty liver in nondiabetic patients with acute coronary syndromes. Eur J Clin Invest 2013;43(5):429–38.

51. Emre A, Terzi S, Celiker E, et al. Impact of nonalcoholic fatty liver disease on myocardial perfusion in nondiabetic patients undergoing primary percutaneous coronary intervention for ST-segment elevation myocardial infarction. Am J Cardiol 2015;116(12):1810–4.

52. Matteoni CA, Younossi ZM, Gramlich T, et al. Nonalcoholic fatty liver disease: a spectrum of clinical and pathological severity. Gastroenterology 1999;116(6):1413–9.

53. Ekstedt M, Franzén LE, Mathiesen UL, et al. Long-term follow-up of patients with NAFLD and elevated liver enzymes. Hepatol Baltim Md 2006;44(4):865–73.

54. Rafiq N, Bai C, Fang Y, et al. Long-term follow-up of patients with nonalcoholic fatty liver. Clin Gastroenterol Hepatol 2009;7(2):234–8.

55. Domanski JP, Park SJ, Harrison SA. Cardiovascular disease and nonalcoholic fatty liver disease: does histologic severity matter? J Clin Gastroenterol 2012;46(5):427–30.

56. Psychari SN, Rekleiti N, Papaioannou N, et al. Epicardial fat in nonalcoholic fatty liver disease: properties and relationships with metabolic factors, cardiac structure, and cardiac function. Angiology 2016;67(1):41–8.

57. VanWagner LB, Wilcox JE, Colangelo LA, et al. Association of nonalcoholic fatty liver disease with subclinical myocardial remodeling and dysfunction: a population-based study. Hepatol Baltim Md 2015;62(3):773–83.

58. Kim NH, Park J, Kim SH, et al. Non-alcoholic fatty liver disease, metabolic syndrome and subclinical cardiovascular changes in the general population. Heart Br Card Soc 2014;100(12):938–43.

59. Fallo F, Dalla Pozza A, Sonino N, et al. Non-alcoholic fatty liver disease is associated with left ventricular diastolic dysfunction in essential hypertension. Nutr Metab Cardiovasc Dis NMCD 2009;19(9):646–53.

60. Wong VW-S, Wong GL-H, Yeung JC-L, et al. Long-term clinical outcomes after fatty liver screening in patients undergoing coronary angiogram: a prospective cohort study. Hepatol Baltim Md 2016;63(3):754–63.

61. Targher G, Bertolini L, Rodella S, et al. Nonalcoholic fatty liver disease is independently associated with an increased incidence of cardiovascular events in type 2 diabetic patients. Diabetes Care 2007;30(8):2119–21.

62. Hamaguchi M, Kojima T, Takeda N, et al. Nonalcoholic fatty liver disease is a novel predictor of cardiovascular disease. World J Gastroenterol 2007;13(10):1579–84.

63. Targher G, Bertolini L, Poli F, et al. Nonalcoholic fatty liver disease and risk of future cardiovascular events among type 2 diabetic patients. Diabetes 2005;54(12):3541–6.

64. Baktır AO, Şarlı B, Altekin RE, et al. Non alcoholic steatohepatitis is associated with subclinical impairment in left ventricular function measured by speckle tracking echocardiography. Anatol J Cardiol 2015;15(2):137–42.

Current Treatment of Nonalcoholic Fatty Liver Disease/Nonalcoholic Steatohepatitis

 CrossMark

Chun Kit Hung, MD[a], Henry C. Bodenheimer Jr, MD[b],*

KEYWORDS

- NAFLD • NASH • Treatment • Pharmacotherapy

KEY POINTS

- Body weight loss via physical activity and dieting is the mainstay of treatment of nonalcoholic fatty liver disease (NAFLD).
- Bariatric and endoscopic weight loss surgery can be effective in obese patients with NAFLD, with and without metabolic complications.
- There is no currently approved pharmacotherapy; vitamin E and pioglitazone are available medications with the most evidence of efficacy in the treatment of patients with NAFLD but have side effects and limitations.
- Treatment of NAFLD should be individualized to each patient's comorbidities and unique situation.

The goal of treatment of nonalcoholic fatty liver disease (NAFLD) and nonalcoholic steatohepatitis (NASH) is to stop the progression of hepatic inflammation and necrosis, which result in fibrosis, cirrhosis, and liver failure. It is also important to improve patient quality of life, the need for hospitalizations and health care utilization, and NAFLD-associated cardiovascular and metabolic complications. Therapy is directed toward patients with NASH. This is because those with NAFLD alone, without steatohepatitis, have a relatively benign course and good prognosis.[1] Currently there are no Food and Drug Administration–approved therapies for NAFLD/NASH. This article examines the role of lifestyle modifications, including diet and exercise, which are the

Disclosure Statement: C.K. Hung has nothing to disclose. H.C. Bodenheimer has served as a consultant for Intercept Pharmaceutcals and Takeda Pharmaceuticals and is principal investigator in a clinical research grant (GFT505B-216-1) from Genfit Pharmaceuticals.
[a] Division of Gastroenterology, Department of Medicine, Northwell Health, 270-05 76th, Avenue, New Hyde Park, NY 11040, USA; [b] Department of Medicine, Zucker Hofstra Northwell School of Medicine, Sandra Atlas Bass Center for Liver Diseases, Northwell Health, 400 Community Drive, Manhasset, NY 11030, USA
* Corresponding author.
E-mail address: hbodenhei1@northwell.edu

Clin Liver Dis 22 (2018) 175–187
http://dx.doi.org/10.1016/j.cld.2017.08.012
1089-3261/18/© 2017 Elsevier Inc. All rights reserved.

liver.theclinics.com

mainstay of treatment. In addition, the role of weight loss surgery and available pharmacologic therapies is discussed.

LIFESTYLE MODIFICATIONS

Intentional weight loss via lifestyle modifications, through a combination of increased physical exercise and calorie-restricted dieting, is currently the mainstay of treatment of NAFLD and is recommended by the American Association for the Study of Liver Diseases and the American Gastroenterological Association.[1] Body weight loss of at least 3% to 5% is required before improvement in hepatic steatosis is seen.[2,3] Using improvement in histology as an endpoint, Promrat and coworkers showed a 2.4-point improvement in NASH fibrosis score (NAS)[4] in the successful weight loss group, from 4.4 at baseline to 2.[5] The amount of weight loss correlated with the degree of histologic improvement. The magnitude of weight loss correlates proportionally with NAS, especially when body weight loss is above 7%. A meta-analysis of 8 randomized clinical trials of weight loss, by Musso and coworkers,[6] confirmed that 7% weight loss resulted in improved NAS, with 2 other trials suggesting that 10% or more did not result in further benefit. Even though weight loss is effective in improving NAS, fewer than half of patients are able to achieve such goals.[6] Although hepatic steatosis, ballooning, lobular inflammation, and NAS are improved, these trials did not show improvement in hepatic fibrosis. A prospective cohort study by Vilar-Gomez and coworkers,[7] in 2015, confirmed that a weight loss of 7% to 10% improved NAS in 100% and steatohepatitis resolution in 90%. Fibrosis regression, in contrast to previous studies, was documented in 45% of those who were able to lose more than 10% body weight.[7] Clinical practice guidelines currently recommend a weight loss of at least 7% to 10% to achieve histologic improvement in steatohepatitis and necroinflammation.[1]

Exercise and Physical Activity

Physical activity is one of the best methods to achieve weight loss. By itself, exercise is an effective method of decreasing hepatic steatosis, even in the absence of body weight loss.[8-10] Metabolic profiles of patients improve, decreasing overall cardiovascular disease risk. Both aerobic exercise and resistance training are effective. A positive effect on hepatic steatosis, as demonstrated by MRI, can be seen with only 8 weeks of strength training.[11] At least 60 minutes of aerobic exercise shows benefit, but longer durations, up to 150 minutes per week, were optimal. Studies of exercise and its effects on NAFLD are limited by small samples sizes. Given the low cost of exercise and the health risks of increasingly sedentary lifestyles, however, physical activity and weight loss should be one of the first interventions in the treatment of NAFLD.

Dieting and Nutrition

Compared with healthy individuals, those with NAFLD consume a diet higher in certain fats and cholesterol, excessive in calories and fructose, while lacking in vitamins and fiber.[12] The type of dietary fats that are associated with NASH are saturated fats and cholesterols.[13-15] Clear evidence for a direct causal relationship, however, between these macronutrients and NAFLD/NASH, in humans, is lacking. Trans–fatty acids and monounsaturated fatty acids have been studied only in animal models; thus, their association with NAFLD in humans is not proven.[16-18] Other fats, namely omega-3 fatty acids or n-3 polyunsaturated fatty acids (PUFAs) might be protective.[19,20] Randomized trials with histologic improvement as an endpoint have not shown significant improvement in NAS,[21,22] and PUFA supplementation is not currently recommended as treatment of established NAFLD. Given the increased consumption of processed foods containing fructose, the identification of this sugar as a risk factor for NAFLD is important.[23] Several studies have associated biopsy-proved NASH with fructose intake, especially in the form of soft drinks.[12,24–26] Despite these associations, a meta-analysis found insufficient evidence to prove fructose alone is a causative culprit, especially given confounding risks, such as a concomitant high-calorie diet.[27,28]

Current evidence points to calorie restriction as an effective therapy in the treatment of NAFLD rather than a specific alteration of macronutrients. Two interventions, 1 limiting carbohydrate intake to less than 20 g/d and the other a caloric deficit of 30%, were beneficial in achieving improvements in NAS[29] and hepatic lipids, respectively.[30] Therefore, a caloric deficit of 500 kcal/d to 750 kcal/d is an appropriate therapeutic intervention for NAFLD. Women are suggested to eat a 1200 kcal/d to 1500 kcal/d diet and men a slightly higher amount of 1500 kcal/d to 1800 kcal/d, with adjustments based on their physical activity and habitus.[31]

There are currently no large-scale studies comparing diet to exercise or a combination of the two in treating NAFLD.[32] It is sensible, however, to combine the two in optimizing weight loss and in achieving a healthier lifestyle. Given the current limited evidence, dietary modification in the treatment of NAFLD/NASH should be aimed at adjusting the ratios of macronutrients that are deficient or overrepresented, to achieve weight loss and to reduce metabolic risk. Patient anthropomorphic parameters, including weight, body mass index (BMI), and waist circumference, should be routinely monitored because they are associated with hepatic fibrosis.[33,34] When available, an interdisciplinary approach, including the use of registered dieticians and physical trainers, can be useful.[35] Laboratory tests, including serum liver enzymes, glycosylated hemoglobin, and lipid panels, are also important to assess.[36] Food diaries and electronic apps are generally available and may help track daily caloric intake and energy expenditure. Given the high rate of failure to lose body weight, serial visits are key to monitor progress as well as to escalate therapy if necessary.

INTERVENTIONAL WEIGHT LOSS SURGERY

Given the association of obesity and metabolic syndrome with NAFLD/NASH and the difficulty associated with voluntary calorie restriction, many patients consider surgery a potential treatment option. Surgery can not only treat obesity but also may improve diabetes, hypertension, dyslipidemia, and sleep apnea in a majority of well-chosen patients. In experienced centers, bariatric surgery has low mortality rates, ranging from 0.1% to 1.1%, depending on the type of surgery.[37] Unfortunately, no randomized controlled trials have been done in surgical patients specifically for the treatment of NASH. The effects of weight loss surgery on liver disease have only been observed in study cohorts during the treatment of obesity.

Bariatric Surgery

Candidates for bariatric surgery are divided into categories by their BMI and medical comorbidities. Patients with a BMI over 40 kg/m^2 even in the absence of any other comorbidities should be considered, as should patients with at least 1 serious comorbidity and a BMI between 35 kg/m^2 and 39.9 kg/m^2 (**Table 1**). NAFLD or NASH is one of the qualifying comorbidities. Although there is limited long-term evidence, those patients with a lower BMI between 30 kg/m^2 and 34.9 kg/m^2 with uncontrolled diabetes and/or metabolic syndrome could also be considered for surgery.[38]

The techniques of bariatric surgery are divided into 2 types: restrictive surgery, in the form of gastric banding and sleeve gastrectomy, and bypass surgery, most commonly

Table 1
Associated comorbidities used for consideration for bariatric surgery in patients by body mass index category

Body Mass Index Greater Than or Equal to 40 kg/m²	Body Mass Index Greater Than or Equal to 35 kg/m²	Body Mass Index 30 kg/m² to 34.9 kg/m² (Limited Evidence)
No coexisting medical problems needed	Type 2 diabetes mellitus	Type 2 diabetes mellitus
	Hypertension	Metabolic syndrome
	Hyperlipidemia	
	Obstructive sleep apnea	
	Obesity hypoventilation syndrome	
	Pickwickian syndrome	
	NAFLD/NASH	
	Pseudotumor cerebri	
	Gastroesophageal reflux disease	
	Asthma	
	Venous stasis	
	Severe urinary incontinence	
	Debilitating arthritis	
	Impaired quality of life	

Data from Raynor HA, Champagne CM. Position of the academy of nutrition and dietetics: interventions for the treatment of overweight and obesity in adults. J Acad Nutr Diet 2016;116(1):129–47.

the Roux-en-Y gastric bypass. The most commonly performed operation is bypass surgery, followed by the sleeve gastrectomy, adjustable gastric banding, and biliopancreatic diversion and duodenal switch.[39] All these procedures improve steatohepatitis, but the degree of improvement is highest with bypass surgery.[40] Although gastric banding and sleeve gastrectomy are purely restrictive procedures that limit the size of the stomach, the Roux-en-Y gastric bypass uses both restriction and bypass. The resulting altered anatomy causes weight loss through the metabolic alterations, called BRAVE effects (**Box 1**).

Collectively these effects lead to an increase in hormones, such as GLP-1 and adiponectin, which decrease lipogenesis, improve lipid metabolism, and increase insulin sensitivity. Changes in gut microbiome from an altered anatomy might also reduce bacterial production of certain fatty acids.[41] A decrease in inflammation is associated

Box 1
Mechanisms generating altered metabolism and resultant weight loss with bariatric surgery

BRAVE effects of bariatric surgery:
1. Bile flow alteration
2. Restriction of gastric size
3. Alteration in flow of nutrients
4. Vagal manipulation
5. Enteric gut and adipose hormone modification.

Data from Ashrafian H, Bueter M, Ahmed K, et al. Metabolic surgery: an evolution through bariatric animal models. Obes Rev 2010;11(12):907–20.

with reduction of multiple interleukins, C-reactive protein, and tumor necrosis factor (TNF)-α.[42] All these collective effects may be instrumental in improving liver histology in NAFLD/NASH patients undergoing bariatric surgery.

The initial perioperative mortality risk from surgery is estimated to be 0.3% at 30 days.[42] Lifelong mortality risk is reduced in patients undergoing bariatric surgery through lowering the rates of diabetes, cancer, and heart disease.[43] Bariatric surgery leads to an improvement in liver enzyme values.[44] Prospective studies show that NAS parameters and hepatic fibrosis stage improve. Liver biopsies in 1 study of 381 patients were taken during the initial operation, then again at 1 and 5 years. There was a sustained improvement in NAS and hepatic steatosis over 5 years.[45] Surgically induced rapid weight loss may induce an increase in fibrosis. This is not, however, progressive because a vast majority of patients (95.7%) had only stage 1 or stage 0 fibrosis in the long term. Improvement of fibrosis was seen in 14 of 23 reviewed studies, with 3 showing worsening, whereas 6 show no change.[46] Scarring may improve in patients who already have cirrhosis at baseline.[47] Bariatric surgery is a potentially useful option in properly selected overweight patients.

Endoscopic Weight Loss

With the advent of endoscopic options for induction of weight loss, there is a small but growing body of literature on the efficacy of endoscopic procedures for weight loss in the treatment of patients with NAFLD. Endoscopic procedures may be restrictive, such as the intragastric balloon and endoscopic sleeve gastrectomy, or affect intestinal absorption, as in duodenal-jejunal bypass liners and duodenal mucosal resurfacing.[48,49] The most studied modality is the endoscopic gastric balloon. Gastric balloons, as in traditional bariatric surgery, have significant impact on parameters of NAFLD, such as serum aspartate aminotransferase (AST) and alanine aminotransferase (ALT) activities.[50–52] Lee and coworkers[53] evaluated the intragastric balloon and its effects on NAS in 18 patients. Along with significant weight loss, his study demonstrated a decrease in NAS at 6 months, although this result was not statistically significant. It is also unclear if there is sustained improvement after removal of the balloon.[53] Further studies are warranted to establish the long-term safety and efficacy of endoscopic weight loss procedures in the treatment of NAFLD.

PHARMACOLOGIC THERAPIES

To date, there are no Food and Drug Administration–approved pharmacologic therapies for the treatment of NAFLD or NASH. Treatment is available for associated metabolic disorders. These agents are being evaluated for their effect on NAFLD. The agent of choice should be tailored toward a patient's comorbidities and unique situation.

Dietary Supplements

Given the active inflammation associated with NASH, the antioxidant vitamin E has been studied as a possible treatment. Vitamin E is shown, in animals, to be an antioxidant that modulates cell signaling and can prevent damage caused by free radicals.[54,55] The largest human trial studying vitamin E is the PIVENS trial, which compared pioglitazone, vitamin E, and placebo in 247 nondiabetic patients. There was significant improvement, compared with placebo, in steatosis, lobular inflammation, ballooning, and NAFLD activity score in subjects receiving 800 IU/d of vitamin E for 96 weeks. Treated subjects also showed improvement in ALT activities and liver histology. The resolution of NASH in 36% of vitamin E–treated patients, however, compared with 21% of placebo recipients was not statistically significant ($P = .05$), and, most importantly, fibrosis did not improve.[56] In the TONIC trial, where vitamin E was compared with metformin and placebo in pediatric patients, improvements in ballooning and NAS and histologic resolution of NASH were demonstrated. Serum ALT and hepatic fibrosis, however, did not meet the primary endpoint of 50% improvement.[57] Although vitamin E is well tolerated, meta-analyses show a small increase in mortality (relative risk 1.04; CI, 1.01–1.07).[58] Others have also associated the use of vitamin E with an increased risk of prostate cancer and hemorrhagic stroke (relative risk 1.2; $P = .5$).[59,60] The use of vitamin E should thus be tailored toward individuals with histologically proven NASH. Patients should be made aware of these associated potential adverse events.

The herbal supplement milk thistle (*Silybum marianum*) is readily available and purported to have anti-inflammatory properties that may be beneficial in NAFLD.[61] A randomized trial for its use in NASH has been performed, where milk thistle in a combination form with vitamin E and phospholipids was compared with placebo. Although there were improvements in homeostatic serum markers, liver enzyme levels, and histology in the intervention group, it is unclear if the benefit is from milk thistle or vitamin E.[62] Further studies are warranted to assess the efficacy of this herbal supplement.

Other dietary supplements studied in the treatment of NASH include coffee, probiotics, and omega-3 fatty acids. Coffee use is associated with a decreased risk of cirrhosis, hepatocellular carcinoma, and mortality. Phenolic and chlorogenic acids among many other chemicals in coffee are postulated to be beneficial.[63] Studies of the effects of coffee consumption of more than 3 cups per day on sonographic and serologic evidence of steatosis have been mixed.[64–66] In a cohort study of 306 patients that utilized liver biopsy specimens, those subjects with mild disease (F0-1 disease) consumed significantly more coffee than those with more advanced disease (F2-4).[67] To date, no randomized controlled trials on the effects of coffee on NAFLD are available. The gut microbiota has also been postulated to have a role in obesity and the development of metabolic syndrome. A few small studies have evaluated noninvasive measures of steatosis and their relationship to administration of probiotics but with unclear and conflicting results.[68–70]

Insulin Sensitizers

Given the association of diabetes with NAFLD as well as the associated increased systemic inflammation and insulin resistance, medications used for the treatment of impaired glucose metabolism are of particular interest. The antidiabetic medication thiazolidinedione (glitazone) has been the most studied. In addition to improving insulin sensitivity and adiponectin production, it leads to the increased uptake of fatty acids in adipose tissue, thus potentially drawing fat deposition away from the liver.[71] In the largest randomized PIVENS trial, pioglitazone was used at a dose of 30 mg daily for 96 weeks in patients without diabetes. As with vitamin E, improvements in steatosis, lobular cellular inflammation, ballooning, NAFLD activity score, and insulin resistance all met statistical significance. The resolution of definite NASH also was significant, 47% in pioglitazone users compared with 21% in placebo recipients ($P = .001$). Hepatic fibrosis, however, did not decrease.[57] Side effects were more common in subjects given pioglitazone compared with those on vitamin E. On average, subjects receiving pioglitazone showed a weight gain of 4.7 kg during the

PIVENS study. Improvements in serum aminotransferase values and insulin resistance were not sustained after cessation of therapy.[72] Even with continued therapy, the benefits may plateau. A study with rosiglitazone showed no changes in NAS but improved hepatic steatosis within the first year of therapy, which was sustained but did not exhibit further benefit during an additional 2 years of therapy.[73] Other adverse events, such as the black box warning of rare episodes of congestive failure, can occur. There was concern for an increased risk of neoplasm, especially bladder cancer associated with pioglitazone, but large-scale cohort studies do not show evidence for this.[74] Especially in patients who need treatment of their diabetes, the use of pioglitazone can be individualized in patients with concurrent NASH.

Metformin, in the biguanide class of antidiabetic medications, has been studied but with disappointing results. In several studies, including randomized trials, metformin seemed to have some beneficial effect on ALT and NASH activity score likely due to weight loss and not the drug itself.[75,76] A meta-analysis of 4 trials using metformin did not show any significant changes in hepatic steatosis, ballooning, inflammation, fibrosis, or ALT.[77] Current clinical guidelines recommend against using metformin for the treatment of NASH.[1]

Miscellaneous Agents

Several other currently available medications have been studied for utility in patients with NAFLD, but none of the following has been shown to have any definite benefits regarding liver disease. Orlistat, which is a gastrointestinal lipase inhibitor for weight loss, was shown to decrease serum ALT and sonographic hepatic steatosis in one study[78] but failed to improve histology or measures of insulin resistance in another.[79]

Pentoxifylline, via its attenuation of TNF-α effect, has been studied as a possible treatment of NASH. Two randomized trials, both using liver histology as an endpoint, were done using a dose of 400 mg of pentoxifylline three times daily. One study showed an improvement in hepatic steatosis and ballooning,[80] whereas the other did not show any significant differences compared with placebo.[81] The administration of pentoxifylline was associated with significant nausea. Ursodeoxycholic acid, which has been used in patients with cholestatic liver diseases, has also been studied in patients with NAFLD. The only randomized trial to evaluate ursodeoxycholic acid at a dose of 13 mg/kg/d to 15 mg/kg/d in NASH patients did not show any difference in histology in treated patients compared with placebo recipients.[82]

Statins are shown to be safe in most patients even with elevated liver enzymes.[83,84] There are 2 prospective, randomized studies on the use of statins for the treatment of NASH. A meta-analysis of the findings shows a decrease in serum ALT levels and sonographic hepatic echogenicity, but liver histology was not assessed.[85] Other retrospective or cohort studies failed to show any benefit in fibrosis. Although statins are clearly beneficial for persons at risk of cardiovascular disease and should be used for such, clinical practice guidelines recommend against using statins specifically for NASH.[1]

A summary of treatment options discussed in this article is provided in **Fig. 1**. The use of these agents should be highly individualized to each individual's specific circumstance and comorbidities. Careful counseling should be provided when starting any of these treatments, with patients made aware of potential side effects and of the off-label use of these medications for NASH. The need to develop additional drugs with proved efficacy in patients with NASH is clear, especially with the increasing prevalence of NAFLD and NASH and their complications.

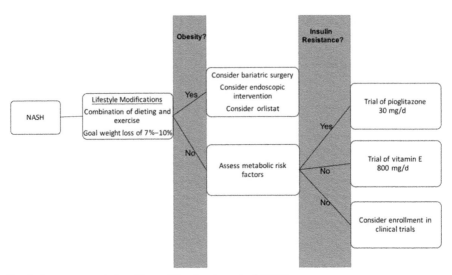

Fig. 1. Summary and algorithm of the treatment of NASH.

SUMMARY

Knowledge of effective treatments of NASH is still in its infancy and remains a challenge. Even though there is yet to be any approved or effective pharmacotherapy, weight loss, dieting, and exercise are effective. The few drugs that have been studied, both prescription and supplement, offer providers a limited number of evidence-based tools in the treatment of this disease. It is important to consider patients with NASH for enrollment in clinical trials. Additional treatment options are on the horizon for this prevalent disease of epidemic proportion.

REFERENCES

1. Chalasani N, Younossi Z, Lavine JE, et al. The diagnosis and management of non-alcoholic fatty liver disease: practice guideline by the American Gastroenterological Association, American Association for the Study of Liver Disease, and American College of Gastroenterology. Gastroenterology 2012;142:1592–609.
2. Patel NS, Doycheva I, Peterson MR, et al. Effect of weight loss on magnetic resonance imaging estimation of liver fat and volume in patients with nonalcoholic steatohepatitis. Clin Gastroenterol Hepatol 2015;13(3):561–8.
3. Wong VW, Chan RS, Wong GL, et al. Community-based lifestyle modification programme for non-alcoholic fatty liver disease: a randomized controlled trial. J Hepatol 2013;59(3):536–42.
4. Kleiner DE, Brunt EM, Van Natta M, et al. Design and validation of a histological scoring system for nonalcoholic fatty liver disease. Hepatology 2005;41(6):1313–21.
5. Promrat K, Kleiner DE, Niemeier HM, et al. Randomized controlled trial testing the effects of weight loss on nonalcoholic steatohepatitis. Hepatology 2010;51:121–9.
6. Musso G, Cassader M, Rosina F, et al. Impact of current treatments on liver disease, glucose metabolism and cardiovascular risk in non-alcoholic fatty liver disease (NAFLD): a systematic review and meta-analysis of randomised trials. Diabetologia 2012;55(4):885–904.

7. Vilar-Gomez E, Martinez-Perez Y, Calzadilla-Bertot L, et al. Weight loss through lifestyle modification significantly reduces features of nonalcoholic steatohepatitis. Gastroenterology 2015;149:367–78.

8. Johnson NA, Sachinwalla T, Walton DW, et al. Aerobic exercise training reduces hepatic and visceral lipids in obese individuals without weight loss. Hepatology 2009;50:1105–12.

9. Perseghin G, Lattuada G, De Cobelli F, et al. Habitual physical activity is associated with intrahepatic fat content in humans. Diabetes Care 2007;30:683–8.

10. George St, Bauman A, Johnston A, et al. Independent effects of physical activity in patients with nonalcoholic fatty liver disease. Hepatology 2009;50:68–76.

11. Hallsworth K, Fattakhova G, Hollingsworth KG, et al. Resistance exercise reduces liver fat and its mediators in non-alcoholic fatty liver disease independent of weight loss. Gut 2011;60:1278–83.

12. Zelber-Sagi S, Nitzan-Kaluski D, Goldsmith R, et al. Long term nutritional intake and the risk for non-alcoholic fatty liver disease (NAFLD): a population based study. J Hepatol 2007;47(5):711–7.

13. Musso G, Gambino R, De Michieli F, et al. Dietary habits and their relations to insulin resistance and postprandial lipemia in nonalcoholic steatohepatitis. Hepatology 2003;37(4):909–16.

14. Enjoji M, Yasutake K, Kohjima M, et al. Nutrition and nonalcoholic fatty liver disease: the significance of cholesterol. Int J Hepatol 2012;2012:925807.

15. Yasutake K, Nakamuta M, Shima Y, et al. Nutritional investigation of non-obese patients with non-alcoholic fatty liver disease: the significance of dietary cholesterol. Scand J Gastroenterol 2009;44:471–7.

16. Machado RM, Stefano JT, Oliveira CP, et al. Intake of trans fatty acids causes nonalcoholic steatohepatitis and reduces adipose tissue fat content. J Nutr 2010;140(6):1127–32.

17. Tetri LH, Basaranoglu M, Brunt EM, et al. Severe NAFLD with hepatic necroinflammatory changes in mice fed trans fats and a high-fructose corn syrup equivalent. Am J Physiol Gastrointest Liver Physiol 2008;295:G987–95.

18. Hussein O, Grosovski M, Lasri E, et al. Monounsaturated fat decreases hepatic lipid content in non-alcoholic fatty liver disease in rats. World J Gastroenterol 2007;13:361–8.

19. Tanaka N, Sano K, Horiuchi A, et al. Highly purified eicosapentaenoic acid treatment improves nonalcoholic steatohepatitis. J Clin Gastroenterol 2008;42(4):413–8.

20. Capanni M, Calella F, Biagini MR, et al. Prolonged n-3polyunsaturated fatty acid supplementation ameliorates hepatic steatosis in patients with non-alcoholic fatty liver disease: a pilot study. Aliment Pharmacol Ther 2006;23(8):1143–51.

21. Argo CK, Patrie JT, Lackner C, et al. Effects of n-3 fish oil on metabolic and histological parameters in NASH: a double-blind, randomized, placebo-controlled trial. J Hepatol 2015;62(1):190–7.

22. Desarathy S, Dasarathy J, Khiyami A, et al. Double-blind randomized placebo-controlled clinical trial of omega 3 fatty acids for the treatment of diabetic patients with nonalcoholic steatohepatitis. J Clin Gastroenterol 2015;49(2):137–44.

23. Alwahsh SM, Gebhardt R. Dietary fructose as a risk factor for non-alcoholic fatty liver disease (NAFLD). Arch Toxicol 2017;91(4):1545–63.

24. Abdelmalek MF, Suzuki A, Guy C, et al. Nonalcoholic Steatohepatitis Clinical Research Network. Increased fructose consumption is associated with fibrosis severity in patients with nonalcoholic fatty liver disease. Hepatology 2010;51(6):1961–71.

25. Abid A, Taha O, Nseir W, et al. Soft drink consumption is associated with fatty liver disease independent of metabolic syndrome. J Hepatol 2009;51(5):918–24.
26. Assy N, Nasser G, Kamayse I, et al. Soft drink consumption linked with fatty liver in the absence of traditional risk factors. Can J Gastroenterol 2008;22(10):811–6.
27. Chun M, Ma J, Patel K, et al. Fructose, high-fructose corn syrup, sucrose and non-alcoholic fatty liver disease or indexes of liver health: a systematic review and meta-analysis. Am J Clin Nutr 2014;100:833–49.
28. Hannah WN Jr, Harrison SA. Effect of weight loss, diet, exercise and bariatric surgery on nonalcoholic fatty liver disease. Clin Liver Dis 2016;20(2):339–50.
29. Tendler D, Lin S, Vancy WS Jr, et al. The effect of a low-carbohydrate, ketogenic diet on nonalcoholic fatty liver disease: a pilot study. Dig Dis Sci 2007;52:589–93.
30. Haufe S, Engeli S, Kast P, et al. Randomized comparison of reduced fat and reduced carbohydrate hypocaloric diets on intrahepatic fat in overweight and obese human subjects. Hepatology 2011;53(5):1504–14.
31. Marchesini G, Petta S, Dalle Grave R. Diet, weight loss, and liver health in nonalcoholic fatty liver disease: pathophysiology, evidence, and practice. Hepatology 2016;63(6):2032–43.
32. Thomas C, Day CP, Trenell MI. Lifstyle interventions for the treatment of nonalcoholic fatty liver disease in adults: a systematic review. Hepatology 2012; 56(1):255–66.
33. Ong JP, Elariny H, Collantes R, et al. Predictors of nonalcoholic steatohepatitis and advanced fibrosis in morbidly obese patients. Obes Surg 2005;15(3):310–5.
34. Zelber-Sagi S, Shoham D, Zvibel I, et al. Predictors for advanced fibrosis in morbidly obese non-alcoholic fatty liver patients. World J Hepatol 2017;9(2):91–8.
35. Raynor HA, Champagne CM. Position of the academy of nutrition and dietetics: interventions for the treatment of overweight and obesity in adults. J Acad Nutr Diet 2016;116(1):129–47.
36. Pimentel CFMG, Lai M. Nitrition interventions for chronic liver diseases and nonalcoholic fatty liver disease. Med Clin North Am 2016;100:1303–27.
37. Buchwald H, Avidor Y, Braunwald E. Bariatric surgery: a systematic review and meta-analysis. JAMA 2004;291(14):1724–37.
38. Mechanick JL, Youdim A, Jones DB, et al. Clinical practice guidelines for the perioperative nutritional, metabolic, and nonsurgical support of the bariatric surgery patient-2013 update: cosponsored by American Association of Clinical Endocrinologists, the Obesity Society, and American Society for Metabolic & Bariatric Surgery. Obesity (Silver Spring) 2013;21(Suppl1):S1–27.
39. Buchwald H, Oien DM. Metabolic/bariatric surgery worldwide 2011. Metabolic/bariatric surgery worldwide 2011. Obes Surg 2013;23(4):427–36.
40. Mattar SG, Velcu LM, Rabinovitz M, et al. Surgically-induced weight loss significantly improves nonalcoholic fatty liver disease and the metabolic syndrome. Ann Surg 2005;242(4):610–7.
41. Bower G, Toma T, Harling L, et al. Bariatric surgery and non-alcoholic fatty liver disease: a systemic review of liver biochemistry and histology. Obes Surg 2015;25:2280–9.
42. Longitudinal assessment of bariatric surgery (LABS) Consortium. Perioperative safety in the longitudinal assessment of bariatric surgery. N Engl J Med 2009; 361:445–54.
43. Adams TD, Gress RE, Smith SC, et al. Long-term mortality after gastric bypass surgery. N Engl J Med 2007;357(8):753–61.

44. Burza MA, Romero S, Kotronen A, et al. Long-term effect of bariatric surgery on liver enzymes in the Swedish Obese Subjects (SOS) study. PLoS One 2013;8(3): e60495.

45. Mathurin P, Hollebecque A, Arnalsteen L, et al. Prospective study of the long-term effects of bariatric surgery on liver injury in patients without advanced disease. Gastroenterology 2009;137(2):532–40.

46. Bower G, Athanasiou T, Isla AM, et al. Bariatric surgery and nonalcoholic fatty liver disease. Eur J Gastroenterol Hepatol 2015;27(7):755–68.

47. Kral JG, Thung SN, Biron S, et al. Effects of surgical treatment of the metabolic syndrome on liver fibrosis and cirrhosis. Surgery 2004;135(1):48–58.

48. Abu Dayyeh BK, Thompson CC. Obesity and bariatrics for the endoscopist: new techniques. Therap Adv Gastroenterol 2011;4(6):433–42.

49. Choi HS, Chun HJ. Recent trends in endoscopic bariatric therapies. Clin Endosc 2017;50(1):11–6.

50. Ricci G, Bersani G, Rossi A, et al. Bariatric therapy with intragastric balloon improves liver dysfunction and insulin resistance in obese patients. Obes Surg 2008;18(11):1438–42.

51. De Jonge C, rensen SS, Koek GH, et al. Endoscopic duodenal-jejunal bypass liner rapidly improves plasma parameters of nonalcoholic fatty liver disease. Clin Gastroenterol Hepatol 2013;11(11):1517–20.

52. Popov VB, Thompson CC, Kumar N, et al. Effect of intragastric balloons on liver enzymes: a systemic review and meta-analysis. Dig Dis Sci 2016;61(9):2477–87.

53. Lee YM, Low HC, Lim LG, et al. Intragastric balloon significantly improves nonalcoholic fatty liver disease activity score in obese patients with nonalcoholic steatohepatitis: a pilot study. Gastrointest Endosc 2012;76(4):756–60.

54. Sokol RJ, McKim JM Jr, Goff MC, et al. Vitamin E reduces oxidant injury to mitochondria and the hepatotoxicity of taurochenodeoxycholic acid in the rat. Gastroenterology 1998;114:164–74.

55. Morante M, Sandoval J, Gomez-Cabrea MC, et al. Vitamin E deficiency induces liver nuclear factor-κB DNA binding activity and changes in related genes. Free Radic Res 2005;39(10):1127–38.

56. Sanyal AJ, Chalasani N, Kowdley KV, et al. Pioglitazone, vitamin E, or placebo for nonalcoholic steatohepatitis. N Engl J Med 2010;362(18):1675–85.

57. Lavine JE, Schwimmer JB, Van Natta ML, et al. Effect of vitamin E or metformin for treatment of nonalcoholic fatty liver disease in children and adolescents. JAMA 2011;305(16):1659–68.

58. Bjelakovic G, Nikolova D, Gluud LL, et al. Mortality in randomized trials of antioxidant supplements for primary and secondary prevention: systematic review and meta-analysis. JAMA 2007;297:842–57.

59. SchÜrks M, Glynn RJ, Rist PM, et al. Effects of vitamin E on stroke subtypes: meta-analysis of randomized controlled trials. BMJ 2010;341:c5702.

60. Klein EA, Thompson IM Jr, Tangen CM, et al. Vitamin E and the risk of prostate cancer. The Selenium and vitamin E cancer prevention trial (SELECT). JAMA 2011;306:1549–56.

61. Hossain N, Kanwar P, Mohanty SR. A comprehensive updated review of pharmaceutical and nonpharmaceutical treatment for NAFLD. Gastroenterol Res Pract 2016;2016:7109270.

62. Loguercio C, Andreone P, Brisc C, et al. Silybin combined with phosphatidylcholine and vitamin E in patients with nonalcoholic fatty liver disease: a randomized controlled trial. Free Radic Biol Med 2012;52(9):1658–65.

63. Hannah WN Jr, Harrison SA. Lifestyle and dietary interventions in the management of nonalcoholic fatty liver disease. Dig Dis Sci 2016;61:1365–74.
64. Gutierrez-Grobe Y, Chavez-Tapia N, Sanchez-Valle V, et al. High coffee intake is associated with lower grade nonalcoholic fatty liver disease: the role of peripheral antioxidant activity. Hepatol 2012;11:350–5.
65. Zelber-Sagi S, Salomone F, Webb M, et al. Coffee consumption and nonalcoholic fatty liver onset: a prospective study in the general population. Transl Res 2015; 165:428–36.
66. Graeter T, Niedermayer PC, Mason RA, et al. Coffee consumption and NAFLD: a community based study on 1223 subjects. BMC Res Notes 2015;8:640.
67. Molloy JW, Calcagno CJ, Williams CD, et al. Association of coffee and caffeine consumption with fatty liver disease, nonalcoholic steatohepatitis, and degree of hepatic fibrosis. Hepatology 2012;55(2):429–36.
68. Eslamparast T, Poustchi H, Zamani F, et al. Synbiotic supplementation in nonalcoholic fatty liver disease: a randomized, double-blind, placebo-controlled pilot study. Am J Clin Nutr 2014;99:535–42.
69. Alisi A, Bedogni G, Baviera G, et al. Randomized clinical trial: the beneficial effects of VSL#3 in obese children with non-alcoholic steatohepatitis. Aliment Pharmacol Ther 2014;39:1276–85.
70. Wong VW, Won GL, Chim AM, et al. Treatment of nonalcoholic steatohepatitis with probiotics. A proof-of-concept study. Ann Hepatol 2013;12:256–62.
71. Ratziu V, Goodman Z, Sanyal A. Current efforts and trends in the treatment of NASH. Hepatol 2015;62:S65–75.
72. Lutchman G, Modi A, Kleiner DE, et al. The effects of discontinuing pioglitazone in patients with nonalcoholic steatohepatitis. Hepatology 2010;51:445–53.
73. Ratziu V, Charlotte F, Bernhardt C, et al. Long-term efficacy of rosiglitazone in nonalcoholic steatohepatitis: results of the fatty liver improvement rosiglitazone therapy (FLIRT 2) extension trial. Hepatology 2010;51:445–53.
74. Levin D, Bell S, Sund R, et al. Pioglitazone and bladder cancer risk: a multipopulation pooled, cumulative exposure analysis. Diabetologia 2015;58:493–504.
75. Haukeland JW, Konopski Z, Eggesbo HB, et al. Metformin in patients with nonalcoholic fatty liver disease: a randomized, controlled trial. Scand J Gastroenterol 2009;44(7):853–60.
76. Loomba R, Lutchman G, Kleiner DE, et al. Clinical trial: pilot study of metformin for the treatment of non-alcoholic steatohepatitis. Aliment Pharmacol Ther 2009; 29(2):172–82.
77. Rakoski MO, Singal AG, Rogers MA, et al. Meta-analysis: insulin sensitizers for the treatment of non-alcoholic steatohepatitis. Aliment Pharmacol Ther 2010; 32(10):1211–21.
78. Zelber-Sagi S, Kessler A, Brazowsky E, et al. A double-blind randomized placebo-controlled trial of orlistat for the treatment of nonalcoholic fatty liver disease. Clin Gastroenterol Hepatol 2006;4(5):639–44.
79. Harrison SA, Fecht W, Brunt EM, et al. Orlistat for overweight subjects with nonalcoholic steatohepatitis: a randomized, prospective trial. Hepatology 2009;49(1): 80–6.
80. Zein CO, Yerian LM, Gogate P, et al. Pentoxifylline improves nonalcoholic steatohepatitis: a randomized placebo-controlled trial. Hepatolgy 2011;54(5):1610–9.
81. Van Wagner LB, Koppe SW, Brunt EM, et al. Pentoxyfylline for the treatment of non-alcoholic steatohepatitis: a randomized controlled trial. Ann Hepatol 2011; 10(3):277–86.

82. Lindor KD, Kowdley KV, Heathcote EJ, et al. Ursodeoxycholic acid for treatment of nonalcoholic steatohepatitis: results of a randomized trial. Hepatology 2004; 39(3):770–8.

83. Chalasani N, Aljadhey H, Kesterson J, et al. Patients with elevated liver enzymes are not at higher risk for statin hepatotoxicity. Gastroenterology 2004;128: 1287–92.

84. Vuppalanchi R, Teal E, Chalasani N. Patients with elevated baseline liver enzymes do not have higher frequency of hepatotoxicity from lovastatin than those with normal baseline liver enzymes. Am J Med Sci 2005;329:62–5.

85. Tziomalos K, Athyros VG, Paschos P, et al. Nonalcoholic fatty liver disease and statins. Metabolism 2015;64(10):1215–23.

Emerging Treatments for Nonalcoholic Fatty Liver Disease and Nonalcoholic Steatohepatitis

Samer Gawrieh, MD*, Naga Chalasani, MD*

KEYWORDS

- NAFLD • NASH • Obeticholic acid • Elafibranor • Liraglutide • Cenicriviroc
- Selonsertib

KEY POINTS

- There is a dramatic increase in the number of clinical trial testing various compounds that target different important molecules and pathways in nonalcoholic steatohepatitis (NASH) pathogenesis.
- Obeticholic acid, elafibranor, and liraglutide have demonstrated variable beneficial effects on NASH histology in phase II randomized controlled trials.
- The 1-year, midstudy interim analysis of cenicriviroc's phase IIb study showed an encouraging improvement in hepatic fibrosis. Completed results after an additional 1 year of therapy are expected later this year.
- Promising results from a phase II study of selonsertib provided impetus for initiating 2 large phase III trials to assess the efficacy of selonsertib in patients with NASH with bridging fibrosis or cirrhosis.
- Cysteamine bitartrate and long-chain polyunsaturated fatty acids did not achieve the primary end point of histologic improvement in high-quality phase II randomized controlled trials.

Disclosures: Dr S. Gawrieh has ongoing participations in safety committees for TREAT (NIH-sponsored Translational Research and Emerging Therapies for Alcoholic Hepatitis) and Trans-Medics. Dr S. Gawrieh receives research grant support from Cirius (Octeta) Therapeutics, Galmed, and Zydus, where his institution receives the funding. Dr N. Chalasani has had ongoing consulting with NuSirt, AbbVie, Eli Lilly, Afimmune (DS Biopharma), Tobira (Allergan), Madrigal, Shire, Cempra, Ardelyx, Gen Fit, and Amarin. Dr N. Chalasani receives research grant support from Intercept, Lilly, Gilead, Galectin Therapeutics, and Cumberland where his institution receives the funding. Over the last decade, Dr N. Chalasani has served as a paid consultant to more than 30 pharmaceutical companies, and these outside activities have regularly been disclosed to his institutional authorities.

Division of Gastroenterology and Hepatology, Indiana University School of Medicine, 702 Rotary Circle, Suite 225, Indianapolis, IN 46202, USA
* Corresponding authors.
E-mail addresses: sgawrieh@iu.edu (S.G.); nchalasa@iu.edu (N.C.)

Clin Liver Dis 22 (2018) 189–199
http://dx.doi.org/10.1016/j.cld.2017.08.013
1089-3261/18/© 2017 Elsevier Inc. All rights reserved.

INTRODUCTION

The public health burden of nonalcoholic fatty liver disease (NAFLD) is now widely recognized. NAFLD is the most common liver disease in children and adults in the United States.[1–3] End-stage liver disease and hepatocellular carcinoma secondary to NAFLD are now the second leading indications for liver transplantation in the United States, an alarming trend that is expected to culminate in NAFLD replacing hepatitis C as the most common indication for liver transplantation in the next decade.[4–6]

The increase of the prevalence and importance has been paralleled by a better understanding of NAFLD pathophysiology (please see Vignan Manne and colleagues's article "Pathophysiology of Nonalcoholic Fatty Liver Disease/Nonalcoholic Steatohepatitis," in this issue). Numerous molecules and pathways driving the progression of NAFLD are currently the targets of emerging therapies. The intense interest in finding treatments for NAFLD and nonalcoholic steatohepatitis (NASH) is best highlighted by the dramatic increase in registered phase II and III clinical trials for NAFLD and NASH over the past 10 years (**Fig. 1**).

Goals of NAFLD and NASH therapy include improving or stabilizing liver histologic injury and fibrosis, prevention of liver-related poor outcomes and death, and improving or not worsening associated cardio-metabolic comorbidities. With the many pathways and molecules involved in NAFLD-NASH pathogenesis, it is likely that a combination of drugs targeting different molecules and pathways may be used in the future to achieve these goals. Because therapy for NAFLD and NASH is probably going to be chronic, the drugs used will not only need to be efficacious but also have a favorable profile on safety, tolerance, and cardio-metabolic comorbidities.

For a discussion on current treatments of NAFLD and NASH please see Chun Kit Hung and Henry C. Bodenheimer's article "Current Treatment of Nonalcoholic Fatty Liver Disease/Nonalcoholic Steatohepatitis," in this issue. In this article, the authors review completed phase II randomized controlled trials (RCTs) with high quality published positive results (**Table 1**). The authors also review the available preliminary data on cenicrivroc and selonsertib, with or without simtuzumab's phase II studies, which have histologic end points (**Table 2**). Finally, the authors touch on compounds that

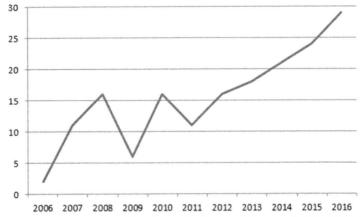

Fig. 1. Registered phase II and III clinical trials for NAFLD-NASH from 2006 to 2016. Search of clinicaltrials.gov as of February 8, 2017 for *NAFLD; interventional studies; phase II, III; studies received from 01/01/2006 to 01/01/2017.*

Table 1
Summary of drugs with published phase II trials with evidence of effect on NASH histology

Drug	Mechanism	Study Size (n)	Route of Administration	Effect on Histology	Common Side Effects
Obeticholic acid	FXR agonist	283	Oral	Improvement in NAS, steatosis, ballooning, lobular inflammation, and fibrosis	Pruritus, weight loss, temporary increase in alkaline phosphatase, temporary changes in lipoprotein profile
Elafibranor	PPAR-α and δ agonist	276	Oral	In subjects with NAS ≥4 elafibranor 120 mg resulted in higher proportion of NASH resolution, improved ballooning, lobular inflammation, and NAS by 2 points; no significant effect on steatosis or fibrosis	Mild increase in serum creatinine in 7.1% of subjects on elafibranor 120 mg
Liraglutide	GLP-1 analogue	52	Subcutaneous	Resolution of NASH with no worsening of fibrosis; improved steatosis	Gastrointestinal symptoms, weight loss

Abbreviations: FXR, farnesoid X receptor; GLP-1, glucagonlike peptide-1; PPAR-α, peroxisome proliferator activated receptor.

have been tested and failed to meet the primary end point of histologic improvement and had high-quality published articles.

Promising Emerging Drugs from Completed Phase II Randomized Controlled Trials

Obeticholic acid

As an agonist of the bile acid nuclear receptor farnesoid X receptor, obeticholic acid (OCA) regulates of bile acids synthesis and transport and modulates lipid and glucose homeostasis and hepatic inflammation.[7,8]

The efficacy of OCA in treating NASH was tested in the *Farnesoid X Receptor Ligand Obeticholic Acid In NASH Treatment* (FLINT) trial.[9] In this trial, 283 subjects with histologically confirmed NASH but without cirrhosis were randomized to receive OCA 25 mg orally daily or matching placebo for 72 weeks. Type 2 diabetes was present in 53% of the OCA and 52% of the control groups. The primary outcome was a decrease in the NAFLD fibrosis score (NAS) by at least 2 points without worsening of fibrosis from baseline to the end of treatment. A planned interim analysis showed significant improvement in liver histology in subjects receiving OCA, which led to modifying the study protocol and not pursuing end-of-treatment liver biopsy on the last 64 subjects. In an intention-to-treat analysis, 45% of subjects in the OCA group versus

Table 2
Summary of preliminary studies of antifibrotic agents, cenicriviroc and selonsertib-simtuzumab

	Cenicriviroc[20]	Selonsertib 18 mg (±Simtuzumab), Selonsertib 6 mg (±Simtuzumab), Simtuzumab alone[24]
Mechanism	Antagonist of C-C chemokine receptors 2 and 5	Inhibitor of ASK1 (selonsertib) Humanized monoclonal antibody to LOX-like 2 (simtuzumab)
Route of administration	Oral	Oral (selonsertib) Subcutaneous (simtuzumab)
Size of initial study	289	72
Diabetic subjects included	Yes	Yes
% Improvement in fibrosis ≥1 stage without worsening of steatohepatitis	20	37, 30, 20
Interval histologic effect observed	1 y	6 mo
Ongoing clinical trials	Current IIb with 289 subjects for 2 y	2 ongoing phase III trials Selonsertib vs placebo (NASH with bridging fibrosis or cirrhosis), each with 800 subjects for 240 wk

Abbreviation: ASK1, apoptosis signal-regulating kinase.
   Data from Refs.[20,24]

21% in the placebo group achieved the study primary outcome (relative risk 1.9, 95% confidence interval [CI] 1.3–2.8; $P = .0002$). OCA was also associated with significant improvement in fibrosis (35% vs 19%, $P = .004$), hepatocyte ballooning (46% vs 31%, $P = .03$), steatosis (61% vs 38%, $P = .001$), and lobular inflammation (53% vs 35%, $P = .006$). There was no significant difference in the frequency of NASH resolution with OCA versus placebo (22% vs 13%, $P = .08$).

OCA was associated with a significant reduction in alanine aminotransferase (ALT) (-38 vs -18 U/L, $P<.0001$), aspartate aminotransferase (AST) (-27 vs -10 U/L, $P = .0001$), gamma-glutamyltransferase (-37 vs -6, $P<.0001$), and bilirubin (-1.0 vs 0.6 µmol/L, $P = .002$) but an increase in alkaline phosphatase (12 vs -6, $P<.0001$). These changes resolved 24 weeks after study drug cessation, at which point no significant difference in liver biochemistries were noted between those on OCA versus placebo.

Subjects on OCA experienced significant weight loss compared with placebo (-2.3 vs 0.0 kg, $P = .008$) and higher insulin (29 vs 10 pmol/L, $P = .02$) and Homeostatic model assessment-insulin resistance (HOMA-IR) (15 vs 4, $P = .01$). Significant changes in serum lipoproteins were also observed with OCA versus placebo: increase in total cholesterol (0.16 vs -0.19 mmol/L, $P = .0009$), low-density lipoprotein (0.22 vs -0.22 mmol/L, $P<.0001$), and a decrease in high-density lipoprotein (HDL) (-0.02 vs 0.03 mmol/L, $P = .01$). These changes attenuated while on the drug but were not sustained after completion of the study.

OCA therapy was associated with pruritus in 23% of subjects versus 6% of those on placebo. Pruritus was also more severe with OCA and led to stopping OCA in one subject and using antipruritic therapies and holding OCA briefly in other subjects.

There were 5 severe or life-threatening adverse events that were thought to be related to OCA. These events included severe pruritus (n = 3), hyperglycemia (n = 1), and possible cerebral ischemia (n = 1). On the other hand, there were 4 severe or life-threatening adverse events in subjects on placebo (abdominal pain, headache, weakness, vertigo with nausea and vomiting). Two deaths occurred during the study duration: one from congestive heart failure and sepsis and one from myocardial ischemia or infarction; both were in subjects receiving OCA but were deemed not to be related to OCA.

Subsequently, a large phase III RCT of OCA has been launched (NCT02548351). A target of 2000 subjects with biopsy-proven NASH will be randomized to OCA 10 mg daily, OCA 25 mg daily, or matching placebo for 18 months. The primary end points are (a) reduction in fibrosis without worsening of NASH, (b) resolution of NASH, and (c) all-cause mortality and liver-related clinical outcomes spanning 6 years from the start of the study. This study is currently recruiting in centers around the world.

Elafibranor

Elafibranor (GFT505) is a dual agonist of the nuclear peroxisome proliferator activated receptors α and δ. It has been shown to improve insulin sensitivity, lipid handling, and inflammation.[10,11] Elafibranor improved liver histology in different animal models of NASH.[11-13]

In a large phase II RCT, 276 subjects with biopsy-proven NASH without cirrhosis were randomized to receive elafibranor 80 mg versus elafibranor 120 mg versus placebo for 52 weeks. In the intention-to-treat group, 40% had type 2 diabetes. NASH resolution without worsening of fibrosis was the primary end point. This end point was not achieved, as there was no significant difference in the primary end point between the 3 study groups. There was no significant effect for either dose of elafibranor on steatosis, lobular inflammation, or hepatocyte ballooning in the primary analysis. A post hoc analysis was then performed looking at patients with NASH and NAS of 4 or greater, which showed that, in this subgroup, elafibranor 120 mg resulted in a higher proportion of NASH resolution versus placebo (20% vs 11%; odds ratio = 3.16; 95% CI: 1.22–8.13; P = .018), in addition to improving steatosis, ballooning, lobular inflammation, and NAS by 2 points. There was no effect for elafibranor on fibrosis in the primary analysis. In the post hoc analysis, those with NAS of 4 or greater who received the 120-mg dose and had NASH resolution showed significant improvement in fibrosis as well as other histologic features compared with those on the same dose without NASH resolution.

Patients receiving either dose of elafibranor had significant improvement in liver enzymes, lipoproteins, triglycerides, and circulating markers of inflammation (haptoglobin and fibrinogen). There was significant improvement in HOMA-IR fasting glucose level and hemoglobin A1c only in diabetic subjects in the elafibranor 120-mg arm.

No cardiovascular events or deaths occurred in subjects receiving elafibranor. There was no effect on body weight. A mild increase in serum creatinine was noted in the elafibranor arms in 7 subjects (6 in the 120-mg arm) who had elevated creatinine and decreased glomerular filtration rate at baseline, which led to discontinuation of the drug with subsequent improvement in creatinine in most but not all subjects. Serious adverse events occurred in 15 (16.1%) patients in the 80-mg, 14 (15.8%) patients in the 120-mg, and 11 (12.0%) patients in the placebo arms. There were 8 treatment-related serious adverse events: 2 in the 80-mg elafibranor group (spontaneous abortion, ataxia, fasciculation, and tremor), in 2 in the elafibranor 120-mg group (acute pancreatitis, Parkinson disease), and in 4 patients from the placebo arm (renal cancer, breast cancer, bladder cancer, and pancreatic cancer). In addition, one bladder cancer occurred in the elafibranor 80-mg arm. All cancers were assessed to be unlikely related to study drug.

There is currently an ongoing phase III RCT of elafibranor (NCT02704403) in patients with biopsy-proven NASH without cirrhosis. The target enrollment is 2000 subjects who will be randomized to elafibranor 120 mg versus placebo for 72 weeks. Resolution of NASH without worsening of fibrosis as well as clinical outcomes (all-cause death and liver-related events over a 4-year period) will be the primary outcome measures.

Liraglutide

Liraglutide is a glucagonlike peptide-1 (GLP-1) analogue that is used for glycemic control in patients with type 2 diabetes. GLP-1 has many biological effects that make it an attractive option to treat NASH. It reduces glucagon secretion, increases insulin secretion, suppresses hepatic de novo lipogenesis, increases fatty acid oxidation, and delays gastric emptying. These effects result in insulin sensitivity and weight loss.[14] Preliminary human data suggested the GLP-1 analogues may improve liver histology in patients with NASH.[15,16]

More recently, a phase II RCT examined the effects of liraglutide on biopsy-proven NASH.[17] The *Liraglutide Efficacy and Action in Non-alcoholic steatohepatitis* (LEAN) trial randomized 52 patients with histologically proven NASH to receive either 1.8 mg/d of liraglutide subcutaneously or placebo for 48 weeks. Subjects with type 2 diabetes and compensated cirrhosis were not excluded from the study. A similar proportion of patients with type 2 diabetes were included in the liraglutide group versus placebo (35% vs 32%), but a lower proportion of subjects on liraglutide had advanced hepatic fibrosis (Kleiner stage 3 and 4) (46% vs 58%) and cirrhosis (8% vs 15%) compared with placebo. The primary end point of this trial was resolution of NASH with no worsening of fibrosis at the end of the study. More subjects receiving liraglutide achieved the primary end point compared with placebo (39% vs 9% relative risk 4·3 [95% CI 1·0–17·7]; $P = .019$). Improvement of steatosis was more common on liraglutide (83% vs 45%, $P = .009$), and worsening of fibrosis was less frequent on liraglutide (9% vs 36%, $P = .04$) (**Fig. 2**). No significant differences were noted in the frequency of improvement in NAS or lobular inflammation, but the improvement of

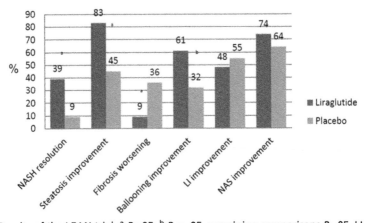

Fig. 2. Results of the LEAN trial. [a] $P<.05$; [b] $P = .05$, remaining comparisons $P>.05$. LI, lobular inflammation.

hepatocyte ballooning showed a trend toward significance on liraglutide (61% vs 32%, $P = .05$).

There was significant improvement in hemoglobin A1c and HDL on liraglutide. There was a numeric but nonstatistically significant improvement in ALT, AST, and keratin-18 on liraglutide. Importantly, there was more weight loss in subjects on liraglutide versus placebo (−5.5 kg vs −0.6 kg, $P = .003$).

Gastrointestinal side effects (eg, nausea, diarrhea, abdominal pain, loss of appetite, and so forth) were most common in both study arms (81% in liraglutide arm vs 65% in placebo arm) and more common in the liraglutide arm than controls. Constipation occurred in 27% of subjects on liraglutide but in none of the subjects on placebo. There were 2 severe adverse events (tuberculosis and migraine) in the liraglutide arm that were deemed not related to the study drug. The drug withdrawal rate was similar between the 2 groups (19%).

To the authors' knowledge, there is no registered phase III RCT for liraglutide in NASH.

Drugs in Phase II Studies with Biopsy End Points

Cenicriviroc

The chemokine C-C ligand type 2 and 5 (CLL2 and CLL5) play an important role in macrophage recruitment and migration to the liver and are overexpressed in the livers of obese patients with NASH.[18] Cenicriviroc is an oral antagonist of C-C chemokine receptors 2 and 5. In animal models of different liver diseases, cenicriviroc exhibited antiinflammatory and antifibrotic effects.[19]

The preliminary 1-year results of a phase IIb RCT (CENTAUR) were recently presented at the 2016 liver meeting.[20] In this trial, 289 subjects with biopsy-proven NASH were randomized to receive cenicriviroc 150 mg daily versus placebo for 2 years. In total, 52% had type 2 diabetes, 72% metabolic syndrome, and 67% stage 2 to 3 fibrosis. The primary outcome is a 2 or more point improvement in NAS, and secondary end points include complete resolution of steatohepatitis without worsening of fibrosis and improvement in hepatic fibrosis by 1 stage or more. In this midstudy interim analysis, the proportion of subjects achieving the primary end point was not different between the two groups (16% vs 19% for cenicriviroc vs placebo, $P = .5$); however, 20% of subjects on cenicriviroc achieved improvement in fibrosis by 1 stage or more without worsening of steatohepatitis compared with 10% of those on placebo ($P = .023$) (see **Table 2**). Treatment-emergent adverse events of grade 2 or greater severity at a frequency 2% or greater included fatigue (2.8%) and diarrhea (2.1%) for cenicriviroc and headache (3.5%) for placebo.

These results are exciting, and the final effects of cenicriviroc on liver histology at the end of the trial (an additional 1 year of therapy) are awaited.

Selonsertib and simtuzumab

Inhibition of apoptosis signal-regulating kinase (ASK1) in mice and monkeys with diet-induced NAFLD results in improvement in hepatic fibrosis, inflammation, steatosis, and insulin sensitivity.[21,22] Selonsertib (GS-4997) is a selective oral inhibitor of ASK1. In a recent randomized phase II clinical trial, selonsertib's safety and efficacy in human NASH were tested in combination with simtuzumab, an injectable humanized monoclonal antibody to lysyl oxidase (LOX)-like 2, which exhibits antifibrotic effects.[23,24]

In this study, 72 subjects with histologically proven NASH with NAS of 5 or greater and stage 2 to 3 fibrosis were randomized to receive selonsertib 6 mg or 18 mg orally once daily, with or without simtuzumab 125 mg subcutaneously once weekly, or just simtuzumab 125 mg subcutaneously once weekly for 24 weeks. Diabetes was present in 70.8% of all subjects. All subjects had a repeat biopsy at the end of the study. In addition, fibrosis and fat were assessed by magnetic resonance (MR) elastography (MRE) and proton density fat fraction (MR-PDFF) at baseline, 12 weeks, and the end of the study. Fibrosis improvement by 1 stage or greater and progression to cirrhosis were the primary histologic efficacy end points, whereas a 15% or greater reduction in MRE-measured liver stiffness and 30% or greater reduction in MR-PDFF–measured hepatic fat were the MR-based efficacy end points. Fibrosis improvement by 1 stage or greater without worsening of steatohepatitis was observed in 37%, 30%, and 20%, whereas progression to cirrhosis was observed in 3%, 7%, and 20%, in the selonsertib 18 mg (±simtuzumab), selonsertib 6 mg (±simtuzumab), and simtuzumab-alone groups, respectively (see **Table 2**). MRE-stiffness reduction of 15% or greater was noted in 20%, 32%, and 0%, whereas MR-PDFF fat reduction of 30% or greataer was noted in 26%, 13%, and 10% in the selonsertib 18-mg (±simtuzumab), selonsertib 6-mg (±simtuzumab), and simtuzumab-alone groups, respectively. Stability or improvement in NAS and lobular inflammation and reduction of fibrosis as measured by morphometric hepatic collagen per 1% decrease and MRE stiffness per 1-kPa decrease were associated with improvement in the pathologist's assessment of fibrosis. No deaths occurred during the study. Five serious adverse events were reported in the selonsertib ± simtuzumab groups versus none in the simtuzumab group, with only 1 serious adverse event deemed related to the study drug. Treatment was discontinued because of adverse events in 3 subjects (4.8%) in the selonsertib ± simtuzumab groups versus none in the simtuzumab group.

The safety and efficacy of selonsertib versus placebo is currently being tested in 2 phase III RCTs in adults with bridging fibrosis (STELLAR 3, NCT03053050) or compensated cirrhosis (STELLAR 4, NCT03053063) due to NASH. Each study plans to recruit 800 subjects, and the study duration will be 240 weeks. Two phase II clinical trials in patients with NASH and bridging fibrosis (NCT01672866) or cirrhosis (NCT01672879) evaluating intravenous simtuzumab's efficacy and safety have been terminated.

Drugs That Have Been Tested in Phase II Trials Without Achieving Primary Histologic End Point

Cysteamine bitartrate
As a precursor to glutathione, cysteamine has the advantage of crossing cellular membranes more efficiently than glutathione. Its efficacy at protecting against acetaminophen-induced liver injury has been demonstrated in prior studies in humans.[25,26]

A recent RCT in 169 children with NAFLD activity scores of 4 or greater (*C*ysteamine Bitartrate Delayed-Release for the Treatment of *N*onalcoholic Fatty Liver Disease in *C*hildren [CyNCh]) randomized subjects to receive weight-based cysteamine or placebo twice daily for 52 weeks.[27] A decrease in NAS of 2 points or greater without worsening fibrosis was the primary outcome. Despite a significant improvement in liver enzymes (ALT -53 ± 88 U/L vs -8 ± 77 U/L; $P = .02$, AST -31 ± 52 vs -4 ± 36 U/L; $P = .008$) and lobular inflammation (36% vs 21%; $P = .03$) on cysteamine compared with placebo, the primary end point was not achieved. In subgroup analyses, children younger than 13 years showed histologic improvement with cysteamine (observed in 43% [16 of 37] versus 21% [8 of 39]; relative risk, 2.3; 95% CI, 1.0 to 5.2; $P = .04$). Children weighing 65 kg or less also showed histologic improvement and achieved the primary outcome on cysteamine versus placebo (observed in 50% [12 of 24] versus 13%

[3 of 23]; relative risk, 4.0; 95% CI, 1.3–12.3; P = .005), which was due to improvement in lobular inflammation (54% vs 22%, relative risk, 2.6; 95% CI, [1.1–6.0]; P = .02) and hepatocyte ballooning (33% vs 4%, relative risk, 8.3; 95% CI, 1.0–71.3; P = .01).

Validation of the effects of cysteamine on NASH histology per age and weight will require adequately powered RCT to measure any potential effect. To the authors' knowledge, there is currently no registered future clinical trial for cysteamine.

Long-chain polyunsaturated fatty acids

Long-chain polyunsaturated fatty acids (LC-PUFAs) are abundant in fish and fish oil supplements and exhibit beneficial metabolic and antiinflammatory effects, including improvement in insulin sensitivity and reduction in serum triglycerides, endothelial dysfunction, and adipose tissue inflammation.[28–30]

Earlier reports of favorable effects on liver enzymes and hepatic steatosis with LC-PUFAs were not substantiated by larger phase II RCTs.[31–34] One RCT randomized 103 subjects with NAFLD to receive docosahexaenoic acid and eicosapentaenoic acid (EPA) (4 g/d) for 15 to 18 months.[35] There was no significant change in hepatic steatosis or noninvasive markers of fibrosis at the end of the study. The largest RCT of LC-PUFAs randomized 243 subjects with histologically confirmed NASH to receive EPA 1800 mg/d, EPA 2700 mg/d, or placebo for 12 months.[36] Subjects on EPA showed no significant change in liver enzymes, markers of fibrosis, insulin resistance, or liver histology compared with those on placebo. These data suggest that LC-PUFAs are not an effective therapy for NASH.

SUMMARY

The intense interest in NASH therapeutics has translated in a significant increase in clinical trials. Of the emerging promising compounds, OCA, elafibranor, and liraglutide have evidence from phase II RCTs of variable beneficial effects on NASH histology. Exciting preliminary results from a small phase II study have led to the launch of 2 large phase III trials to assess the efficacy of selonsertib in patients with NASH with bridging fibrosis or cirrhosis. OCA and elafibranor have now moved to be tested in ongoing large phase III RCTs. These RCTs are slated to provide the largest efficacy and safety data in NASH therapeutic trials to date and will also collect hard clinical outcomes. The data from the completed cenicrivoc phase II RCT is expected in the next year, which may provide impetus for yet another large phase III RCT. For all these promising compounds and others in different stages of development, the establishment of long-term safety, efficacy, and tolerability will be key for their approvals as therapies for patients with NASH.

REFERENCES

1. Browning JD, Szczepaniak LS, Dobbins R, et al. Prevalence of hepatic steatosis in an urban population in the United States: impact of ethnicity. Hepatology 2004; 40(6):1387–95.

2. Schwimmer JB, Deutsch R, Kahen T, et al. Prevalence of fatty liver in children and adolescents. Pediatrics 2006;118(4):1388–93.

3. Vernon G, Baranova A, Younossi ZM. Systematic review: the epidemiology and natural history of non-alcoholic fatty liver disease and non-alcoholic steatohepatitis in adults. Aliment Pharmacol Ther 2011;34(3):274–85.

4. Wong RJ, Aguilar M, Cheung R, et al. Nonalcoholic steatohepatitis is the second leading etiology of liver disease among adults awaiting liver transplantation in the United States. Gastroenterology 2015;148(3):547–55.

5. Charlton MR, Burns JM, Pedersen RA, et al. Frequency and outcomes of liver transplantation for nonalcoholic steatohepatitis in the United States. Gastroenterology 2011;141(4):1249–53.

6. Goldberg D, Ditah IC, Saeian K, et al. Changes in the prevalence of hepatitis C virus infection, nonalcoholic steatohepatitis, and alcoholic liver disease among patients with cirrhosis or liver failure on the waitlist for liver transplantation. Gastroenterology 2017;152(5):1090–9.e1.

7. Adorini L, Pruzanski M, Shapiro D. Farnesoid X receptor targeting to treat nonalcoholic steatohepatitis. Drug Discov Today 2012;17(17–18):988–97.

8. Mazuy C, Helleboid A, Staels B, et al. Nuclear bile acid signaling through the farnesoid X receptor. Cell Mol Life Sci 2015;72(9):1631–50.

9. Neuschwander-Tetri BA, Loomba R, Sanyal AJ, et al. Farnesoid X nuclear receptor ligand obeticholic acid for non-cirrhotic, non-alcoholic steatohepatitis (FLINT): a multicentre, randomised, placebo-controlled trial. Lancet 2015;385(9972):956–65.

10. Cariou B, Zaïr Y, Staels B, et al. Effects of the new dual PPAR alpha/delta agonist GFT505 on lipid and glucose homeostasis in abdominally obese patients with combined dyslipidemia or impaired glucose metabolism. Diabetes Care 2011;34(9):2008–14.

11. Quintero P, Arrese M. Nuclear control of inflammation and fibrosis in nonalcoholic steatohepatitis: therapeutic potential of dual peroxisome proliferator-activated receptor alpha/delta agonism. Hepatology 2013;58(6):1881–4.

12. Cariou B, Staels B. GFT505 for the treatment of nonalcoholic steatohepatitis and type 2 diabetes. Expert Opin Investig Drugs 2014;23(10):1441–8.

13. Staels B, Rubenstrunk A, Noel B, et al. Hepatoprotective effects of the dual peroxisome proliferator-activated receptor alpha/delta agonist, GFT505, in rodent models of nonalcoholic fatty liver disease/nonalcoholic steatohepatitis. Hepatology 2013;58(6):1941–52.

14. Baggio LL, Drucker DJ. Biology of incretins: GLP-1 and GIP. Gastroenterology 2007;132(6):2131–57.

15. Kenny PR, Brady DE, Torres DM, et al. Exenatide in the treatment of diabetic patients with non-alcoholic steatohepatitis: a case series. Am J Gastroenterol 2010;105(12):2707–9.

16. Eguchi Y, Kitajima Y, Hyogo H, et al. Pilot study of liraglutide effects in non-alcoholic steatohepatitis and non-alcoholic fatty liver disease with glucose intolerance in Japanese patients (LEAN-J). Hepatol Res 2015;45(3):269–78.

17. Armstrong MJ, Gaunt P, Aithal GP, et al. Liraglutide safety and efficacy in patients with non-alcoholic steatohepatitis (LEAN): a multicentre, double-blind, randomised, placebo-controlled phase 2 study. Lancet 2016;387(10019):679–90.

18. Bertola A, Bonnafous S, Anty R, et al. Hepatic expression patterns of inflammatory and immune response genes associated with obesity and NASH in morbidly obese patients. PLoS One 2010;5(10):e13577.

19. Lefebvre E, Moyle G, Reshef R, et al. Anti-fibrotic and anti-inflammatory activity of the dual CCR2 and CCR5 antagonist cenicriviroc in a mouse model of NASH. Hepatology 2013;58(S1):219A–22A.

20. Friedman S, Sanyal A, Goodman Z, et al. Efficacy and safety study of cenicriviroc for the treatment of non-alcoholic steatohepatitis in adult subjects with liver fibrosis: CENTAUR phase 2b study design. Contemp Clin Trials 2016;47:356–65.

21. Xiang M, Wang PX, Wang AB, et al. Targeting hepatic TRAF1-ASK1 signaling to improve inflammation, insulin resistance, and hepatic steatosis. J Hepatol 2016;64(6):1365–77.

22. Wang PX, Ji YX, Zhang XJ, et al. Targeting CASP8 and FADD-like apoptosis regulator ameliorates nonalcoholic steatohepatitis in mice and nonhuman primates. Nat Med 2017;23(4):439–49.
23. Van Bergen T, Marshall D, Van de Veire S, et al. The role of LOX and LOXL2 in scar formation after glaucoma surgery. Invest Ophthalmol Vis Sci 2013;54(8):5788–96.
24. Loomba R, et al. GS-4997, an inhibitor of apoptosis signal-regulating kinase (ASK1), alone or in combination with simtuzumab for the treatment of nonalcoholic steatohepatitis (NASH): a randomized, phase 2 trial. Hepatology 2016;64(6):1119a–20a.
25. Prescott LF, Newton RW, Swainson CP, et al. Successful treatment of severe paracetamol overdosage with cysteamine. Lancet 1974;1(7858):588–92.
26. Prescott LF, Sutherland GR, Park J, et al. Cysteamine, methionine, and penicillamine in the treatment of paracetamol poisoning. Lancet 1976;2(7977):109–13.
27. Schwimmer JB, Lavine JE, Wilson LA, et al. In children with nonalcoholic fatty liver disease, cysteamine bitartrate delayed release improves liver enzymes but does not reduce disease activity scores. Gastroenterology 2016;151(6):1141–54.e9.
28. Flachs P, Rossmeisl M, Bryhn M, et al. Cellular and molecular effects of n-3 polyunsaturated fatty acids on adipose tissue biology and metabolism. Clin Sci (Lond) 2009;116(1):1–16.
29. Flachs P, Rossmeisl M, Kopecky J. The effect of n-3 fatty acids on glucose homeostasis and insulin sensitivity. Physiol Res 2014;63(Suppl 1):S93–118.
30. Wu JH, Cahill LE, Mozaffarian D. Effect of fish oil on circulating adiponectin: a systematic review and meta-analysis of randomized controlled trials. J Clin Endocrinol Metab 2013;98(6):2451–9.
31. Capanni M, Calella F, Biagini MR, et al. Prolonged n-3 polyunsaturated fatty acid supplementation ameliorates hepatic steatosis in patients with non-alcoholic fatty liver disease: a pilot study. Aliment Pharmacol Ther 2006;23(8):1143–51.
32. Tanaka N, Sano K, Horiuchi A, et al. Highly purified eicosapentaenoic acid treatment improves nonalcoholic steatohepatitis. J Clin Gastroenterol 2008;42(4): 413–8.
33. Sofi F, Giangrandi I, Cesari F, et al. Effects of a 1-year dietary intervention with n-3 polyunsaturated fatty acid-enriched olive oil on non-alcoholic fatty liver disease patients: a preliminary study. Int J Food Sci Nutr 2010;61(8):792–802.
34. Nobili V, Alisi A, Della Corte C, et al. Docosahexaenoic acid for the treatment of fatty liver: randomised controlled trial in children. Nutr Metab Cardiovasc Dis 2013;23(11):1066–70.
35. Scorletti E, Bhatia L, McCormick KG, et al. Effects of purified eicosapentaenoic and docosahexaenoic acids in non-alcoholic fatty liver disease: results from the *WELCOME study. Hepatology 2014;60(4):1211–21.
36. Sanyal AJ, Abdelmalek MF, Suzuki A, et al. No significant effects of ethyl-eicosapentaenoic acid on histologic features of nonalcoholic steatohepatitis in a phase 2 trial. Gastroenterology 2014;147(2):377–84.e1.

Nonalcoholic Fatty Liver Disease/Nonalcoholic Steatohepatitis and Hepatocellular Carcinoma

Omar Massoud, MD[a], Michael Charlton, MD, FRCP[b],*

KEYWORDS

- Nonalcoholic steatohepatitis • Obesity • Hepatocellular carcinoma
- Metabolic syndrome

KEY POINTS

- The progressive increase in the prevalence of nonalcoholic fatty liver disease and nonalcoholic steatohepatitis are likely to make nonalcoholic fatty liver disease/nonalcoholic steatohepatitis the most common predisposing factor of hepatocellular carcinoma in the upcoming decades.
- The frequency of nonalcoholic fatty liver disease/nonalcoholic steatohepatitis –related hepatocellular carcinoma in the absence of cirrhosis is unclear.
- Screening and surveillance for hepatocellular carcinoma should, for now, be limited to patients thought to have cirrhosis.
- Obesity can make screening for hepatocellular carcinoma in patients with nonalcoholic steatohepatitis cirrhosis challenging, increasing the technical failure rate of ultrasound scan as a screening method.
- The delay in the diagnosis of hepatocellular carcinoma in the setting of nonalcoholic fatty liver disease/nonalcoholic steatohepatitis and the presence of multiple comorbidities in this population negatively impacts prognosis.

INTRODUCTION

The incidence of hepatocellular carcinoma (HCC) in the United States has tripled over the last 3 decades. A recent study using the Surveillance, Epidemiology and End Result (SEER) database found an increase in the incidence rate of HCC from 1.6 per 100000 in 1975 to 4.9 per 100000 in 2000.[1] HCC is the fastest growing cause of

The authors have nothing to disclose.
[a] Division of Gastroenterology and Hepatology, University of Alabama, 1720 2nd Avenue South, BDB 380, Birmingham, AL 35233, USA; [b] Division of Gastroenterology and Hepatology, University of Chicago, Center for Liver Diseases, The University of Chicago Biological Sciences, 5841 South Maryland Avenue, Room M-454, Chicago, IL 60637, USA
* Corresponding author.
E-mail address: mcharlton@medicine.bsd.uchicago.edu

cancer death in the United States male population.[2] The primary risk factor for HCC is cirrhosis, which is present in 70% to 90% of cases.[2] The most common causes of cirrhosis are viral hepatitis (hepatitis B and hepatitis C), alcoholic hepatitis, and nonalcoholic steatohepatitis (NASH), the most common cause of liver disease in the West and globally.[3–10] However, 15% to 50% of HCC cases occur in patients with cryptogenic cirrhosis without other known chronic liver disease.[2] Further, there is a growing body of literature showing that HCC can develop from noncirrhotic NASH or even simple hepatic steatosis.[11] In addition, obesity has been established as a risk factor for the development of a variety of malignancies, including liver cancer.[12–14] This review discusses the association between HCC and NASH cirrhosis, noncirrhotic NASH/nonalcoholic fatty liver disease (NAFLD), diabetes, obesity, and metabolic syndrome. This review also discusses the pathogenesis of HCC in cirrhosis and noncirrhosis and reviews the challenges of surveillance for HCC in NASH/NAFLD population.

HEPATOCELLULAR CARCINOMA AND NONALCOHOLIC FATTY LIVER DISEASE/NONALCOHOLIC STEATOHEPATITIS–RELATED CIRRHOSIS

The first report on HCC complicating NASH with cirrhosis was published in the 1990s. Further studies indicated that NASH is a risk factor for the development of cirrhosis and HCC.[15] Although most cases of HCC occur in the setting of hepatitis C virus (HCV) or alcoholic cirrhosis, in 15% to 50% of cases, HCC occurs in the setting of cryptogenic cirrhosis.[2,10] It is widely believed that cryptogenic cirrhosis represents "burnt out" NASH, bearing metabolic features of metabolic syndrome but no longer having the classic biopsy features of NASH, such as steatosis, which dissipates with more advanced liver disease.[14,16] The risk of HCC in NASH-related cirrhosis seems to be lower than in viral or alcohol-related cirrhosis.[17] In a large cohort study, HCC was significantly more common in HCV than in NAFLD (6.8% vs 2.4% overall, respectively).[18] The perception that HCC is less common in NASH-related cirrhosis has, however, recently been challenged. In a report from England, the overall incidence of HCC increased 1.8-fold from 2000 to 2010 with more than 10-fold increase in HCC associated with NAFLD, accounting for 34.8% of all the cases in 2010 and making it the single most common underlying etiology.[19] The lower incidence of HCC with NASH cirrhosis may be outweighed by the progressive increase in NASH-related cirrhosis.[17]

Ascha and colleagues[20] compared the incidence of HCV- and NASH-related cirrhosis. Among 510 patients with cirrhosis, 196 had underlying NASH, whereas 315 had cirrhosis secondary to HCV. Median follow-up of 3.2 years found an annual cumulative HCC incidence of 2.6% for NASH-related cirrhosis compared with 4% for HCV-related cirrhosis cases. Despite the estimated low HCC incidence rate of 2.6% in patients with NASH-related cirrhosis, the surge in the number of cases with NAFLD is projected to lead to an increase in the number of patients with NASH-related HCC.[10] A recent study found a 4-fold increase in the prevalence of NASH-related HCC among liver transplant recipients since the implementation of the model for end-stage liver disease in 2002. In this large US population-based study, which used the United Network for Organ Sharing database from 2002 to 2012, Wong and colleagues[21,22] reported 10,061 patients with HCC among 61,868 liver transplant recipients. To achieve a more accurate assessment of the true prevalence of NASH, the investigators created a modified NASH category, which included patients with a formal diagnosis of NASH and obese patients (body mass index [BMI] more than 30 kg/m^2) with cryptogenic cirrhosis and obese patients with unknown etiology of HCC. The proportion of HCC patients undergoing liver transplantation increased from 3.3% in 2000 to 13.5% in 2012 (**Table 1**). Although HCV remained the leading

Table 1
The etiologies of liver disease among hepatocellular carcinoma–related liver transplant recipients after the implementation of MELD in 2002

Etiology of HCC	2002	2007	2012
HCV (%)	43.4	46.3	49.9
NASH (%)	0	4	6
Modified NASH (%)	8.3	10.3	13.5

etiology of HCC, NASH was found to be the second leading cause of HCC in patients undergoing liver transplantation.

With the growing burden of obesity and diabetes mellitus (DM) in the developed countries leading to NAFLD and NASH, there is cumulative evidence suggesting that NASH may account for a large portion of idiopathic or cryptogenic cirrhosis.[16,23] NASH-related HCC patients undergoing liver transplantation have significantly higher rates of DM and higher BMI.[22] Similar to the NASH population, patients with cryptogenic cirrhosis have a high prevalence of obesity and DM. Additionally, a significant number of liver transplant recipients with cryptogenic cirrhosis go on to have NAFLD (25.4%) or NASH (15.7%) within 2 years after transplant surgery.[24] This finding provides further support that patients with end-stage or burnt out NASH are potentially being misclassified with cryptogenic cirrhosis.[25]

HEPATOCELLULAR CARCINOMA AND NONCIRRHOTIC NONALCOHOLIC FATTY LIVER DISEASE/NONALCOHOLIC STEATOHEPATITIS

NAFLD, the most common liver disorder in the United States and other industrialized countries, affects between 25% and 45% of the US population. NASH affects 5% of the population.[26–29] Although HCC almost always occurs in adults in the setting of cirrhosis, there is growing evidence that HCC can develop in the setting of noncirrhotic NAFLD.[11] Since 2004, several reports have described the development of HCC in non-cirrhotic NAFLD.[14,30–43] The largest study was from Japan and included 87 patients who had HCC in the setting of NAFLD. Forty-three of these patients did not have cirrhosis.[43] In 2008 Guzman and colleagues[37] published a small case series of 3 patients with noncirrhotic HCC in the setting of NAFLD. All had at least 2 features of metabolic syndrome with a mean BMI of 33.5. More recently, Perumpail and colleagues[26] published a case series of 9 patients who had HCC in the absence of cirrhosis. Of these, 1 patient had chronic hepatitis B virus (HBV), 1 had chronic HCV infection, and 1 had the fibrolamellar variant of HCC. Six patients (66.7%) had either NASH/NAFLD or at least 2 features of metabolic syndrome without underlying liver disease. The mean age of the 6 patients was 72 ± 8 years. One patient had NASH, 2 had NAFLD, and 3 had no known liver disease. All 6 patients had at least 2 of the features of metabolic syndrome; all 6 had hypertension, and 5 had dyslipidemia. All 6 had either type II diabetes or evidence of insulin resistance. The mean BMI was 29.4, with 2 patients meeting criteria for severe obesity (BMI, 35–39.9), 1 for obesity (BMI, 30–34.9), 2 for overweight (BMI, 25–29.9), and 1 for normal weight. Patients with HCC in the setting of noncirrhotic NAFLD were older in age and mostly men.[26] HCC was more likely to be well differentiated, and many developed in a preexisting liver cell adenoma.[38] Although the growing body of evidence suggesting HCC can develop in the setting of NAFLD without cirrhosis deserves particular attention, current guidelines recommend HCC screening *only* in patients with cirrhosis, with the exception of patients with chronic HBV.[14]

HEPATOCELLULAR CARCINOMA AND OBESITY, DIABETES, AND METABOLIC SYNDROME

The prevalence of obesity, type II diabetes, and metabolic syndrome has been increasing at alarming rates, both in the United States and worldwide. Obesity affects more than one-third of the population of the USA.[44] Type II diabetes affects one in ten middle-aged adults.[27,45] Metabolic syndrome, as defined by the presence of at least 3 of the following risk factors: central obesity, elevated triglycerides, hypertension, impaired fasting glucose, and reduced high-density lipoprotein cholesterol, affects up to 25% of the US population.[46,47]

In a prospectively studied population of more than 900,000 US adults, who were free from cancer at enrollment in 1982, Calle and colleagues[13] identified 57,145 deaths from cancer during 16 years of follow-up. The investigators examined the relation in men and women between the BMI in 1982 and the risk of death from all cancers and from cancers at individual sites, while controlling for other risk factors in multivariate and proportional-hazards models. The study found that individuals with BMI of at least 40 had death rates from all cancers combined of 52% higher (for men) and 62% higher (for women) than the rates in men and women of normal weight. The relative risk of death was 1.52 for men and 1.62 for women. In both men and women, BMI was significantly associated with higher rates of death from cancer of the esophagus, colon and rectum, liver, gallbladder, pancreas, and kidney. On the basis of associations observed in this study, the authors estimated that current patterns of overweight and obesity in the United States could account for 14% of all deaths from cancer in men and 20% of those in women. Other studies confirmed the association between obesity and the increase in the risk of cancer. In a Swedish population-based cohort of 28,129 hospital patients, Wolk and colleagues[48] reported a 33% increase in the incidence of cancer in obese persons compared with nonobese persons. In a Danish cohort of 43,965 obese persons, Moller and colleagues[49] observed increased incidences of liver cancer (58 cases; relative risk, 1.9) compared with the general population. In a prospective study of 771 French patients with well-compensated alcoholic and hepatitis C–related cirrhosis, BMI was found to have a positive linear relationship with incidence of HCC over the follow-up period of up to 7 years. In this study, BMI between 25 and 30 kg/m^2 was associated with a hazard ratio of 2, whereas BMI of 30 kg/m^2 or greater was associated with a hazard ratio of 2.8.[50]

An association between HCC and diabetes has been reported as early as 1986.[51,52] El-Serag and colleagues,[53] in a study that included 823 patients, found an increase in the risk of HCC in diabetics. In a large prospective study, investigators found that patients with diabetes were more than twice as likely as controls to have chronic nonalcoholic liver disease or HCC.[54] A large population-based study, which used the SEER database, showed a 2.87 odds ratio of HCC among older patients with DM without other risk factors for chronic liver disease.[55] Diabetes was also found to be an independent risk factor for HCC in the setting of cryptogenic cirrhosis.[16] The association between HCC and diabetes was confirmed in many other studies.[14,16,56,57] A systematic review and meta analysis of the studies published between 1966 and 2005 also found a significant association of diabetes and HCC in 9 of 13 case-controlled studies (pooled odds ratio, 2.5) and 7 of 13 cohort studies (pooled odds ratio, 2.5).[55]

The association between HCC and metabolic syndrome is more difficult to assess because of the lack of uniform diagnostic criteria for the metabolic syndrome. The most widely used criteria for diagnosis are those set by the US National Cholesterol Education Program Adult Treatment Panel III (NCEP ATP III) (**Table 2**).[58]

Table 2
National Cholesterol Education Program Adult Treatment Panel III definition for metabolic syndrome (2001)

	Three or More of the Following Risk Factors
Fasting plasma glucose	≥5.6 mmol/L (100 mg/dL)
Blood pressure	≥130/≥85 mm Hg
Triglycerides	≥1.7 mmol/L (150 mg/dL)
High-density lipoprotein cholesterol	Men: <1.03 mmol/L (40 mg/dL) Women: <1.29 mmol/L (50 mg/dL)
Obesity	Men: waist circumference >102 cm Women: waist circumference >88 cm

Data from Expert Panel on Detection, Evaluation, and Treatment of High Blood Cholesterol in Adults. Treatment of high blood cholesterol in, executive summary of the third report of The National Cholesterol Education Program (NCEP) expert panel on detection, evaluation, and treatment of high blood cholesterol in adults (Adult Treatment Panel III). JAMA 2001:285(19);2486–97.

In a population-based study, using the SEER-Medicare database, Welzel and colleagues[59] identified 3649 HCC cases. Metabolic syndrome, defined by the NCEP ATP III, was significantly more common among persons who had HCC (37.1%) than the comparison group (17.1%; $P<.0001$). In an adjusted multiple logistic regression analysis, metabolic syndrome remained significantly associated with increased risk of HCC (odds ratio, 2.13; confidence interval, 1.96–2.31; $P<.0001$).[59] More recently, Perumpail and colleagues[26] published a case series of 6 patients who had HCC in the absence of cirrhosis, HBV, or HCV infection. All 6 patients had at least 2 or more features of metabolic syndrome; all 6 had hypertension, all 6 had either type 2 diabetes or evidence of insulin resistance, and 5 had dyslipidemia.

MECHANISM OF HEPATOCELLULAR CARCINOMA IN THE SETTING OF NONALCOHOLIC FATTY LIVER DISEASE/NONALCOHOLIC STEATOHEPATITIS

The mechanism of HCC arising in the setting of cirrhosis has been extensively studied. It is generally characterized by cycles of hepatocellular death and compensatory regeneration, accompanied by constant cell growth and proliferation that favor tumor development.[16] The mechanisms of HCC in the setting of NAFLD, in the absence of cirrhosis, are less well understood. These mechanisms involve 3 groups of factors: proinflammatory cytokines, diet and gut microbiomes, and genetic factors.

Proinflammatory Cytokines

Insulin resistance, in the setting of obesity, is characterized by low-grade inflammation that is associated with macrophage activation with release of proinflammatory cytokines including tumor necrosis factor alpha (TNF-α) and interleukin 6 (IL-6).[60] TNF-α interacts with the nuclear factor kappa-B kinase beta subunit (NF-κB) to promote apoptosis, inflammation, proliferation, and angiogenesis.[61] IL-6 activates the signal transducer and activator of transcription 3 (STAT3), which promotes cell growth and differentiation. STAT3 is also involved in other tumor pathogenesis.[62]

Diet and Gut Microbiome

A diet with high fat content increases the expression of TNF-α and IL-6 and activates NF-κB. All are involved in angiogenesis and cell differentiation.[63] Fructose stimulates hepatic lipogenesis, which amplifies lipotoxic injury. Lipogenesis downregulates the expression of sirtuin-1, which is involved in the regulation of cellular survival.[64] Obesity is associated with changes in composition of the gut microbiota, which produces reactive oxygen species leading to DNA damage and release of senescence-associated secretory phenotype from hepatic stellate cells.[65]

Genetic Factors

Romeo and colleagues[66] described a single-nucleotide polymorphism in the patatin-like phospholipase domain–containing 3 (PNPLA3) gene, which encodes the triglycerides lipase adiponutrin. The PNPLA3 rs738409 [G] risk allele increases the risk of HCC development by 12-fold. Further, GG homozygosity is associated with the development of HCC in younger age, and more diffuse nature at the diagnosis.[67]

SURVEILLANCE FOR HEPATOCELLULAR CARCINOMA IN THE SETTING OF NONALCOHOLIC FATTY LIVER DISEASE/NONALCOHOLIC STEATOHEPATITIS

US and European societies recommend regular surveillance for HCC in patients with cirrhosis every 6 months.[68,69] Ultrasound scan is the recommended method of surveillance.[68–70] There are data suggesting that HCC surveillance in cirrhotic patients in general is inadequate[71] but much less used in patients with cirrhosis secondary to NASH.[72] A retrospective analysis of a cohort with 1500 HCC patients from Veterans Administration hospitals found that patients with NAFLD HCC underwent less frequent surveillance (43.3%) in the 3 years before HCC diagnosis than patients with alcohol-(59.8%) or HCV-induced (86.7%) HCC.[73] The basis for the lower frequency of screening among patients with NAFLD cirrhosis is not clear. The lower US screening rate is compounded by the higher technical failure rate of US examinations of the liver in patients with BMI greater than 25 kg/m^2. The fact that HCC can develop in the absence of cirrhosis adds uncertainty to who should undergo surveillance. Another challenge of surveillance in patients with NASH is that obesity can reduce the sensitivity of ultrasound examination. An Italian study found that a BMI greater than 25 was significantly associated with ultrasound surveillance failure.[74] Computed tomography scans or MRIs are more accurate in this setting, but they may not be cost effective or appropriate for initial surveillance.[75] A recent study suggested that alpha-fetoprotein has a better sensitivity and specificity in NAFLD cirrhosis patients than in HCV cirrhosis patients with a sensitivity of 89.7% and a specificity of 85.1% at a cutoff value of 20 ng/mL in NAFLD patients.[76] Whether noncirrhotic NAFLD/NASH patients should be screened for HCC and the best method for screening are still to be determined.

PREVENTION

Metformin may have antineoplastic effects through both insulin-dependent and insulin-independent mechanisms.[77] A meta-analysis including 22,650 cases of HCC in 334,307 patients with type 2 diabetes concluded that incidence of HCC was reduced by 50% with metformin use, increased with sulfonylurea or insulin, and unchanged with glitazones.[78] Statins may also decrease the risk of cancers through antiproliferative, proapoptotic, anti-angiogenic, and immunomodulatory effects.[17] A systematic meta-analysis of 26 randomized controlled trials, including almost 1.5 million patients and 4298 cases of HCC, found that the use of statins was associated with a 37% reduction in HCC incidence after adjusting for potential confounders.[79] It is conceivable that controlling risk factors for metabolic syndrome would decrease the risk of HCC. The role of bariatric surgery in reducing the risk of HCC is to be determined.

SUMMARY

The progressive increase in the prevalence of NAFLD and NASH are likely to make NAFLD/NASH the most common predisposing factor of HCC in the upcoming decades. The frequency of NAFLD/NASH-related HCC in the absence of cirrhosis is unclear. Screening and surveillance for HCC should, for now, be limited to patients thought to have cirrhosis. Obesity can make screening for HCC in patients with NASH cirrhosis challenging, increasing the technical failure rate of ultrasound scan as a screening method. The delay in the diagnosis of HCC in the setting of NAFLD/NASH and the presence of multiple comorbidities in this population negatively impacts prognosis. A better understanding of the mechanisms involved in the development of NAFLD/NASH-related HCC will allow the discovery of new targets for therapeutic and preventive intervention.

REFERENCES

1. Altekruse SF, McGlynn KA, Reichman ME. Hepatocellular carcinoma incidence, mortality, and survival trends in the United States from 1975 to 2005. J Clin Oncol 2009;27(9):1485–91.
2. El-Serag HB, Rudolph KL. Hepatocellular carcinoma: epidemiology and molecular carcinogenesis. Gastroenterology 2007;132(7):2557–76.
3. Rinella M, Charlton M. The globalization of non-alcoholic fatty liver disease - prevalence and impact on World Health. Hepatology 2016;64(1):19–22.
4. Davila JA, Morgan RO, Shaib Y, et al. Hepatitis C infection and the increasing incidence of hepatocellular carcinoma: a population-based study. Gastroenterology 2004;127(5):1372–80.
5. El-Serag HB, Mason AC. Risk factors for the rising rates of primary liver cancer in the United States. Arch Intern Med 2000;160(21):3227–30.
6. Hassan MM, Frome A, Patt YZ, et al. Rising prevalence of hepatitis C virus infection among patients recently diagnosed with hepatocellular carcinoma in the United States. J Clin Gastroenterol 2002;35(3):266–9.
7. Kulkarni K, Barcak E, El-Serag H, et al. The impact of immigration on the increasing incidence of hepatocellular carcinoma in the United States. Aliment Pharmacol Ther 2004;20(4):445–50.
8. Fattovich G, Stroffolini T, Zagni I, et al. Hepatocellular carcinoma in cirrhosis: incidence and risk factors. Gastroenterology 2004;127(5 Suppl 1):S35–50.
9. Montalto G, Cervello M, Giannitrapani L, et al. Epidemiology, risk factors, and natural history of hepatocellular carcinoma. Ann N Y Acad Sci 2002;963:13–20.
10. Gomaa AI, Khan SA, Toledano MB, et al. Hepatocellular carcinoma: epidemiology, risk factors and pathogenesis. World J Gastroenterol 2008;14(27):4300–8.
11. White DL, Kanwal F, El-Serag HB. Association between nonalcoholic fatty liver disease and risk for hepatocellular cancer, based on systematic review. Clin Gastroenterol Hepatol 2012;10(12):1342–59.e2.
12. Davila JA, Morgan RO, Shaib Y, et al. Diabetes increases the risk of hepatocellular carcinoma in the United States: a population based case control study. Gut 2005;54(4):533–9.
13. Calle EE, Rodriguez C, Walker-Thurmond K, et al. Overweight, obesity, and mortality from cancer in a prospectively studied cohort of U.S. adults. N Engl J Med 2003;348(17):1625–38.
14. Regimbeau JM, Colombat M, Mognol P, et al. Obesity and diabetes as a risk factor for hepatocellular carcinoma. Liver Transpl 2004;10(2 Suppl 1):S69–73.

15. Adams LA, Lymp JF, St Sauver J, et al. The natural history of nonalcoholic fatty liver disease: a population-based cohort study. Gastroenterology 2005;129(1): 113–21.

16. Bugianesi E, Leone N, Vanni E, et al. Expanding the natural history of nonalcoholic steatohepatitis: from cryptogenic cirrhosis to hepatocellular carcinoma. Gastroenterology 2002;123(1):134–40.

17. Marengo A, Rosso C, Bugianesi E. Liver cancer: connections with obesity, fatty liver, and cirrhosis. Annu Rev Med 2016;67:103–17.

18. Bhala N, Angulo P, van der Poorten D, et al. The natural history of nonalcoholic fatty liver disease with advanced fibrosis or cirrhosis: an international collaborative study. Hepatology 2011;54(4):1208–16.

19. Dyson J, Jaques B, Chattopadyhay D, et al. Hepatocellular cancer: the impact of obesity, type 2 diabetes and a multidisciplinary team. J Hepatol 2014;60(1): 110–7.

20. Ascha MS, Hanouneh IA, Lopez R, et al. The incidence and risk factors of hepatocellular carcinoma in patients with nonalcoholic steatohepatitis. Hepatology 2010;51(6):1972–8.

21. Wong RJ, Aguilar M, Cheung R, et al. Nonalcoholic steatohepatitis is the second leading etiology of liver disease among adults awaiting liver transplantation in the United States. Gastroenterology 2015;148(3):547–55.

22. Wong RJ, Cheung R, Ahmed A. Nonalcoholic steatohepatitis is the most rapidly growing indication for liver transplantation in patients with hepatocellular carcinoma in the U.S. Hepatology 2014;59(6):2188–95.

23. Starley BQ, Calcagno CJ, Harrison SA. Nonalcoholic fatty liver disease and hepatocellular carcinoma: a weighty connection. Hepatology 2010;51(5):1820–32.

24. Ong J, Younossi ZM, Reddy V, et al. Cryptogenic cirrhosis and posttransplantation nonalcoholic fatty liver disease. Liver Transpl 2001;7(9):797–801.

25. Khan FZ, Perumpail RB, Wong RJ, et al. Advances in hepatocellular carcinoma: nonalcoholic steatohepatitis-related hepatocellular carcinoma. World J Hepatol 2015;7(18):2155–61.

26. Perumpail RB, Wong RJ, Ahmed A, et al. Hepatocellular carcinoma in the setting of non-cirrhotic nonalcoholic fatty liver disease and the metabolic syndrome: US experience. Dig Dis Sci 2015;60(10):3142–8.

27. Williams CD, Stengel J, Asike MI, et al. Prevalence of nonalcoholic fatty liver disease and nonalcoholic steatohepatitis among a largely middle-aged population utilizing ultrasound and liver biopsy: a prospective study. Gastroenterology 2011;140(1):124–31.

28. Rinella ME. Nonalcoholic fatty liver disease: a systematic review. JAMA 2015; 313(22):2263–73.

29. Chalasani N, Younossi Z, Lavine JE, et al. The diagnosis and management of non-alcoholic fatty liver disease: practice guideline by the American Association for the Study of Liver Diseases, American College of Gastroenterology, and the American Gastroenterological Association. Hepatology 2012;55(6):2005–23.

30. Benchequroun R, Duvoux C, Luciani A, et al. Hepatocellular carcinoma without cirrhosis in a patient with nonalcoholic steatohepatitis. Gastroenterol Clin Biol 2004;28(5):497–9 [in French].

31. Bullock RE, Zaitoun AM, Aithal GP, et al. Association of non-alcoholic steatohepatitis without significant fibrosis with hepatocellular carcinoma. J Hepatol 2004; 41(4):685–6.

32. Gonzalez L, Blanc JF, Sa Cunha A, et al. Obesity as a risk factor for hepatocellular carcinoma in a noncirrhotic patient. Semin Liver Dis 2004;24(4):415–9.

33. Cuadrado A, Orive A, García-Suárez C, et al. Non-alcoholic steatohepatitis (NASH) and hepatocellular carcinoma. Obes Surg 2005;15(3):442–6.

34. Hai S, Kubo S, Shuto T, et al. Hepatocellular carcinoma arising from nonalcoholic steatohepatitis: report of two cases. Surg Today 2006;36(4):390–4.

35. Ichikawa T, Yanagi K, Motoyoshi Y, et al. Two cases of non-alcoholic steatohepatitis with development of hepatocellular carcinoma without cirrhosis. J Gastroenterol Hepatol 2006;21(12):1865–6.

36. Hashizume H, Sato K, Takagi H, et al. Primary liver cancers with nonalcoholic steatohepatitis. Eur J Gastroenterol Hepatol 2007;19(10):827–34.

37. Guzman G, Brunt EM, Petrovic LM, et al. Does nonalcoholic fatty liver disease predispose patients to hepatocellular carcinoma in the absence of cirrhosis? Arch Pathol Lab Med 2008;132(11):1761–6.

38. Paradis V, Zalinski S, Chelbi E, et al. Hepatocellular carcinomas in patients with metabolic syndrome often develop without significant liver fibrosis: a pathological analysis. Hepatology 2009;49(3):851–9.

39. Kawada N, Imanaka K, Kawaguchi T, et al. Hepatocellular carcinoma arising from non-cirrhotic nonalcoholic steatohepatitis. J Gastroenterol 2009;44(12):1190–4.

40. Chagas AL, Kikuchi LO, Oliveira CP, et al. Does hepatocellular carcinoma in non-alcoholic steatohepatitis exist in cirrhotic and non-cirrhotic patients? Braz J Med Biol Res 2009;42(10):958–62.

41. Takuma Y, Nouso K. Nonalcoholic steatohepatitis-associated hepatocellular carcinoma: our case series and literature review. World J Gastroenterol 2010; 16(12):1436–41.

42. Ikura Y, Mita E, Nakamori S. Hepatocellular carcinomas can develop in simple fatty livers in the setting of oxidative stress. Pathology 2011;43(2):167–8.

43. Yasui K, Hashimoto E, Komorizono Y, et al. Characteristics of patients with nonalcoholic steatohepatitis who develop hepatocellular carcinoma. Clin Gastroenterol Hepatol 2011;9(5):428–33 [quiz: e50].

44. Flegal KM, Carroll MD, Ogden CL, et al. Prevalence and trends in obesity among US adults, 1999-2008. JAMA 2010;303(3):235–41.

45. Torres DM, Williams CD, Harrison SA. Features, diagnosis, and treatment of nonalcoholic fatty liver disease. Clin Gastroenterol Hepatol 2012;10(8):837–58.

46. Ford ES, Giles WH, Mokdad AH. Increasing prevalence of the metabolic syndrome among U.S. Adults Diabetes Care 2004;27(10):2444–9.

47. Alberti KG, Zimmet P, Shaw J. Metabolic syndrome–a new world-wide definition. A Consensus statement from the International Diabetes Federation. Diabet Med 2006;23(5):469–80.

48. Wolk A, Gridley G, Svensson M, et al. A prospective study of obesity and cancer risk (Sweden). Cancer Causes Control 2001;12(1):13–21.

49. Moller H, Mellemgaard A, Lindvig K, et al. Obesity and cancer risk: a Danish record-linkage study. Eur J Cancer 1994;30A(3):344–50.

50. N'Kontchou G, Paries J, Htar MT, et al. Risk factors for hepatocellular carcinoma in patients with alcoholic or viral C cirrhosis. Clin Gastroenterol Hepatol 2006;4(8): 1062–8.

51. Lawson DH, Gray JM, McKillop C, et al. Diabetes mellitus and primary hepatocellular carcinoma. Q J Med 1986;61(234):945–55.

52. Adami HO, Chow WH, Nyrén O, et al. Excess risk of primary liver cancer in patients with diabetes mellitus. J Natl Cancer Inst 1996;88(20):1472–7.

53. El-Serag HB, Richardson PA, Everhart JE. The role of diabetes in hepatocellular carcinoma: a case-control study among United States Veterans. Am J Gastroenterol 2001;96(8):2462–7.

54. El-Serag HB, Tran T, Everhart JE. Diabetes increases the risk of chronic liver disease and hepatocellular carcinoma. Gastroenterology 2004;126(2):460–8.

55. El-Serag HB, Hampel H, Javadi F. The association between diabetes and hepatocellular carcinoma: a systematic review of epidemiologic evidence. Clin Gastroenterol Hepatol 2006;4(3):369–80.

56. Caldwell SH, Oelsner DH, Iezzoni JC, et al. Cryptogenic cirrhosis: clinical characterization and risk factors for underlying disease. Hepatology 1999;29(3):664–9.

57. Poonawala A, Nair SP, Thuluvath PJ. Prevalence of obesity and diabetes in patients with cryptogenic cirrhosis: a case-control study. Hepatology 2000;32(4 Pt 1):689–92.

58. Expert Panel on Detection, Evaluation, and Treatment of High Blood Cholesterol in Adults. Treatment of high blood cholesterol in, executive summary of the third report of The National Cholesterol Education Program (NCEP) Expert Panel on Detection, Evaluation, And Treatment of High Blood Cholesterol In Adults (Adult Treatment Panel III). JAMA 2001;285(19):2486–97.

59. Welzel TM, Graubard BI, Zeuzem S, et al. Metabolic syndrome increases the risk of primary liver cancer in the United States: a study in the SEER-Medicare database. Hepatology 2011;54(2):463–71.

60. Shoelson SE, Herrero L, Naaz A. Obesity, inflammation, and insulin resistance. Gastroenterology 2007;132(6):2169–80.

61. Hirosumi J, Tuncman G, Chang L, et al. A central role for JNK in obesity and insulin resistance. Nature 2002;420(6913):333–6.

62. Hodge DR, Hurt EM, Farrar WL. The role of IL-6 and STAT3 in inflammation and cancer. Eur J Cancer 2005;41(16):2502–12.

63. Vanni E, Bugianesi E. Obesity and liver cancer. Clin Liver Dis 2014;18(1):191–203.

64. Donnelly KL, Smith CI, Schwarzenberg SJ, et al. Sources of fatty acids stored in liver and secreted via lipoproteins in patients with nonalcoholic fatty liver disease. J Clin Invest 2005;115(5):1343–51.

65. Dongiovanni P, Romeo S, Valenti L. Hepatocellular carcinoma in nonalcoholic fatty liver: role of environmental and genetic factors. World J Gastroenterol 2014;20(36):12945–55.

66. Romeo S, Kozlitina J, Xing C, et al. Genetic variation in PNPLA3 confers susceptibility to nonalcoholic fatty liver disease. Nat Genet 2008;40(12):1461–5.

67. Krawczyk M, Stokes CS, Romeo S, et al. HCC and liver disease risks in homozygous PNPLA3 p.I148M carriers approach monogenic inheritance. J Hepatol 2015;62(4):980–1.

68. Bruix J, Sherman M, American Association for the Study of Liver Diseases. Management of hepatocellular carcinoma: an update. Hepatology 2011;53(3):1020–2.

69. Bruix J, Sherman M, Llovet JM, et al. Clinical management of hepatocellular carcinoma. Conclusions of the Barcelona-2000 EASL conference. European Association for the Study of the Liver. J Hepatol 2001;35(3):421–30.

70. Forner A, Reig M, Bruix J. Alpha-fetoprotein for hepatocellular carcinoma diagnosis: the demise of a brilliant star. Gastroenterology 2009;137(1):26–9.

71. Davila JA, Morgan RO, Richardson PA, et al. Use of surveillance for hepatocellular carcinoma among patients with cirrhosis in the United States. Hepatology 2010;52(1):132–41.

72. Mittal S, Sada YH, El-Serag HB, et al. Temporal trends of nonalcoholic fatty liver disease-related hepatocellular carcinoma in the veteran affairs population. Clin Gastroenterol Hepatol 2015;13(3):594–601.e1.

73. Younossi ZM, Otgonsuren M, Henry L, et al. Association of nonalcoholic fatty liver disease (NAFLD) with hepatocellular carcinoma (HCC) in the United States from 2004 to 2009. Hepatology 2015;62(6):1723–30.
74. Del Poggio P, Olmi S, Ciccarese F, et al. Factors that affect efficacy of ultrasound surveillance for early stage hepatocellular carcinoma in patients with cirhhosis. Clin Gastroenterol Hepatol 2014;12:1927e2–33e2.
75. Thompson Coon J, Rogers G, Hewson P, et al. Surveillance of cirrhosis for hepatocellular carcinoma: a cost-utility analysis. Br J Cancer 2008;98(7):1166–75.
76. Gopal P, Yopp AC, Waljee AK, et al. Factors that affect accuracy of alphafetoprotein test in detection of hepatocellular carcinoma in patients with cirrhosis. Clin Gastroenterol Hepatol 2014;12(5):870–7.
77. Chen HP, Shieh JJ, Chang CC, et al. Metformin decreases hepatocellular carcinoma risk in a dose-dependent manner: population-based and in vitro studies. Gut 2013;62(4):606–15.
78. Zhang H, Gao C, Fang L, et al. Metformin and reduced risk of hepatocellular carcinoma in diabetic patients: a meta-analysis. Scand J Gastroenterol 2013;48(1):78–87.
79. Singh S, Singh PP, Singh AG, et al. Statins are associated with a reduced risk of hepatocellular cancer: a systematic review and meta-analysis. Gastroenterology 2013;144(2):323–32.

Nonalcoholic Fatty Liver Disease/Nonalcoholic Steatohepatitis in Liver Transplantation

Danielle Carter, MD*, Douglas T. Dieterich, MD,
Charissa Chang, MD

KEYWORDS

- Nonalcoholic steatohepatitis • Nonalcoholic fatty liver disease • Liver transplant
- Metabolic syndrome • Recurrent NAFLD

KEY POINTS

- Nonalcoholic fatty liver disease (NAFLD)/nonalcoholic steatohepatitis (NASH) is emerging as one of the leading causes of liver transplant in the United States.
- Given the association of NAFLD with metabolic syndrome, patients are often older, obese, and have more cardiac risk factors than other transplant candidates.
- Patients transplanted for NASH have excellent long-term patient and graft survival but they are at risk for increased early mortality caused by cardiac disease.
- Posttransplant metabolic syndrome increases risk for recurrent NAFLD and NASH but with rare progression to cirrhosis or graft failure.

INTRODUCTION

Liver transplant is a resource-intensive procedure reserved for patients with severe acute or chronic liver disease. According to Organ Procurement and Transplantation Network (OPTN) data, 7841 liver transplants were performed in the United States in 2016. Proper selection of transplant candidates and advances in immunosuppressive therapy have resulted in 5-year survival rates of 75% and 84% for recipients of deceased and living donors, respectively.[1] Chronic hepatitis C virus (HCV) is the most common cause of hepatic decompensation leading to hepatocellular carcinoma (HCC) and transplant. In recent years, nonalcoholic fatty liver disease

Disclosure: Dr C. Chang is a consultant for Gilead Sciences. Drs D. Carter and D.T. Dieterich have nothing to disclose.
Division of Liver Diseases, Icahn School of Medicine at Mount Sinai, 17 East 102nd Street, 2nd Floor, New York, NY 10029, USA
* Corresponding author.
E-mail address: dcarter93@gmail.com

(NAFLD)/nonalcoholic steatohepatitis (NASH) has emerged as a major cause of chronic liver disease fueled in part by the increase in obesity and metabolic syndrome. By 2025 it is estimated that 25million Americans will have NASH,[2] of whom 20% are expected to develop cirrhosis or HCC.[3] Because direct-acting antivirals are curing more patients with HCV, it is expected that NASH will increase to become the leading indication for liver transplant.[4] NAFLD/NASH is frequently described as the hepatic manifestation of metabolic syndrome. As a result, patients with NASH carry a distinct set of comorbidities and risk factors that deserve special attention in the pretransplant and posttransplant settings.

In 2001, United Network for Organ Sharing (UNOS) began including NASH among the list of primary diagnoses for liver transplant registrants. Since that time the number of patients undergoing liver transplant for NASH increased from 1.2% of recipients in 2001 to 9.7% in 2009. NASH is currently the third most common indication for liver transplant in the United States.[5] This ranking includes patients transplanted for cirrhotic decompensation and HCC. Although the risk of HCC in patients with NASH cirrhosis is lower than with other causes, it has become a growing indication for liver transplant listing. In 2012, NASH cirrhosis accounted for 13.5% of HCC-related transplants, which represented a 4-fold increase from 2002. Although HCV remains the leading cause of HCC-related transplants (HCV comprises 50% of HCC cases listed for transplant), by comparison there was only a 2.25-fold increase during the same time frame.[6] Part of the increase in liver transplants for NASH can be attributed to more accurate diagnosis of patients previously labeled as cryptogenic cirrhosis. Given that histologic features of steatosis may disappear in end-stage NASH, patients with clinical features of metabolic syndrome and pathologic findings of cryptogenic cirrhosis are recognized as having underlying NASH.[6,7]

A more up-to-date prevalence of patients with end-stage NASH is reflected in the numbers of patients added to the transplant wait-list. In 2015 there were 10,630 candidates added to the wait-list, with a median wait time of 11 months.[1] NASH is the second leading cause of liver disease among patients newly added to the transplant list. Between 2004 and 2013 the number of new registrants with NASH increased by 170% compared with a 14% increase in HCV and 45% for patients with alcoholic liver disease (ALD)[8] (Fig. 1). Although the number of wait-list registrants with NASH is rapidly increasing, not all of these patients proceed to transplant. O'Leary

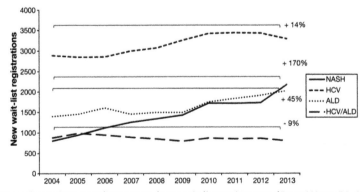

Fig. 1. Annual trends in new liver transplant wait-list registrants. (*From* Wong RJ, Aguilar M, Cheung R, et al. Nonalcoholic steatohepatitis is the second leading etiology of liver disease among adults awaiting liver transplantation in the United States. Gastroenterology 2015;148(3):547–55; with permission.)

and colleagues[9] found that, especially among patients listed with Model for End-Stage Liver Disease (MELD) score less than 15, patients with NASH were less likely to receive a transplant than patients with HCV. Patients with NASH had a slower progression of disease, increasing only 1.3 MELD points per year compared with 3.2 points in patients with HCV. As a result, patients with NASH were more likely to die or be delisted (likely because of progression of their comorbidities) while awaiting transplant. Even when adjusted for MELD score, patients with HCV and ALD were more likely than patients with NASH to receive a transplant off the wait-list at 90 days and 1 year.[8]

PRETRANSPLANT CONSIDERATIONS

Patients evaluated for liver transplant undergo extensive medical, surgical, and psychosocial assessments to identify factors that may hinder a successful outcome. Patients with severe chronic medical conditions that confer an unacceptably high perioperative risk or who are unlikely to achieve long-term benefit are excluded from transplant. Compared with recipients for other causes, patients with NASH are more likely to be female, older, and obese with higher average body mass indices (BMIs). They have higher rates of diabetes, dyslipidemia, hypertension, and cardiac disease.[5,6,8,10–12] Many of these features are independently associated with increased perioperative risk and long-term complications. Pretransplant assessment of patients with NASH should focus on how best to optimize these conditions when possible.

Obesity

Obesity (defined as BMI >30 kg/m^2) is present among approximately 20% to 30% of liver transplant candidates.[13,14] In the perioperative setting, obesity has been associated with increased risk of complications, including poor wound healing, infection, deep vein thrombus, and pulmonary and cardiac disease.[15,16] Guidelines from the American Association for the Study of Liver Diseases (AASLD) have listed BMI greater than 40 kg/m^2 as a relative contraindication for liver transplant and suggest pretransplant dietary counseling for all patients with BMI greater than 30 kg/m^2.[17] Earlier research on the effects of BMI and obesity using the UNOS database found that morbid obesity (BMI >40 kg/m^2) was an independent predictor of mortality following liver transplant. Morbidly obese patients had higher 30-day, 1-year, and 5-year mortalities, whereas severely obese patients (BMI, 35–39 kg/m^2) only had significantly higher 5-year mortality.[18] However, more recent studies have shown that BMI alone does not worsen posttransplant outcomes (**Table 1**).

In a retrospective study of obese patients undergoing liver transplant using the National Institute of Diabetes and Digestive and Kidney Diseases (NIDDK) liver transplant database, BMI was not a predictor of graft survival or overall survival once correction for ascites was taken into account. Correction of BMI for ascites led to reclassification of patients into a lower BMI category; there were no differences in early or late complications based on corrected BMI.[13] A more recent meta-analysis of pooled data from 13 studies also found that there was no difference in long-term survival between obese and nonobese patients but did observe decreased survival rates among obese patients in short-term follow-up of less than 5 years.[19] Even among the morbidly obese (BMI >40 kg/m^2), long-term survival over a median of 2 years was equivalent to that of obese patients with lower BMI. Obese patients are at greater risk for immediate surgical-related complications, including wound infections requiring reoperation, intra-abdominal infections, venous thrombosis, and biliary complications.[16] As a result, they have a longer overall length of stay with decreased likelihood of being

Table 1
Effects of body mass index on posttransplant outcomes

Source	Size	Study Design	Conclusions
Nair et al,[18] 2002	N = 18,172	Retrospective analysis of UNOS database 3877 (21.3%) with BMI >30	22% 1-y mortality in morbidly obese (BMI >40) vs 16% in normal-weight patients. Higher mortality in morbidly obese group at all time points. Severely obese and morbidly obese had higher 5-y mortality
Pelletier et al,[14] 2007	N = 4488	Retrospective analysis of SRTR data 1498 (33%) with BMI >30	Posttransplant mortality HR: class I obese, 0.84 (0.68–1.03) vs class II, 1.04 (0.80–1.34) vs class III, 1.16 (0.80–1.68). No difference in mortality among patients with higher BMI compared with normal-weight transplant recipients
Leonard et al,[13] 2008	N = 1313	Prospective, multicenter 280 (21.3%) with BMI >30	11% 1-y mortality in normal weight vs 10% in class II obese. No difference in mortality or graft survival
LaMattina et al,[16] 2012	N = 813	Single-center, retrospective review 306 (38%) with BMI >30	94% 1-y survival in normal weight vs 91% in class II obese. Class II obese patients had lower survival than normal-weight patients. No difference seen in class I or class III obese. BMI class was not independent predictor of patient or graft survival
Singhal et al,[20] 2015	N = 12,445	Retrospective analysis of SRTR BMI >40 (316) vs BMI <40 (12,029)	Perioperative mortality 4.1% for BMI <40 vs 4.8% for patients with BMI >40 kg/m². No difference in perioperative mortality or long-term survival

Obesity classes (BMI in kg/m²): I, 30.0–34.9; II, 35.0–39.9; III, greater than or equal to 40.
Abbreviations: HR, hazard ratio; SRTR, Scientific Registry of Transplant Recipients.

discharged home. However, despite these potential setbacks, their mortality decreases after undergoing transplant as opposed to remaining on the wait-list.[14,20]

Although the evidence suggests that obesity alone should not be prohibitive to transplant, many programs aim to optimize the BMIs of recipients to promote the best outcomes. Bariatric surgery has long been proved to be an effective weight loss strategy that also reduces obesity-related complications and can improve liver histology for patients with NAFLD.[21,22] In properly selected patients, bariatric surgery can be used to improve eligibility and posttransplant outcomes. Patients with early-stage liver disease can undergo bariatric surgery without significant increased risk of complications,[23] but the procedure may be too risky in patients with more advanced disease. In a retrospective analysis of nationwide data, patients with decompensated cirrhosis undergoing bariatric surgery had a 20-fold higher mortality than patients without cirrhosis. When the procedure was performed at low-volume bariatric centers (<50 procedures per year) patients with decompensated cirrhosis had a 41% mortality, whereas no deaths were recorded at high-volume centers (>100 procedures per year).[24] More recent smaller prospective studies at academic tertiary care centers have shown favorable outcomes for patients undergoing bariatric surgery in the pretransplant and peritransplant settings. Both Roux-en-Y gastric bypass and sleeve gastrectomy are effective weight loss procedures for patients with liver disease,[25] but, for transplant candidates, sleeve gastrectomy is often the preferred operative procedure. It is less technically challenging, has a shorter average operative time than gastric bypass, and preserves endoscopic access to the upper gastrointestinal and biliary tracts. Sleeve gastrectomy also avoids potential vitamin deficiency and malabsorption complications that come with bypass surgery. A pilot trial at the University of California, San Francisco, performed sleeve gastrectomy in liver and kidney transplant candidates who would otherwise have been excluded from the procedure because of increased BMI ($\geq$40 kg/m^2). Patients presented for laparoscopic sleeve gastrectomy with an average BMI of 48.3 kg/m^2 and average MELD score of 11. Complications following sleeve gastrectomy included superficial wound infection, encephalopathy, and transient renal insufficiency. One patient had a staple line leak that was further complicated by development of chronic fistula. He died 4 years later. Of the 20 patients with end-stage liver disease who underwent sleeve gastrectomy, 6 proceeded to successful transplant after an average of 16.6 months. At the time of transplant the average BMI improved to 31.4 kg/m^2 and patients continued to show weight loss over the first postoperative year. Among those with diabetes, 61% saw improvement in glucose control following bariatric surgery.[26]

Simultaneous sleeve gastrectomy at the time of liver transplant potentially reduces surgical risks and the technical challenges of undergoing 2 separate procedures. In a single-institution program, liver transplant candidates with BMI greater than 35 kg/m^2 were enrolled in an aggressive noninvasive weight management program. Seven patients who were unable to achieve target BMI underwent combined liver transplant with sleeve gastrectomy. The group had an average MELD score of 32 with most having a primary or secondary diagnosis of NASH. Following liver transplant, these patients had sustained weight loss reaching an average BMI of 29 kg/m^2 at follow-up. One patient had early graft dysfunction and gastric staple line leak that required a prolonged hospitalization; however, there were no postoperative deaths or need for retransplant. None of the patients developed diabetes or had evidence of steatosis on ultrasonography. In contrast, those who achieved the target pretransplant weight on a noninvasive protocol had higher rates of posttransplant diabetes and steatosis, with 60% patients having BMI greater than 35 kg/m^2.[27]

Cardiovascular Disease

Cardiovascular disease is a leading cause of posttransplant mortality, responsible for up to 42% of non–graft-related deaths.[28] NAFLD is recognized as an independent predictor of cardiovascular disease[29,30] and is associated with pathologic changes such as increased intima media thickness and plaque,[31] endothelial dysfunction,[32] coronary artery calcifications,[33] and ventricular dysfunction.[34,35] Although the link between NAFLD and cardiovascular disease exists independently of metabolic syndrome, many of the baseline characteristics seen in patients with NASH overlap with traditional cardiac risk factors (**Table 2**). Preoperative cardiac assessment of patients with NASH is crucial to identify high-risk candidates who require medical optimization or may have severe disease prohibitive to listing. All patients should undergo noninvasive pharmacologic stress testing because most would not be able to tolerate exercise testing. Dobutamine stress echocardiography is often preferred because of its negative predictive value in being able to identify low-risk candidates who can safely proceed to transplant surgery. Coronary angiography is recommended for those with equivocal or positive results on noninvasive testing as well as patients with a high pretest probability of cardiac disease based on medical history.[36,37] Revascularization procedures should be considered in patients with significant stenosis detected on angiography, although there are no clear guidelines for these interventions in the end-stage liver disease population. A small cohort study has shown that percutaneous coronary intervention with bare metal stenting can be both safe and effective in the pretransplant population. There were no bleeding complications even while receiving dual antiplatelet therapy and all patients were cleared for transplant 1 month after their procedures.[38] Bare metal stents require a shortened course of antiplatelet therapy compared with drug-eluting stents and may be a better choice in this population. For lesions not amenable to percutaneous intervention, surgical revascularization may be indicated. Patients who require surgical revascularization to treat coronary artery disease are often at prohibitively high risk for operative interventions because of underlying cirrhosis and are therefore usually excluded from transplant.

Diabetes

The percentage of patients with NASH with a pretransplant diagnosis of diabetes ranges from 40% to 70%.[8,10,12,39–41] Diabetic patients have higher posttransplant mortality, longer in-hospital length of stay, higher 30-day readmission rates, and lower 5-year survival (67% vs 75%) compared with nondiabetics.[42] When stratified by insulin dependence and non–insulin dependence, only patients requiring insulin have significantly lower survival rates and are 40% more likely to die within 5 years of transplant than nondiabetics.[43] The presence of pretransplant diabetes also serves as an independent risk factor for increased cardiovascular mortality and decreased patient

Table 2	
Factors to consider in assessing risk for cardiac disease	
Traditional Cardiovascular Risk Factors	**Coronary Heart Disease Risk Equivalents[a]**
Age	Clinical coronary heart disease
Sex	Symptomatic carotid artery disease
Total cholesterol	Peripheral arterial disease
HDL cholesterol	Abdominal aortic aneurysm
Systolic blood pressure	Diabetes mellitus
Use of antihypertensive medications	Chronic kidney disease
Current tobacco use	
Diabetes mellitus	

[a] Risk for major coronary event equal to that of established coronary heart disease (>20% per 10 years).

Data from Refs.[84–86]

survival.[44] The combination of coronary artery disease and diabetes imparts a greater mortality risk than either factor alone.[43] There is no evidence to suggest that tightly controlled diabetes results in improved survival rates, although patients with uncontrolled disease and secondary complications are less likely to be discharged home following liver transplant.[42]

Renal Disease

Chronic kidney disease affects approximately 14% of adult Americans and is a major risk factor for development of end-stage renal disease and cardiovascular disease.[45] Features of metabolic syndrome such as type-2 diabetes and hypertension frequently coexist with kidney disease and often serve as underlying causes. NAFLD is associated with increased risk for development of chronic kidney disease in both diabetic and nondiabetic patients.[46] In a meta-analysis, presence of NASH and advanced fibrosis was associated with greater prevalence of chronic kidney disease and a more severe disease stage compared with simple steatosis.[47] Transplant candidates with NASH cirrhosis tend to present with higher serum creatinine levels,[10,48] and a greater percentage of patients require renal replacement therapy compared with HCV and cholestatic causes of liver disease.[49] Pretransplant renal impairment reduces long-term survival rates,[50] especially in patients with NASH, in whom the need for hemodialysis confers a 150% increased mortality risk.[51] Patients with hemodialysis-dependent disease coupled with a BMI greater than 35 kg/m^2 have a 3-year posttransplant survival rate of 40%.[51] NASH has become the most rapidly growing indication for patients undergoing simultaneous liver-kidney transplants, having increased more than 200% in a 10-year period. Between 2002 and 2011, 9.1% of NASH transplants included simultaneous kidney transplants, a proportion that is higher than all other recorded causes.[52] NASH is also an independent risk factor for posttransplant renal dysfunction at both short-term and long-term follow-up.[53] Two years after transplant, 31.2% of patients with NASH developed advanced renal dysfunction (chronic kidney disease stage III) compared with only 8.3% of matched non-NASH controls.[54] Given the high medical costs associated with renal disease and its asymptomatic early stages, transplant candidates with NASH should be evaluated for chronic kidney disease and offered kidney transplants if indicated.

OUTCOMES

Patients undergoing liver transplant for NASH-related cirrhosis or HCC have overall long-term outcomes that are comparable with those of patients being transplanted for other causes, with 1-year and 3-year survival rates of 84% and 78%, respectively.[5] Sepsis and cardiovascular disease are leading causes of non–liver-related posttransplant mortality.[11,12,50,55,56] However, because of their comorbidities, patients with NASH have a higher incidence of postoperative cardiac complications and, as a result, a higher immediate and 30-day mortality.[47,55,57] Within the first year of transplant, approximately 25% of patients with NASH had an adverse cardiac event compared with only 8% of patients with alcoholic cirrhosis. Patients with NASH are susceptible to acute pulmonary edema, new-onset atrial fibrillation, and cardiac arrest independent of traditional cardiac risk factors.[56] Higher immediate mortalities were secondary to increased rates of sudden cardiac arrest, which was the cause of death in 53% of patients with NASH who died within the first 30 days following transplant.[49] Patients with high-risk characteristics of obesity, diabetes mellitus, hypertension, and age greater than 60 years had an immediate mortality of 25% and 1-year mortality of 50%.[11] The metabolic factors promoting cardiac disease persist beyond the immediate postoperative period and patients with NASH are overall more likely to die from cardiac causes than recurrent liver disease or graft failure.[10,49,57,58] In data from the UNOS database, 8.6% of patients with NASH died of graft failure compared with 16.6% of patients with other causes of liver disease.[10]

Metabolic Syndrome and Posttransplant Nonalcoholic Fatty Liver Disease

Posttransplant metabolic syndrome is a common occurrence, affecting up to 50% of liver transplant recipients.[59,60] The prevalence of hypertension increases from between 10% and 15% to between 60% and 70% in the posttransplant period and hyperlipidemia is seen in 50% to 70% of transplanted patients.[59–62] Weight gain is also common, with up to one-third of patients becoming obese.[59–61,63] In one study, average BMI increased from 24.8 kg/m^2 to 28.1 kg/m^2 at 2 years posttransplant.[64] Immunosuppressive medications have long been implicated as a contributing factor in the development of metabolic syndrome[59,65] (see **Table 2**). Corticosteroids are often tapered in the first 3 to 6 months following transplant and therefore have only a transient impact. However, long-term treatment with calcineurin inhibitors is associated with high rates of hypertension, diabetes, and dyslipidemia (mainly hypertriglycerides).[61] Tacrolimus and cyclosporine seem to have equal impacts on the development of metabolic syndrome but mediate different components. Cyclosporine is associated with higher rates of hypertension and hyperlipidemia,[59] whereas the use of tacrolimus increases the rate of new-onset diabetes by 27%.[66]

Many patients with NASH are likely to have worsening of underlying metabolic syndrome following liver transplant (**Table 3**). Over an average 3-year follow-up, 39.8% of patients with NASH developed de-novo diabetes compared with 27% of controls transplanted for other causes. Although most were diagnosed within 1 year of transplant, patients with NASH were 1.47 times more likely to develop diabetes at any time period. Even after controlling for other pretransplant factors, including components of metabolic syndrome, NASH remained an independent risk for de-novo diabetes.[67] New-onset diabetes following transplant confers a worse overall patient and graft survival even compared with patients with a diagnosis of pretransplant diabetes.[68,69]

The ongoing presence of metabolic syndrome also places patients with NASH at risk for recurrent disease in their graft livers. Various studies using protocol biopsy have observed a prevalence of posttransplant steatosis ranging from 16% to as high as 70% after a follow-up period of 18 months.[39,51,70,71] In one retrospective analysis of patients transplanted for NASH and/or cryptogenic cirrhosis, all assessable patients had evidence of fatty liver after 5 years.[7] Suspicion for recurrent disease cannot

Table 3 Metabolic syndrome–related side effects of immunosuppressive agents	
Corticosteroids	Increased insulin resistance Obesity Hyperlipidemia (long-term use) Hypertension
Calcineurin inhibitors	Decreased insulin production (tacrolimus > cyclosporine) Hyperlipidemia (cyclosporine > tacrolimus) Hypertension (cyclosporine > tacrolimus) Nephrotoxicity
mTOR inhibitors	Increased insulin resistance Hypertriglyceridemia

Abbreviation: mTOR, mammalian target of rapamycin.

be based on clinical findings alone because up to one-third of patients with recurrent NASH had normal liver enzyme levels at time of biopsy.[39] The presence of dyslipidemia, posttransplant weight gain, and development of new-onset diabetes were all more common in patients who developed recurrent steatosis.[57] Of those who do develop steatosis, between 20% and 50% may progress to steatohepatitis. As in the nontransplanted population, NASH increases the probability of developing bridging fibrosis or cirrhosis compared with patients with simple steatosis.[57] Despite the high rates of recurrent disease, it seems to have little impact on long-term outcomes or need for retransplant. Patients with NASH have a 3-year graft survival of 76% to 81%[40,70] with retransplant for recurrent disease extremely rare to nonexistent based on existing data. Survival rates for patients with recurrent NAFLD or NASH are similar to those for patients without evidence of steatosis on posttransplant biopsy.[11,39,70,71] Although current evidence does not suggest a significant impact of recurrent NASH on posttransplant outcomes, more long-term studies are needed. Considering the association with metabolic syndrome, patients may succumb to cardiovascular disease or other comorbidities as a part of their recurrent disease before clinically significant graft failure occurs.

De-Novo Nonalcoholic Fatty Liver Disease

De-novo NAFLD has been seen in 30% to 40% of patients without NASH, with a higher incidence among those transplanted for alcoholic cirrhosis.[72,73] The development of NAFLD increases over time, with one study reporting a 47.6% prevalence 10 years after transplant.[74] Patients who developed steatosis had features of metabolic syndrome and were more often obese, with increased rates of hyperlipidemia, hypertension, and diabetes compared with their counterparts.[72,73,75] Patients with a higher pretransplant weight and those who gained more than 10% of their pretransplant weight were at risk for developing de-novo steatosis.[75,76] In one study, tacrolimus was independently associated with a greater risk of de-novo steatosis compared with cyclosporine, likely as a result of its increased diabetogenic effects.[72] Donor characteristics also affect the development of de-novo NAFLD, with higher rates in patients who received organs with preexisting graft steatosis.[72,73] In a series of 131 patients with posttransplant NAFLD, 30% had received grafts with steatosis (defined as >5% steatosis). Compared with the group of patients without posttransplant NAFLD, only 12% had initial graft steatosis.[72] Despite high rates of de-novo NAFLD, its presence does not seem to affect long-term patient or graft survival rates. In a retrospective study comparing patients with significant steatosis (grade 2 or 3) with patients with little or no steatosis (grade 0 or 1), long-term survival times were equivalent and the severity of steatosis had no bearing on rates of graft loss.[74] Progression from NAFLD to NASH is uncommon, occurring in only 5% to 8% of patients with posttransplant allograft steatosis, although studies in this area are limited.[72,73,75] In one study, 2% of patients progressed to cirrhosis with no reports of retransplant or graft failure. There is no current medical therapy to prevent development of posttransplant steatosis but use of an angiotensin-converting enzyme inhibitor was protective in 1 study.[75] Given the close association with obesity and metabolic syndrome, preventive interventions should focus on lifestyle modifications promoting weight loss and healthy eating.

Patatinlike Phospholipase 3 Mutation

Genetic factors also affect the development of steatosis. Recent genome-wide association studies have identified a single nucleotide polymorphism, rs738409, in the PNPLA3 gene where a C to G substitution is associated with increased hepatic fat content and liver enzyme levels.[77] The patinin-like phospholipase 3 (PNPLA3) gene encodes for adiponutrin, a membrane-bound protein that is primarily expressed in adipose tissue. Although the function of adiponutrin has not been fully determined, it is involved in triacylglycerol hydrolysis. The substitution of cytosine to guanine changes codon 148 from isoleucine to methionine, which leads to increased triglyceride storage in hepatocytes.[78] The presence of a G allele of rs738409 in PNPLA3 is associated with higher rates of histologic NAFLD and its related components of steatosis, portal inflammation, and lobular inflammation.[79] Among all patients with NAFLD or NASH, patients with the G allele have more severe disease, measured by higher NAFLD activity and fibrosis scores, and an increased incidence of cirrhosis.[79,80]

In the posttransplant setting, patients with PNPLA3 GG alleles and obesity had a greater than 70% prevalence of de-novo NAFLD compared with 20% prevalence in patients with obesity alone.[81] PNPLA3 is thought to exert its effects via extrahepatic pathways because the development of steatosis is associated with recipient factors rather than donor genotype. In a retrospective study in which steatosis was assessed by computed tomography imaging, the presence of recipient GG allele conferred a 12.6-fold increased risk of steatosis compared with the CC genotype. When stratified by donor genotype, there was no difference in the development of steatosis.[82] The recipient GG genotype also increases risk of posttransplant obesity, with one study reporting 82% obesity (BMI >30) 3 years following transplant. Again there was no association between the donor genotype and obesity, suggesting that liver-specific expression of PNPLA3 is not necessary for the development of steatosis or other features of metabolic syndrome.[83]

SUMMARY

The increasing prevalence of NAFLD coupled with improved curative therapies for hepatitis C means that NASH will soon become the most common indication for liver transplant in the United States. Patients transplanted for NASH have long-term outcomes equivalent to other causes of chronic liver disease but require careful preoperative evaluation. Patients with NASH tend to be older, with higher rates of obesity, cardiac disease, and features of metabolic syndrome. As a result, they are likely to spend more time on the wait-list and are at risk for early postoperative cardiac complications. Obesity as a number alone should not be prohibitive to transplant but, in combination with other cardiometabolic risk factors, may impart a worse prognosis. Steatosis can recur in the graft organ following transplant for NASH or may appear de-novo in patients who develop metabolic syndrome posttransplant. There are rare reports of posttransplant NAFLD progressing to cirrhosis or graft failure but more long-term studies are needed to assess the true impact of recurrent disease. It is possible that patients may succumb to cardiac-related comorbidities before significant disease has time to develop in the graft organ. Future efforts should focus on managing the interaction between genetic and metabolic determinants of NAFLD to promote the best posttransplant outcomes.

REFERENCES

1. Kim WR, Lake JR, Smith JM, et al. OPTN/SRTR 2015 Annual data report: liver. Available at: http://srtr.transplant.hrsa.gov/annual_reports/Default.aspx. Accessed March 8, 2017.
2. Burke A, Lucey MR. Non-alcoholic fatty liver disease, non-alcoholic steatohepatitis and orthotopic liver transplantation. Am J Transpl 2004;4(5):686–93.

3. Ong JP, Younossi ZM. Epidemiology and natural history of NAFLD and NASH. Clin Liver Dis 2007;11(1):1–16, vii.
4. Fleming JA, Kim WR, Brosgart CL, et al. Reduction in liver transplant wait-listing in the era of direct-acting antiviral therapy. Hepatology 2017;65(3):804–12.
5. Charlton MR, Burns JM, Pedersen RA, et al. Frequency and outcomes of liver transplantation for nonalcoholic steatohepatitis in the United States. Gastroenterology 2011;141(4):1249–53.
6. Wong RJ, Cheung R, Ahmed A. Nonalcoholic steatohepatitis is the most rapidly growing indication for liver transplantation in patients with hepatocellular carcinoma in the U.S. Hepatology 2014;59(6):2188–95.
7. Contos MJ, Cales W, Sterling RK, et al. Development of nonalcoholic fatty liver disease after orthotopic liver transplantation for cryptogenic cirrhosis. Liver Transpl 2001;7(4):363–73.
8. Wong RJ, Aguilar M, Cheung R, et al. Nonalcoholic steatohepatitis is the second leading etiology of liver disease among adults awaiting liver transplantation in the United States. Gastroenterology 2015;148(3):547–55.
9. O'Leary JG, Landaverde C, Jennings L, et al. Patients with NASH and cryptogenic cirrhosis are less likely than those with hepatitis C to receive liver transplants. Clin Gastroenterol Hepatol 2011;9(8):700–4.e1.
10. Afzali A, Berry K, Ioannou GN. Excellent posttransplant survival for patients with nonalcoholic steatohepatitis in the United States. Liver Transpl 2012;18(1):29–37.
11. Bhagat V, Mindikoglu AL, Nudo CG, et al. Outcomes of liver transplantation in patients with cirrhosis due to nonalcoholic steatohepatitis versus patients with cirrhosis due to alcoholic liver disease. Liver Transpl 2009;15(12):1814–20.
12. Malik SM, deVera ME, Fontes P, et al. Outcome after liver transplantation for NASH cirrhosis. Am J Transpl 2009;9(4):782–93.
13. Leonard J, Heimbach JK, Malinchoc M, et al. The impact of obesity on long-term outcomes in liver transplant recipients–results of the NIDDK liver transplant database. Am J Transpl 2008;8(3):667–72.
14. Pelletier SJ, Schaubel DE, Wei G, et al. Effect of body mass index on the survival benefit of liver transplantation. Liver Transpl 2007;13(12):1678–83.
15. Choban PS, Flancbaum L. The impact of obesity on surgical outcomes: a review. J Am Coll Surg 1997;185(6):593–603.
16. LaMattina JC, Foley DP, Fernandez LA, et al. Complications associated with liver transplantation in the obese recipient. Clin Transpl 2012;26(6):910–8.
17. Martin P, DiMartini A, Feng S, et al. Evaluation for liver transplantation in adults: 2013 practice guideline by the American Association for the Study of Liver Diseases and the American Society of Transplantation. Hepatology 2014;59(3):1144–65.
18. Nair S, Verma S, Thuluvath PJ. Obesity and its effect on survival in patients undergoing orthotopic liver transplantation in the United States. Hepatology 2002;35(1):105–9.
19. Saab S, Lalezari D, Pruthi P, et al. The impact of obesity on patient survival in liver transplant recipients: a meta-analysis. Liver Int 2015;35(1):164–70.
20. Singhal A, Wilson GC, Wima K, et al. Impact of recipient morbid obesity on outcomes after liver transplantation. Transpl Int 2015;28(2):148–55.
21. Mattar SG, Velcu LM, Rabinovitz M, et al. Surgically-induced weight loss significantly improves nonalcoholic fatty liver disease and the metabolic syndrome. Ann Surg 2005;242(4):610–7 [discussion 618–20].
22. Lassailly G, Caiazzo R, Buob D, et al. Bariatric surgery reduces features of metabolic syndrome in morbidly obese patients. Gastroenterology 2015;149:379–88.

23. Weingarten TN, Swain JM, Kendrick ML, et al. Nonalcoholic steatohepatitis (NASH) does not increase complications after laparoscopic bariatric surgery. Obes Surg 2011;21(11):1714–20.

24. Mosko JD, Nguyen GC. Increased perioperative mortality following bariatric surgery among patients with cirrhosis. Clin Gastroenterol Hepatol 2011;9(10): 897–901.

25. Billeter AT, Senft J, Gotthardt D, et al. Combined non-alcoholic fatty liver disease and type 2 diabetes mellitus: sleeve gastrectomy or gastric bypass? — a controlled matched pair study of 34 patients. Obes Surg 2016;26(8):1867–74.

26. Lin MY, Tavakol MM, Sarin A, et al. Laparoscopic sleeve gastrectomy is safe and efficacious for pretransplant candidates. Surg Obes Relat Dis 2013;9(5):653–8.

27. Heimbach JK, Watt KD, Poterucha JJ, et al. Combined liver transplantation and gastric sleeve resection for patients with medically complicated obesity and end-stage liver disease. Am J Transpl 2013;13(2):363–8.

28. Vogt DP, Henderson M, Carey W, et al. The long-term survival and causes of death in patients who survive at least 1 year after liver transplantation. Surgery 2002;132(4):775–80.

29. Stepanova M, Younossi ZM. Independent association between nonalcoholic fatty liver disease and cardiovascular disease in the US population. Clin Gastroenterol Hepatol 2012;10(6):646–50.

30. Lu H, Liu H, Hu F, et al. Independent association between nonalcoholic fatty liver disease and cardiovascular disease: a systematic review and meta-analysis. Int J Endocrinol 2013;2013:124958.

31. Targher G, Bertolini L, Padovani R, et al. Relations between carotid artery wall thickness and liver histology in subjects with nonalcoholic fatty liver disease. Diabetes Care 2006;29(6):1325–30.

32. Villanova N, Moscatiello S, Ramilli S, et al. Endothelial dysfunction and cardiovascular risk profile in nonalcoholic fatty liver disease. Hepatology 2005;42(2): 473–80.

33. Kim D, Choi SY, Park EH, et al. Nonalcoholic fatty liver disease is associated with coronary artery calcification. Hepatology 2012;56(2):605–13.

34. Fotbolcu H, Yakar T, Duman D. Impairment of the left ventricular systolic and diastolic function in patients with non-alcoholic fatty liver disease. Cardiol J 2012; 17(5):457–63.

35. VanWagner LB, Wilcox JE, Colangelo LA, et al. Association of nonalcoholic fatty liver disease with subclinical myocardial remodeling and dysfunction: a population-based study. Hepatology 2015;62:773–83.

36. Ehtisham J, Altieri M, Salamé E, et al. Coronary artery disease in orthotopic liver transplantation: pretransplant assessment and management. Liver Transp 2010; 16(5):500–57.

37. Raval Z, Harienstein ME, Skaro AI, et al. Cardiovascular risk assessment of the liver transplant candidate. J Am Coll Cardiol 2011;58(3):223–31.

38. Azarbal B, Poommipanit P, Arbit B, et al. Feasibility and safety of percutaneous coronary intervention in patients with end-stage liver disease referred for liver transplantation. Liver Transpl 2001;17(7):809–13.

39. Malik SM, Devera ME, Fontes P, et al. Recurrent disease following liver transplantation for nonalcoholic steatohepatitis cirrhosis. Liver Transpl 2009;15(12): 1843–51.

40. Singal AK, Guturu P, Hmoud B, et al. Evolving frequency and outcomes of liver transplantation based on etiology of liver disease. Transplantation 2013;95(5): 755–60.

41. Barritt AS, Dellon ES, Kozlowski T, et al. The influence of nonalcoholic fatty liver disease and its associated co-morbidities on liver transplant outcomes. J Clin Gastroenterol 2011;45(5):372–8.

42. Hoehn RS, Singhal A, Wima K, et al. Effect of pretransplant diabetes on short-term outcomes after liver transplantation: a national cohort study. Liver Int 2015;35(7):1902–9.

43. Yoo HY, Thuluvath PJ. The effect of insulin-dependent diabetes mellitus on outcome of liver transplantation. Transplantation 2002;74(7):1007–12.

44. Younossi ZM, Stepanova M, Saab S, et al. The impact of type 2 diabetes and obesity on the long-term outcomes of more than 85 000 liver transplant recipients in the US. Aliment Pharmacol Ther 2004;40(6):686–94.

45. Centers for Disease Control and Prevention. Chronic kidney disease surveillance system—United States. Web site. Available at: http://www.cdc.gov/ckd. Accessed March 10, 2017.

46. Targher G, Chonchol M, Zoppini G, et al. Risk of chronic kidney disease in patients with non-alcoholic fatty liver disease: is there a link? J Hepatol 2011; 54(5):1020–9.

47. Musso G, Gambino R, Tabibian JH, et al. Association of non-alcoholic fatty liver disease with chronic kidney disease: a systematic review and meta-analysis. PLoS Med 2014;11(7):e1001680.

48. Park CW, Tsai NT, Wong LL. Implications of worse renal dysfunction and medical comorbidities in patients with NASH undergoing liver transplant evaluation: impact on MELD and more. Clin Transpl 2011;25(6):E606–11.

49. VanWagner LB, Lapin B, Skaro AI, et al. Impact of renal impairment on cardiovascular disease mortality after liver transplantation for nonalcoholic steatohepatitis cirrhosis. Liver Int 2015;35(12):2575–83.

50. Watt KD, Pedersen RA, Kremers WK, et al. Evolution of causes and risk factors for mortality post-liver transplant: results of the NIDDK long-term follow-up study. Am J Transpl 2010;10(6):1420–7.

51. Agopian VG, Kaldas FM, Hong JC, et al. Liver transplantation for nonalcoholic steatohepatitis: the new epidemic. Ann Surg 2012;256(4):624–33.

52. Singal AK, Hasanin M, Kaif M, et al. Nonalcoholic steatohepatitis is the most rapidly growing indication for simultaneous liver kidney transplantation in the United States. Transplantation 2016;100(3):607–12.

53. Fussner L, Charlton M, Heimbach J, et al. The impact of gender and NASH on chronic kidney disease before and after liver transplantation. Liver Int 2014; 34(8):1259–66.

54. Houlihan DD, Armstrong MJ, Davidov Y, et al. Renal function in patients undergoing transplantation for nonalcoholic steatohepatitis cirrhosis: time to reconsider immunosuppression regimens? Liver Transpl 2011;17(11):1292–8.

55. Kennedy C, Redden D, Gray S, et al. Equivalent survival following liver transplantation in patients with non-alcoholic steatohepatitis compared with patients with other liver diseases. HPB (Oxford) 2012;14(9):625–34.

56. Vanwagner LB, Bhave M, Te HS, et al. Patients transplanted for nonalcoholic steatohepatitis are at increased risk for postoperative cardiovascular events. Hepatology 2012;56(5):1741–50.

57. Yalamanchili K, Saadeh S, Klintmalm GB, et al. Nonalcoholic fatty liver disease after liver transplantation for cryptogenic cirrhosis or nonalcoholic fatty liver disease. Liver Transpl 2010;16(4):431–9.

58. Wang X, Li J, Riaz DR, et al. Outcomes of liver transplantation for nonalcoholic steatohepatitis: a systematic review and meta-analysis. Clin Gastroenterol Hepatol 2014;12(3):394–402.e1.

59. Laish I, Braun M, Mor E, et al. Metabolic syndrome in liver transplant recipients: prevalence, risk factors, and association with cardiovascular events. Liver Transpl 2011;17(1):15–22.

60. Laryea M, Watt KD, Molinari M, et al. Metabolic syndrome in liver transplant recipients: prevalence and association with major vascular events. Liver Transpl 2007; 13(8):1109–14.

61. Bianchi G, Marchesini G, Marzocchi R, et al. Metabolic syndrome in liver transplantation: relation to etiology and immunosuppression. Liver Transpl 2008; 14(11):1648–54.

62. Watt KD. Metabolic syndrome: is immunosuppression to blame? Liver Transpl 2011;17(Suppl 3):S38–42.

63. Richards J, Gunson B, Johnson J, et al. Weight gain and obesity after liver transplantation. Transpl Int 2005;18(4):461–6.

64. Everhart JE, Lombardero M, Lake JR, et al. Weight change and obesity after liver transplantation: incidence and risk factors. Liver Transpl Surg 1998;4(4):285–96.

65. Marchetti P, Navalesi R. The metabolic effects of cyclosporine and tacrolimus. J Endocrinol Invest 2000;23(7):482–90.

66. Haddad E, McAlister V, Renouf E, et al. Cyclosporin versus tacrolimus for liver transplanted patients. Cochrane Database Syst Rev 2006;(4):CD005161.

67. Stepanova M, Henry L, Garg R, et al. Risk of de novo post-transplant type 2 diabetes in patients undergoing liver transplant for non-alcoholic steatohepatitis. BMC Gastroenterol 2015;15:175.

68. John PR, Thuluvath PJ. Outcome of patients with new-onset diabetes mellitus after liver transplantation compared with those without diabetes mellitus. Liver Transpl 2002;8(8):708–13.

69. Moon JI, Barbeito R, Faradji RN, et al. Negative impact of new-onset diabetes mellitus on patient and graft survival after liver transplantation: long-term follow up. Transplantation 2006;82(12):1625–8.

70. Charlton M, Kasparova P, Weston S, et al. Frequency of nonalcoholic steatohepatitis as a cause of advanced liver disease. Liver Transpl 2001;7(7):608–14.

71. Dureja P, Mellinger J, Agni R, et al. NAFLD recurrence in liver transplant recipients. Transplantation 2011;91(6):684–9.

72. Dumortier J, Giostra E, Belbouab S, et al. Non-alcoholic fatty liver disease in liver transplant recipients: another story of "seed and soil." Am J Gastroenterol 2010; 105:613–20.

73. Kim H, Lee K, Lee KW, et al. Histologically proven non-alcoholic fatty liver disease and clinically related factors in recipients after liver transplantation. Clin Transpl 2014;28(5):521–9.

74. Hejlova I, Honsova E, Sticova E, et al. Prevalence and risk factors of steatosis after liver transplantation and patient outcomes. Liver Transpl 2016;22(5):644–55.

75. Seo S, Maganti K, Khehra M, et al. De novo nonalcoholic fatty liver disease after liver transplantation. Liver Transpl 2007;13(6):844–7.

76. Lim LG, Cheng CL, Wee A, et al. Prevalence and clinical associations of post transplant fatty liver disease. Liver Int 2007;27(1):76–80.

77. Romeo S, Kozlitina J, Xing C, et al. Genetic variation in PNPLA3 confers susceptibility to nonalcoholic fatty liver disease. Nat Genet 2008;40(12):1461–5.

78. He S, McPhaul C, Li JZ, et al. A sequence variation (I148M) in PNPLA3 associated with nonalcoholic fatty liver disease disrupts triglyceride hydrolysis. J Biol Chem 2010;285(9):6706–15.
79. Rotman Y, Koh C, Zmuda JM, et al. The association of genetic variability in patatin-like phospholipase domain-containing protein 3 (PNPLA3) with histologic severity of nonalcoholic fatty liver disease. Hepatology 2010;52(3):894–903.
80. Salameh H, Hanayneh MA, Masadeh M, et al. PNPLA3 as a genetic determinant of risk for and severity of non-alcoholic fatty liver disease spectrum. J Clin Transl Hepatol 2016;4(3):175–91.
81. Liu ZT, Chen TC, Lu XX, et al. PNPLA3 I148M variant affects non-alcoholic fatty liver disease in liver transplant recipients. World J Gastroenterol 2015;21(34): 10054–6.
82. Finkenstedt A, Auer C, Glodny B, et al. Patinin-like phospholipase domain-containing protein 3 rs738409-G in recipient of liver transplants is a risk factor for graft steatosis. Clin Gastroenterol Hepatol 2013;11(12):1667–72.
83. Watt KD, Dierkhising R, Fan C, et al. Investigation of PNPLA3 and IL28B genotypes on diabetes and obesity after liver transplantation: insight into mechanism of disease. Am J Transpl 2013;13:2450–7.
84. D'Agostino RB, Vasan RS, Penicina MJ, et al. General cardiovascular risk profile for use in primary care. Circulation 2008;117:743–53.
85. Expert Panel on Detection, Evaluation, and Treatment of High Blood Cholesterol in Adults. Executive summary of the Third Report of the National Cholesterol Education Program (NCEP) Expert Panel on Detection, Evaluation, and Treatment of High Blood Cholesterol in Adults (Adult Treatment Panel III). JAMA 2001;285(19): 2486–97.
86. Sarnak MJ, Levey AS, Schoolwerth AC, et al. Kidney disease as a risk factor for development of cardiovascular disease: a statement from the American Heart Association Councils on Kidney in Cardiovascular Disease, High Blood Pressure Research, Clinical Cardiology and Epidemiology and Prevention. Hypertension 2003;42(5):1050–65.

Moving?

Make sure your subscription moves with you!

To notify us of your new address, find your **Clinics Account Number** (located on your mailing label above your name), and contact customer service at:

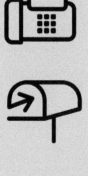

Email: **journalscustomerservice-usa@elsevier.com**

800-654-2452 (subscribers in the U.S. & Canada)
314-447-8871 (subscribers outside of the U.S. & Canada)

Fax number: 314-447-8029

Elsevier Health Sciences Division
Subscription Customer Service
3251 Riverport Lane
Maryland Heights, MO 63043

*To ensure uninterrupted delivery of your subscription, please notify us at least 4 weeks in advance of move.